About the author

Dr Hilary Jones qualified at the Royal Free Hospital School of Medicine, London in 1976. He established himself as Britain's most popular and trusted media doctor following his twice daily 'Doc Spot' on TVam, and he currently appears every weekday morning on GMTV where he provides up-to-date medical information and advice. He has written for numerous medical and national newspapers over the years, and currently has a weekly column in the *News of the World Sunday Magazine*. His first book, *Before You Call The Doctor*, was published in June 1994.

The father of five children, Hilary lives in Hampshire with his wife Sarah, their baby son Dylan, twins Rupert and Samantha and sons Tristan and Sebastian.

Acknowledgements

I am indebted to my wife Sarah for all her encouragement and support whilst the book was being written, and for keeping five delightful but demanding children from disturbing my concentration as I worked. Her own contributions as a health visitor and midwife, and last but by no means least, as an experienced mother, have been considerable. I would also like to thank Consultant Paediatrician Dr Richard Primavesi, who provides expert medical care on the wards and in the Special Care Baby Unit at our local NHS hospital, for acting as Medical Editor for the book and updating, clarifying and emphasising the text where necessary. Finally, I would like to thank my own children whose symptoms over the years have provided me with a wealth of practical knowledge without which my medical qualifications alone would seem woefully inadequate.

Your Child's Health

From Birth to Twelve Years Old

Dr Hilary Jones

Hodder & Stoughton

Copyright © 1996 by Dr Hilary Jones
Illustrations by Rodney Paull

Consultant Paediatrician: Doctor Richard J Primavesi MRCP

Growth charts © Child Growth Foundation: available from
Harlow Printing, Maxwell Street, South Shields NE33 4PU

The right of Dr Hilary Jones to be identified as the Author of the Work
has been asserted by him in accordance with the Copyright, Designs
and Patents Act 1988.

First published in Great Britain in 1996 by Hodder and Stoughton
A division of Hodder Headline PLC

10 9 8 7 6 5 4

ISBN 0 340 65400 7

Typeset by Phoenix Typesetting, Ilkley, West Yorkshire

Printed and bound in Great Britain by
Mackays of Chatham PLC

Hodder and Stoughton Ltd
A Division of Hodder Headline PLC
338 Euston Road
London NW1 3BH

To Sarah, Tristan, Sebastian, Samantha, Rupert and Dylan

CONTENTS

Chapter Seven
SOURCES OF HELP   459

Foreword

'Your book is so brilliant, Hilary!' said I, 'that it scarce needs me to write a Preface!' Anyway, I wrote one just the same, and here, for those of you who want to feel more confident about coping with your children when they are poorly, it is. Afterwards all you need to do is simply turn the page to enter the munificent world of medical malady.

Hilary Jones has dedicated his life through responsible medical journalism to increasing public understanding of medical issues. That combined with his very considerable experience in general practice, has convinced him of the value of enablement and empowerment of child patients and their families.

This book is very much needed because at a time when there is an unquenchable thirst for knowledge about medical matters, the modern nuclear family lacks much of the guidance that came from knowledgeable elders. Its use of an alphabetical, symptom based layout allows easy access to required information, giving a clear explanation of the possible causes of symptoms, what the patient can do at home, and what the doctor might reasonably be expected to do after seeing the child.

I believe every parent would do well to have a copy of *Your Child's Health* in a prominent position on the bookshelf at home.

Doctor Richard J Primavesi MRCP
Loddon NHS Trust, North Hampshire Hospital, Basingstoke.

INTRODUCTION

As a parent of five children myself, I know how harrowing it can be when children in distress throw themselves on your mercy. You want to help. You want more than anything else to put it right and make it better. But that is far from easy, because children's symptoms can be notoriously complex and confusing.

All parents have considered the possibility of meningitis when their child develops a high fever and a headache, and many have been puzzled by their infant's continuous coughing or wheezing at night. Mothers and fathers often agonise over how long to leave their child with tummy pain, and wonder how seriously they should take the child's refusal to eat. But whether it's bed-wetting, breast-feeding or birthmarks, the explanation of the likely cause and its significance will be found within these user-friendly pages.

This book is dedicated to helping worried parents understand the meaning of their children's symptoms. It suggests reasons why a baby might be crying continuously or not sleeping, and the various possibilities when an infant breaks out in a rash, limps or simply looks off colour. The book is intended to aid parents discover the real meaning of their child's behaviour and symptoms, and to advise how urgently the child should be referred to a doctor. The book is not intended to be a substitute in any way for a proper medical consultation and examination. But as a handy reference guide when a doctor may not be immediately contactable, it could be invaluable.

In addition to specific and general symptoms, there are useful sections on growth and development, preventative child health including immunisations, accidents and emergencies. Symptoms, of course, apply to both boys and girls alike, although the word 'he' has been used throughout to keep matters simple. Where lists appear showing the possible causes of a particular symptom, they have been set down in order of commonness as much as possible to keep priorities clear.

I know as well as any other parent that small children who are unwell are unable to tell us exactly what is wrong. It is my heartfelt hope that *Your Child's Health* will help us find out.

CHAPTER ONE

THE FIRST MONTHS OF LIFE

The First Few Days

Expectations

It is a popular myth that a happy, healthy and successful pregnancy always ends, after nine months, with the delivery of a bonny, bouncing baby. Everybody is thrilled, celebrations start and flowers arrive in the arms of hoards of excited friends and relatives. The reality, however, can be somewhat different. Whereas all the parents' expectations will have focused on the physical production of the infant, they will probably have made very little preparation to cope with some of the common discomforts of the first few days. This can be quite a nasty surprise for the first-time mother and it is very easy for her to become rather disillusioned and despondent about the sudden change in her life. It is common, for example, for some mums to feel deserted by friends and family who seem to lose interest after a couple of days, leaving her to cope on her own with the physical and psychological challenges which now appear.

Baby-blues

It would be surprising if the mother of a newborn baby did not feel exhausted and tired. Amazing if she felt no discomfort whatsoever from her breasts, from the afterpains as her uterus contracts again and from stretched perineal muscles down below – especially if she has had to have stitches. With all this going on as well as the responsibility of caring for and feeding the baby, it is little wonder that 85 per cent of all mothers experience the baby-blues on about the third or fourth day after delivery. At this time mums often become emotional and tearful, feel a little low and depressed and may well take out their feelings on those around them and especially those closest and dearest to them. Thankfully it only lasts for a day or two and is not associated with the much more serious condition of postnatal depression which may occur at any time from birth up to the time when the child is some two years of age.

Organisation and Priorities

In the early days parents are having to change nappies several times during the day as well as in the small hours, and have to cope with apparently incessant crying at times too. They are tired, they are distracted by thoughts of getting the nursery finished and paying for all the new equipment they need and it is normal for tension and friction to occur. On top of all this they may get conflicting advice from midwives, health visitors and GPs, not to mention well-meaning mothers and mothers-in-law.

But nobody ever said that coping with a newborn baby in the early days was easy. In fact, when it was discussed in the prenatal classes this was probably the bit most likely to have gone in one ear and straight out of the other. The truth is that it can be, and often is, difficult, despite the unique feelings of joy and wonder that parenthood brings. The baby will undoubtedly change the lives of both parents and therefore they shouldn't try to keep life exactly as it was. When you are tired and there is not enough time in the day to achieve everything you wish, it is important to get your priorities right and grab as much help as you can. Certain tasks can be left until later, such as non-essential housework, and recruiting your partner to do their share is vital, not only to get things done but also to include them in the domestic readjustments.

It is important to remember that there is no right or wrong way of handling a baby. Parents should, however, establish their own rules from the start and then stick to them. It also helps if parents find time to talk to one another. If they can agree on baby policies together, the organisation of each day falls into place more easily and there are fewer disagreements at the times you could most do without them. It is also important for parents to find time purely to enjoy the baby when all the hard work has been done so that actually being with the baby does not become associated with stress and duress. Parents need time on their own together as well to maintain and preserve their relationship, and establishing a regular bedtime routine for the baby from the outset is one way of achieving this.

Reality

I expect we will continue to see ridiculously over-romanticised portrayals of fantastic looking, super-slim, highly capable Super Mothers on television and in magazines, but in my many years as a GP they do not exist. Not unless they have a couple of live-in nannies and frequent holidays without the baby, that is! Mothers – and fathers – who feel they cannot live up to unrealistic expectations are normal and should certainly not be allowed to feel guilty. Everybody has to cope with the challenges and difficulties of early childhood, myself and my wife included, and all of us need help, support and encouragement at the best of times.

Single Mums

Things are particularly hard for single parents. It's true that they may obtain more satisfaction from bringing up a baby alone than with a partner, and for that reason develop a stronger bond with the child. On the other hand, they have to make difficult decisions alone, and it is harder to get help, to make friends and to find time for themselves, for leisure activities and for meeting other people. Money and housing can also be a problem, and babysitting arrangements may be harder to organise because it is difficult for single parents to reciprocate.

Premature Babies

A premature baby is a baby born before 37 weeks of gestation rather than the usual 40; and about five to 10 per cent of babies fit into this category. Although prematurity causes few problems for the mother, the premature baby is much more vulnerable than a full-term baby, and increasingly so the earlier the infant is delivered.

The problem lies in the fact that the newborn is not yet fully developed and may be unable to deal with an independent life outside the womb. Not so long ago, prematurity was a major cause of infant death or disability, but with newer and more sophisticated medical treatments carried out in dedicated special care baby units staffed by highly trained health care professionals, the survival rate and outlook has dramatically improved. My own twins were born prematurely at 28 weeks and it is much to the credit of our local Special Care Baby Unit (SCBU) that they first of all survived at all, and then continued to develop from strength to strength quite normally.

Why Does Premature Labour Happen?

In nearly one half of all cases no reason is ever discovered as to exactly why it happens. In other examples, conditions affecting either the mother, the baby or the placenta are responsible. The commonest cause is twins or higher multiple births which account for about fifteen per cent of all premature births. It seems that the additional load in the womb stretches the membranes and starts up the muscular contractions leading to the onset of labour. Often, to avoid complications, the labour is induced early or a Caesarian is carried out before 37 weeks to attain the safest and best possible result from the pregnancy.

High blood pressure and pre-eclampsia in the mother (where swelling of the fingers and ankles and protein in the urine accompany the high blood pressure), can cause it. So can diabetes, heart and long-standing kidney disorders. Often, to protect the mother from suffering further as a result of these conditions, the obstetrician again decides to deliberately deliver the infant early either by means of an induced labour or a Caesarian section.

Sometimes the membranes surrounding the foetus in the womb rupture early causing anything from a slow trickle of fluid from the vagina right through to the whole of the waters breaking. This can bring on premature labour and so can any infection within the uterus which may follow it. If the placenta itself becomes detached from the lining of the womb, profuse bleeding can occur (antepartum haemorrhage), and this will almost always result in premature labour or urgent delivery by Caesarian to save the baby's life.

Finally, where the uterine cavity is abnormally small (in cases where a congenital abnormality creates a partition within it, effectively separating it into two halves) or where excess amniotic fluid is formed around the baby, the risk of an early delivery is greater too.

The Premature Baby

The premature baby is smaller and lighter than a full-term baby, and because he lacks fat stores under the skin looks typically scrawny and thin. The skin is almost transparent it is so delicate and is covered with fine, downy hair known as lanugo.

The vital internal organs, such as the brain, heart, lungs, liver, and kidneys are also immature so the baby needs to be carefully monitored in a SCBU in hospital until his ability to cope with an independent life has been adequately developed.

The major problems faced by the premature baby are breathing difficulties (Respiratory Distress Syndrome), bleeding into the brain around the time of delivery, jaundice, low blood sugar and infection. The baby is more vulnerable to all of these conditions and cannot, in addition, regulate his own body temperature sufficiently well. Modern SCBUs are specially designed to identify and treat all of these conditions as they arise.

Treatment

When parents are faced with the prospect of their newborn baby being transferred to special care they are understandably upset, confused, frightened and very anxious. Most of the time, the decision is made as a precaution to eradicate any possibility of a problem, and the infant is soon returned to the mother.

In very premature babies however, difficulties are more or less anticipated and the Special Care Baby Unit is the only place they will survive. The baby is placed in a special see-through incubator which is kept at a constant temperature. Artificial ventilation may be used to assist the baby to breathe and because the premature baby is unable to suck or swallow, feeding can be either through a vein or via a tiny tube passed down through the nose into the stomach. Iron and vitamins are given to supplement the specially-enriched milk feeds and the infant is generally kept in hospital until he reaches the weight of about 2.25 kg, is feeding well and growing normally.

The Parents

Having a premature baby looked after in an intensive care incubator in a SCBU is a harrowing experience for any parent as my wife and I know only too well. Your baby (or babies) is attached to all kinds of tubes and other paraphernalia and because of his tiny size and the number of drip lines entering his fragile body, he at times resembles a pathetic pin-cushion. But the staff know what they are doing and every intervention is a necessary one.

The parents often need much reassurance and support at this time, especially if a premature delivery had not been anticipated and came as something of a shock, but SCBU staff are well-trained in providing sympathetic care for the parents, providing any information, explanation and encouragement where needed.

Worries about not being able to properly 'bond' with a premature baby are also unfounded since parents are actively encouraged to take as full a role as possible in caring for the baby, in holding him in their arms, feeding him and dressing him. Even the problems of breast-feeding, which is often impossible in this situation, can be addressed.

Having said that, feelings of resentment that your baby is being cared for by someone else are understandable and natural but there is ultimately still no substitute for the real father and mother. As my wife and I found, it makes the day they are discharged all the more exciting – and we should know, our twins were in special care for 58 days!

The Outlook for Premature Babies

The longer a baby remains in its mother's womb when all is well, the better its chances of survival. So the more premature a baby is at birth, the greater the risk. With modern paediatric techniques and equipment many babies born as early as 23 weeks and weighing as little as 500g survive, and many do well, but some may suffer long-term complications and may face a future with a degree of disability of some kind.

A pregnancy lasting at least 28 weeks is often regarded as something of a milestone since it is known that of all premature babies born at this level of maturity, more than 80% will survive. A great deal depends on the availability and expertise of local SCBUs and survival rates and outcomes certainly vary from region to region.

Sadly, intensive care provision for premature babies is expensive whilst NHS resources are finite, so we remain very dependent on voluntary organisations like BLISS and BLISSLINK who do so much to help through their charitable efforts (see page 464).

Older Children

Another group of mothers who are likely to have a bit of a shock in the first few days after childbirth are mums having a second or third baby. Having two children to look after is not twice as hard as having one but is, in fact, much more than that. The parents' time and attention has to be divided between the two and this in itself can put a strain on the parents. Whilst they have gained experience and confidence from having brought up one child already, they face new problems such as jealousy and resentment in the older sibling. This is not always the case but it is absolutely normal for older children to seek extra time and attention from their parents, becoming particularly clingy or indulging in naughty behaviour as a symptom.

Older children previously dry at night may start to wet the bed and other forms of regression may also be seen. Food refusal and tantrums can to some extent be anticipated. It is important to take the feelings of older children into consideration and to make the necessary adjustments. It is all the more vital to keep to a regular routine and involving older siblings in the baby's welfare as much as possible is a good idea. Explaining what is going on can satisfy the curiosity of an older child, and some – the more gentle ones! – can even be given the responsibility and fun of feeding the baby, provided it is under your careful supervision. It is important, too, to give an older child time on his own with each parent.

Twins

With twins and other multiple births, the problems of having two or more children are slightly different. You haven't got the 'older sibling' problem but if it really is twice as nice, it is definitely double the trouble, as the old adage goes. Extra help and support from friends, relatives and professionals will certainly be required, particularly if the babies are born prematurely, which is common in multiple pregnancies.

Professional Help

However well prepared a parent is, there is no substitute for living through the personal experience of childbirth, and it is not until the problems arise afterwards that parents really understand what has hit them. This is where professional help can be so valuable. Partners, friends and relatives can devote their time and practical help to new parents but the healthcare team is in the best position to maximise the health and well-being of all concerned.

The hospital staff soon pass on the burden of care to the community midwife, the health visitor and the GP. All three liaise together and with the social services when required. In addition, local mother and baby groups and other parent support organisations can be extremely helpful, as can national organisations such as the National Childbirth Trust, Gingerbread which provides self-help for one-parent families and the National Council for One Parent Families which offers free advice to single parents. The social services can also help out where money or housing is a pressing problem and TAMBA – the Twins and Multiple Births Association – can provide information and advice to parents of twins or more, as well as addresses and phone numbers of local twins clubs. (For a complete list of useful organisations, see page 464.)

It is easy for the many little problems that arise in the first few days after childbirth to get on top of you. If you and your child are happy and everything is going fine, terrific. But if things have gone wrong, if you feel you cannot cope or you feel inadequate or guilty in any way and are sinking into a bottomless pit of depression, then do seek help urgently. These feelings are absolutely normal and eminently correctable. The crucial and immediate hurdle to get over is recognising this and seeking help. That help is free, effective and universally available.

Breast-feeding

Advantages

Many mothers find that the close bonding they obtain with their babies during breast-feeding is uniquely rewarding and without parallel. There is no doubt that when it comes to feeding, breast is best for baby. Having said that, what is best for mum is ultimately best for baby and for a proportion of new mothers breast-feeding may not be possible or desirable.

The advantages of breast-feeding for the baby are considerable. Breast milk is natural and is specifically designed to meet the nutritional requirements of your baby. It provides a perfect balance for maximum health and development, is easily digested and contains hormones and other active substances which are not present in formula milks. Constipation is hardly ever seen in breast-fed babies either.

Another major advantage is that maternal antibodies are passed on to the baby, protecting him from infections and disease. Babies who are breast-fed get fewer tummy bugs and if they do they recover more quickly than bottle-fed babies. Breast-fed babies are less likely to develop asthma, eczema, hay fever and other allergies in the future. Premature babies obtain a special advantage from breast-feeding in this respect since their nutritional requirements are greater, as is their need for antibodies.

There are also considerable advantages of breast-feeding for mum herself. Breast-feeding is much more practical since no preparation is required and the milk is always there when needed once the process has been established. Breast milk is always of the right concentration, unlike formula milk which, when made up artificially, may be too strong or too weak. There is also less equipment to worry about – bottles, sterilisers, etc. – by feeding your baby the natural way. It is also cost-free. The act of breast-feeding produces a hormone which speeds up contraction of the uterus, perhaps better known as the womb, and allows it to return to its normal size more quickly. Some mothers find that they get back into general shape more speedily too. This is not always the case, however, since breast-feeding requires quite a lot of energy and a moderate to high calorie diet to sustain it. It depends purely on the individual. There is, in addition, some evidence that breast-feeding can protect the mother against future breast cancer since this form of cancer seems to be more common in mums who did not breast-feed.

Finally, cot death is less likely to occur in babies who are breast-fed, even allowing for the fact that breast-feeding mothers tend to smoke much less than bottle-feeding mothers (smoking is known to be a very important risk factor in cot death).

Disadvantages

Although the various promoters of breast-feeding will probably hate me for saying this, the truth is that breast-feeding just does not suit everybody. Some mothers simply do not like the idea, others find the process unmanageable or uncomfortable and others may have a multiple birth which compounds the difficulties enormously, although breast-feeding is still sometimes possible. It should be of great help to these parents to know that babies who are bottle-fed will grow and develop quite satisfactorily.

When breast-feeding is not going well, it is stressful and harrowing and this distress allied to worry and fatigue can turn off the hormones and reflexes required to produce breast milk. The result is that the whole thing becomes a dreadful hassle. Happily, in almost all cases these problems can be addressed and corrected, but this requires patience, consistent handling and sound and confident professional advice and help which, sadly, is not always available.

Occasionally it may be convenient to express some breast milk into a bottle, enabling your baby to obtain the benefits of the breast milk while you have a break from feeding. This is not a bad idea, anyway, as it allows the baby to become accustomed to the teat of a bottle and gives the father and other members of the family an opportunity to feed the bond with the baby too. Expressed milk can be kept in the fridge in a sterilised capped bottle for up to 24 hours, and if you wish to keep it longer it can be deep-frozen for up to a few weeks.

Problems

One of the commonest difficulties encountered are sore nipples, but unless severe, this is not an absolute reason for abandoning breast-feeding. It is inevitable that the skin over the nipples initially becomes sore as a result of the frequent sucking, mechanical trauma and constant moisture. Keeping the nipples dry and clean and changing breast pads frequently certainly helps. If discomfort continues, nipple shields which fit over your nipples like teats are worth trying. This means that your baby then sucks on the shield rather than on the nipple and these can be used for two or three days without reducing milk production.

Thrush infection, also fairly common, can make things worse as this can further inflame the nipple and the baby's mouth at the same time (see pages 28 and 136). Any thrush infection of the nipple needs to be treated with an anti-fungal cream which should be washed off thoroughly before the infant feeds. Thrush in the baby's mouth is generally treated with antifungal drops.

Another common symptom is engorgement of the breasts. When the milk builds up in the breast tissue the breast becomes swollen, hard and tender. The answer is to feed the baby or at least express some of the milk, and to take a hot bath or apply a hot flannel to the breast to soothe it. A loose but supportive bra is helpful and, if absolutely necessary, a mild painkiller in the form of paracetamol is fine. When the breasts become lumpy as well as sore, some of the milk ducts may have become blocked. Again, a proper feed from the affected breast will help to unblock the tubes and encourage milk flow. Sometimes it is helpful to apply a hot flannel to the lumpy areas while breast-feeding. Expressing milk can also be tried, but if at any time the mother feels unwell or develops a temperature, the doctor should be consulted so that any mastitis can be diagnosed and treated. If neglected, this can lead to a breast abscess, which is very tender and shows itself as a red, painful, localised area under the skin which may well require antibiotics and the immediate discontinuation of breast-feeding.

The Process of Breast-feeding

During pregnancy the breasts are developing all the time. Remember that one of the earliest signs of pregnancy is a tingling sensation in the breast tissue. The milk-producing glands and the milk ducts all enlarge, as does the nipple and the surrounding brown area, the areola, which softens and darkens. As soon as the baby is born, the breasts begin to produce milk in response to the baby suckling at your breast. It is a supply-and-demand situation – the more the baby takes the more milk you produce. Because of this, the amount of milk produced initially may be small and many mothers worry that they will not be able to produce enough. But if the baby is allowed to feed whenever he wants to, milk production should be sufficient to meet his needs. Feeding the baby more often will, in fact, increase the milk supply, and the last thing you should do is supplement the baby's nutrition with bottle feeds if you do not feel your baby is getting enough since this will simply result in less milk being produced.

Since breast-feeding mums tend to produce less milk when they are tired or stressed, it is important that you eat well and often, take enough rest and drink plenty of fluids.

The position you and your baby are in during breast-feeding is very important. The baby has to be in the correct position at the breast to stimulate the let-down reflex which allows the milk to flow down and collect behind the nipple. If the baby is sucking on an empty nipple, he will be restless, the nipple will become sore and no milk will flow through. It is important that the whole of the areola, the brown area at the base of the nipple, is in contact with the baby's mouth.

Mum also needs to be comfortable, sitting well supported and propped up on soft cushions. She should also be free of hassle, anxiety, exhaustion and even embarrassment, which is sometimes encountered in public places where inadequate breast-feeding facilities are available.

It may take a while before breast-feeding falls into a regular pattern with a newborn baby. It will be a day or two before breast-feeding is established, the pace largely being dictated by the baby. A particularly sleepy, jaundiced or restless baby will not suck very often or for very long, and in this situation the answer is to persevere. Then there is the question of for how long the baby should be put to each breast in turn. What you should do is to empty one breast at a time because the last part of the milk, the hind milk, has the greatest calorific value. If the baby is still hungry, he can then be moved to the other breast. If the baby becomes entirely satisfied, lets go of the nipple or falls asleep in the process, so be it. The trick is to start subsequent feeds on alternate breasts so that each breast is drained in turn, reducing the risk of engorgement or the lumpy, tender, breast tissue inflammation known as mastitis.

How Often to Breast Feed

To begin with, a hungry young baby may require lengthy and frequent feeds, often enough to make the weary mother feel that she is doing nothing else. This will improve, however, and a pattern will soon be established where feeds become fulfilling and happy times for mothers to share with their babies, occurring for shorter periods of time and less often. Mothers know that their baby is obtaining enough breast milk if he is putting on weight steadily and producing about half a dozen damp nappies each day. This means that the baby's input and output of fluid are correctly balanced. Difficulties are more likely to arise if the baby is a particularly poor feeder, is exceptionally sleepy for long periods, is gaining weight only very slowly or not at all, or is feeding less than four or five times each day. Professional help should always be consulted if this is the case.

Going Back to Work

Some breast-feeding mothers choose to, and others have no option but to, return to work whilst they are still breast-feeding. When this happens they may combine breast- and bottle-feeding in order that both mother and baby remain satisfied. Ideally, bottle-feeding can be carried out whilst the mother is at work using expressed milk. When this is not possible, formula milk can be substituted, enabling the mother to adapt to a pattern of breast-feeding at times just before and just after her working shift. Practical advice on how best this may be achieved is available from health visitors and any of the appropriate breast-feeding counselling services (see page 464).

Changing Over to Bottle-feeding

When a baby is changed from breast-feeding to bottle-feeding it should ideally be carried out very gradually. A good way to achieve this is to substitute just one feed a day then go on to two feeds a day until eventually all have been changed. Try not to give the first bottle feed when the baby is particularly tired or restless as he will quickly associate the strange, synthetic teat with something he does not really want, and quickly rebel. In fact the teat shape itself seems important and it is worth trying one or two different ones to see which suits your baby best. I recommend special ortho-dontic teats available from Lewis Woolf Griptight Ltd in Worcestershire.

Do not worry if you feel a little guilty at first when your child becomes upset when offered a bottle instead of the breast. This is understandable and normal. It helps if the father can give the first bottle feed as not only is this rewarding for him, but the baby is removed from the smell of the mother's breast, which might be distracting.

Vitamins

All infant formula milks and follow-on milks are fortified with vita-mins A and D, and bottle-fed babies therefore require no vitamin supplements. Babies who are breast-fed do not generally need any vitamin supplements until the age of six months as they will already have acquired enough vitamins from the mother during the pregnancy. For the second six months of the baby's life, however, all breast-fed babies should have vitamin drops containing vitamins A, C and D. Five drops of Department of Health vitamin drops a day is the dose, and this should be continued until the child is about two. Since the action of sunlight on the skin can produce vitamin D naturally, children who spend the majority of their time indoors and who rarely see sunlight are more prone to vitamin D deficiency and some babies, even under the age of six months, are advised to have vitamin D supplements. These tend to be babies born to Asian mothers, babies born in the north of England and Scotland and babies who were born after a pregnancy in the winter months.

Sources of Help

To overcome any difficulties with the establishment and mainte-nance of breast-feeding, there are many sources of advice and help. Your community midwife, health visitor and GP are all there to help you. In addition, breast-feeding counsellors, support groups and local branches of the Natural Childbirth Trust, the La Leche League and the Association of Breast Feeding Mothers are all available (see page 464).

Bottle-Feeding

How Much and How Often?

One of the reasons a tiny sample of blood is taken from a newborn baby is to check the level of glucose. A baby can become fairly distressed during childbirth and the last feed he gets is through the umbilical cord before it is cut. From this time on the baby's blood sugar depends on stored energy reserves. These are often quite low, especially in premature babies and low birth weight babies, and feeding needs to take place fairly soon. Most babies show signs of interest within the first four hours after birth and generally develop the habit of three- to four-hourly feeds thereafter. As a general guide, a baby will require something in the region of 2.5 ounces of milk for every pound the baby weighs in a 24-hour period. In other words, a seven pound baby will be having 17.5 ounces over the course of a day. You will know if your baby is getting enough milk if he is happy and contented and gaining weight normally.

Advantages

One of the great advantages of bottle-feeding is that fathers too can play a part in feeding the baby, thereby reducing pressure on the mother, especially at night, and gaining a closer, more intimate relationship with their child.

Initially there can be problems until a regular pattern is established and it is best not to be tempted to change the type of milk, bottle or teat too quickly. Instead, persevere for a reasonable amount of time and ask advice from your midwife or health visitor if in doubt.

Formula Milk

There are a variety of infant formula milks which fall broadly into three categories. These are:

Whey-dominant infant formula milks are derived from cow's milk but the saturated animal fat has been replaced by vegetable fats. In addition, the cow's milk protein has been modified to make it more suitable for babies.

Casein-dominant infant formula milks have also had the animal fats replaced with vegetable fat but contain unmodified cow's milk protein.

Soya-based milks are used where dietary intolerance or suspected intolerance to cow's milk protein or cow's milk sugar (lactose) is present (see pages 220 to 221). Babies who do not settle after a reasonable length of time on the other types of formula milks are sometimes changed to this one.

By and large, most normal babies will tolerate and enjoy any of the above types of formula milk. What they should never have in the first year of their life is full-fat, semi-skimmed or skimmed cow's milk, goat's milk or ewe's milk. These are difficult for a baby to digest and contain the wrong balance of nutrients and minerals. Sheep and goat's milk may not be pasteurised, either.

Making Up the Feeds

Hygiene is vitally important when making up the feeds, so wash your hands thoroughly and ensure that all work surfaces are spotless before starting the procedure. Follow the instructions on the container to the letter. Never add extra scoops of powder or sugar since this can be harmful to the baby. For convenience, it is perfectly all right to make up enough feeds to cover a 24-hour period provided the bottles and teats have been completely sterilised and the made-up feeds are stored at the right temperature in the fridge. Never store milk for longer than 24 hours as this may lead to the growth of bacteria in the milk that may cause gastroenteritis with all its attendant complications in the newborn infant.

Feeding the Baby

Most babies prefer their milk warmed to body temperature and doing this may be less likely to provoke colic (see pages 24–26). The bottle should be stood in hot water or in a commercial bottle warmer which brings the milk to the correct temperature. It is not recommended to warm milk in a microwave oven as unequal heating of the liquid leads to 'hot spots' which could accidentally burn the baby's mouth. However, for convenience, many people do this, swirling the milk in the bottle several times after heating to mix it.

Before giving the milk to the baby, you should test a drop on your wrist to make sure it is at the right temperature. As the baby starts to feed there may be some frantic struggling until the teat is properly inside the baby's mouth. The baby may even then spit the teat out, squirm or cry. The important thing for the person giving the feed is to be patient and calm, giving the baby time to settle. Some babies will soon doze off only to wake again shortly after for a second go at the bottle. Others will calmly and swiftly drain the bottle in one go. Keep the teat of the bottle full of milk at all times to avoid any air being swallowed, which can lead to the baby bringing up air and curdled milk together. Equally important, the teat should be withdrawn from the baby's mouth at frequent intervals to prevent a vacuum from building up in the bottle, which can lead to the teat collapsing or being sucked inside it. As regards the size of the hole in the teat, this may need to be adjusted. A hole that is too small will frustrate the baby as he will have to suck extremely hard to take in any milk at all. Too big a hole, on the other hand, will overwhelm the baby's capacity to swallow and cause choking and coughing. Under no circumstances should any solids be added to the milk (unless advised by your doctor) as this too is likely to cause choking.

Equipment

The basic equipment needed for bottle-feeding is relatively straightforward. You will need at least half a dozen bottles and a selection of teats. Formula milk can be purchased almost anywhere and the type and brand that is chosen is a matter of individual choice, perhaps guided by the advice of your midwife, health visitor or doctor. It is worth remembering that formula milk may be cheaper to purchase at the baby clinic and that some mothers may be entitled to claim free or low-price milks.

Sterilising

Scrupulously thorough sterilising of equipment is vital to avoid tummy infections in the baby. All milk residues must be completely removed from teats and bottles by washing with ordinary washing-up liquid and then rinsing before sterilising is carried out. This can be done using chemical sterilising tablets or liquids, or alternatively a microwave or steam steriliser. Simply boiling bottles and teats in water for five to ten minutes is equally effective though more time-consuming and less practical. The most economical method is to use sterilising tablets or liquids especially as once the solution has been finished with after 24 hours, it can then be used to sterilise terry nappies.

Further Advice

Various questions may arise during the first few weeks of bottle-feeding to which the parents could do with some answers. The best sources of help are your midwife, health visitor, paediatrician, GP and, of course, the baby's grandmother, though the most current and clued-up experts may well be any other young mums that you may know!

Weaning

As your baby grows and develops he will require more calories than can be supplied by milk alone. The introduction of solid food into your baby's daily feeding routine is known as weaning, and this will provide all the extra calories, minerals and vitamins which your baby increasingly needs. Inevitably, weaning your first baby can create all sorts of problems initially, since you need to build up your confidence in which new foodstuffs and in what quantities to give him. With second or subsequent babies parents are usually much more relaxed about the whole thing and these offspring are expected to fit in much more with the feeding pattern of the rest of the family.

When Does Weaning Start?

Most babies will be entirely breast- or bottle-fed until the age of three months. From this time onwards it is perfectly acceptable to start gently introducing solid foods which can be puréed, mashed or sieved. Most babies will begin weaning at about four months and almost all will have started solid food by the age of six months albeit in addition to their regular bottle or breast feeds. In fact, it is usual for babies to continue with their normal milk feeds until they are aged one year as this helps to maintain their general level of nutrition. Bottle-fed babies should, however, be fully weaned by the age of one since by that time all their energy requirements are obtained from solid food and because the habit of taking milk from a bottle is much harder to break if it is continued beyond that time. These babies can be encouraged to use a feeding cup with a lid initially, in addition to bottle-feeding, but then the bottle feeds should be gradually cut out altogether.

You will know when your baby is ready to start weaning when he still seems to be hungry after taking his milk, even when he has had an extra quantity. Demands for feeds will become more frequent and your baby may well start waking at night again eager for a top up. Sometimes your baby will be increasingly restless or irritable, a sure sign of hunger. If you have any doubts about whether your baby is ready to be weaned, ask your health visitor's advice on the subject.

How to Begin

It's important to remember that all babies are different and will respond to weaning at their own pace. Some will start early, others much later. Some will be happy to consume everything offered to them, others will be much more fussy. But the greater the variety of foods introduced early on the better, since infants will soon become accustomed to the various tastes and textures and this is a useful way of avoiding food fads and food refusal later on. As more and more solid food is gradually introduced, a pattern of feeding more in line with that of the rest of the family will become established, although it may be some years before three main meals a day is achieved.

Initially, babies will find the feel of solid food in their mouths strange and spit it out. This is quite different from difficult behaviour later on when food refusal may represent an attention-seeking device or an attempt to obtain a more tempting sweet dessert earlier than allowed. It may also simply mean that they are just not hungry. As infants begin to learn to feed themselves with a spoon, it's worth being prepared for the inevitable mess that will be caused and to try to spoon in two or three helpings for every one the infant manages. Finally, tempting though it may be, try to avoid keeping half-eaten food for another meal or re-heating food as this is likely to allow bacteria to breed and lead to food-poisoning.

Taking One Stage at a Time

A common way to start weaning is to feed your baby a small amount of fruit or vegetable purée on the tip of your finger or a spoon. A non-wheat cereal is a good alternative, but apple, banana, carrot, potato, rice or baby porridge are the things that most parents begin with. This can be given just after or during a milk feed and, if successful, it can be increased from one to two feeds a day after a week or two. Gradually, the amount of solid food given with each milk feed can be increased. It is probably best to confine cereals to one feed a day (the one closest to breakfast time being the obvious choice) and to introduce different tastes and textures at other times. On the whole, no more than two or three new foods should be started in any one week. The next important food group to introduce will be meat, poultry and fish.

In time, solids can be given before the milk feed. At this stage drinks can come in the form of diluted natural fruit juice rather than milk or water. After this, almost any food commonly consumed by the rest of the family is suitable provided it is of the right consistency (mashed, puréed or sieved). Soon the infant will be chewing, and feeding himself with lumpier foodstuffs such as bread, peeled apple, toast or sandwiches. He will be well on his way to independent feeding.

Food to be Avoided Too Soon

Neither sugar nor salt should be added to baby's foods. Introducing sugar to the baby rapidly leads to the development of a taste for this strong flavour and it will become difficult to get him to eat anything which is not sweet. In addition, there is no doubt that sugar accelerates the rate of tooth decay and this will have profound consequences for your child in the future. Nor can small babies handle salt in large quantities. There is an adequate amount of salt in normal food and milk, and additional salt will make the baby thirsty and possibly even overload the normal excretory function of his kidneys.

Some foods, such as wheat, eggs and citrus fruits, may be responsible for food allergy or food intolerance and therefore should only be introduced gradually in infants over the age of six months. Ideally, they should be introduced in small quantities and one item at a time. If any reaction does ensue the culprit can then be identified easily. Eggs should be cooked thoroughly to reduce the risk of salmonella infection and since the yolk is more digestible than the white, this can be separated out and used for cooking.

Cow's milk in any shape or form should be avoided until the infant has passed the age of one year, and the same applies to goat's and sheep's milk. Goat's milk is particularly low in folic acid, one of the most important vitamins for a growing baby, and neither goat's nor sheep's milk is always pasteurised. Allergies, including those leading to asthma, eczema and hay fever (see page 143), are more likely in children given cow's milk too early on. Finally, nuts are another relatively common form of allergy but even more importantly they can lead to choking if given to babies (or toddlers) whole. If given before the age of one year, they should be in ground-up form after the age of six months.

Colic

What is it?

Incessant crying at particular times of the day, especially in the evening, is often attributed to colic, implying that it is due to abdominal cramps. The trouble is doctors cannot really agree on what this is. Some are convinced it arises from pain within the intestine as it does seem to produce the type of crying that might accompany bouts of tummy pain, the child being extremely distressed and unhappy for a while before stopping momentarily and then starting again. The baby may draw his legs up and become red in the face, a worrying sign for any parent. But other doctors, including those who have had children themselves, believe this is merely the baby picking up on the mother's own tensions. At the end of the day, mum is understandably tired and often irritable, and babies are very astute. If they feel they are getting less attention than during the rest of the day, they will complain and show their anxiety by crying. To support this theory, some doctors claim that this is why first-born babies cry more than subsequent ones. Evidence for this, however, is distinctly lacking.

Another body of opinion which seems to be gaining favour is that colic is the result of some kind of food sensitivity or intolerance. Food allergists claim that babies fed with infant formula milk which does not contain whole cow's milk protein experience colic less often than other babies. They also believe that mothers who breast-feed but drink cow's milk themselves or eat foods likely to produce intolerance such as eggs, chocolate, nuts or fish are more likely to have babies with colic than mothers who avoid these foods. It is always possible that the baby is reacting to all of the various kinds of foreign proteins entering his digestive system and that it takes about three months to adapt to them all. It is also possible that this subtle food sensitivity may continue after the colic has subsided in the form of eczema, asthma or diarrhoea, but again the medical evidence for this remains largely circumstantial.

When all is said and done, medical specialists who argue academically about the cause of colic do not really help the parents of an incessantly crying baby who are at their wits' end. What these parents need most is practical help.

What To Do

Babies cry so much and so often it may just be that they are 'programmed' from birth to do so. But having said this, the first thing a parent who suspects their child is suffering from colic should try to do is to make sure that all other causes of crying are excluded. Make sure that the baby is not hungry, thirsty, wet or uncomfortable for any reason. A fever, earache, sore throat or dehydration can make a baby very miserable indeed and symptoms are often worse in the evening. Another cause of crying after a feed is the reflux of stomach acid into the gullet. This is harder to diagnose but tends to be worse when the baby is lying flat or has had a large feed. Another possible cause is lactose intolerance. If a baby has recently had gastroenteritis with diarrhoea and vomiting there may be a temporary reduction in the amount of an enzyme in the intestine which normally digests the sugar molecules in milk (lactose). Standard medical advice is to give clear fluids to the baby immediately after this kind of tummy bug to enable the bowel to recover, but if milk is reintroduced too quickly the sugar in the milk remains undigested, bacteria flourish as a result and gas and toxins within the intestine accumulate. This can result in discomfort through intestinal distension and colic.

Mothers who are bottle-feeding are often advised to give smaller but more frequent feeds when the baby has colic and breast-feeding mothers can try reducing the size of the morning feed (expressing what remains) and giving additional amounts later in the day if the colic appears in the evenings. Generally speaking, when screaming seems to continue all day, the possibility of it being caused by food intolerance is higher and it is worth discussing this with your GP who can refer you and your baby to a paediatrician. Sometimes, knowing that physical causes have been excluded helps to calm the situation down, allowing the mother to approach the problem more rationally.

Crying

Many parents believe that a happy, contented baby is a quiet baby, that is, a baby that does not cry. But some babies, even though they have absolutely nothing to cry about, will scream anyway. It is all too easy for parents to become worried and upset when they cannot comfort a crying child, but some babies simply have an inborn predisposition to cry much more than others. On the other hand, crying can be the first sign of discomfort or distress and it is well worth running through a list of possible reasons why your baby could be crying more than usual. Here is a simple checklist:

Is Your Baby Uncomfortable?

Check to see that the baby's nappy is not wet or dirty. Not only is this uncomfortable for the baby, but it increases the risk of nappy rash, soreness and irritation of the skin and pain on passing urine. If the baby has missed one of his usual naps during the day he may be over-tired and fractious. This will make him cry louder and longer. Also, some babies quickly become bored and lonely. These are the babies that tend to settle down immediately once you pick them up, talk to them and give them the attention they crave.

Is Your Baby Thirsty?

Sometimes, particularly if the baby has been kept very warm, either in a hot room with too many clothes on or just exposed to particularly summery weather, extra fluid loss can make him more thirsty than usual. Often the baby appears flushed and may have a slight temperature. This all means the baby will be restless and will only settle down when he has taken extra fluids. Milk is usually sufficient, but if you suspect that dehydration is a problem, then it is worth either diluting the milk feeds or giving the baby just plain, boiled, cooled water to try.

Is Your Baby Hungry?

Ask yourself when your baby was last fed. Was it a normal feed or did he take less than usual? Has he been sick and brought up a good proportion of his last feed? There will also come a time when milk alone is not sufficient to satisfy your baby's hunger. Perhaps he is approaching the age of four months and is requiring larger feeds more frequently. This may indicate that it is time to start weaning him onto solid foods (see pages 21–24).

Is He in Pain?

Usually, a baby in pain will scream shrilly rather than cry. He will be restless and distressed, perhaps pulling his ears if he has earache or pulling his knees up towards his tummy with

27

abdominal pain. Soreness at the vaginal lips or the tip of the fore-skin can cause burning pain when passing urine, and this is usually evident if, when you strip off the nappy, you notice that your baby cries specifically when urinating. Some babies cry a lot when teething begins (see pages 382–384). Teething gels and teething rings along with paracetamol may be used to alleviate this.

Is Your Baby Ill?

When your baby has been crying for any length of time and when this is unusual for him, check your baby's temperature. Any slight fever will make him irritable and unwell. Look for any rash on the skin, the first sign of a childhood illness or allergy (see page 278). Is he off his food? Being disinterested in more than one feed is quite unusual and often the first sign that something is wrong. If your baby cries during the actual process of feeding this may point to a throat infection or soreness in the mouth due, for example, to thrush. Does you baby have any other symptoms? Is there any diar-rhoea or vomiting? A runny nose or a cough? Is he wheezing, is he pale, is there any blood in the stools? Listen to the cry itself. Most babies have a characteristic cry, but when the cry is unusual, shrill or high-pitched, it may be a warning sign that something more serious is wrong. Meningitis in a baby will often produce a particularly high-pitched cry. Similarly, if your baby has been crying unusually loudly and long, check to see that he is not becoming excessively drowsy, floppy or limp. These are all signs that a serious infection may be present and certainly warrant the urgent attention of a doctor.

Is He Just a Cross Baby?

Some babies, I'm afraid, are just born bad-tempered. This does not necessarily run in the family because parents with several children often find that some are angelic whilst others are little monsters. There is not really any pattern to it, and many children who cry excessively when they are young become delightful when they are older and vice versa. No doubt you will be given huge amounts of conflicting advice about what might be the cause of bad temper in a child. Allergists will tell you it is due to food intolerance, psychologists will say that your baby is picking up on family tensions. Your mother-in-law might simply tell you it's the way you are bringing him up! The truth is that as long as you do your best to bring up your child the way you want to, and provided you have excluded any illness or source of discomfort, crying is something all parents have to put up with. Having said that, there are certain things that you can do to try to get round the problem.

What You Can Do

Let us assume you have already gone through the checklist of reasons why your baby might be crying and have found nothing at all untoward. The first natural instinct is to pick the baby up, talk to him, sing to him, jiggle or rock him. A breast-feeding mother may wish to let the baby suckle at the breast. Or you might take the baby for a walk in the pram or out for a drive in the car. All babies that I know enjoy this. If you have work to get on with, try putting your baby in a sling so that he moves as you move and knows that he is close to your body, warm and snug. Try playing him some music from the radio or a tape. It does not really matter what it is. One of my own babies liked classical music, another was into rock.

An interesting alternative is the sound of a domestic appliance like the washing machine or the vacuum cleaner. These emit what engineers call 'white noise', a blend of sounds of different frequency which for some peculiar reason is eminently soothing to a crying baby. Perhaps it is similar to the muffled sounds heard by the unborn baby in the womb, some say – who knows? Another indispensable prop for many parents is the dummy. Obviously dummies need to be kept as sterile as possible and they should never be coated with anything sweet as this simply leads to tooth decay in the future. Finally, you could try the warm bath. But whereas some babies will settle straightaway in the bath, others will only be stimulated to scream even louder.

Sometimes it is difficult to know quite what to do for the best. You can try one or all of these techniques and usually the baby will eventually settle down. Coping with a crying baby can be trying and extremely frustrating, especially when you are desperately tired, so when this happens share the burden with your partner or get whatever help you can so that you can have a break.

When You've Simply Had Enough

Incessant crying in a baby can drive a parent mad. When a parent is tired and exhausted the constant noise can make them extremely angry and ready to snap. But this is dangerous, as uncontrolled bouts of rage and bad temper can sometimes be metered out on the innocent baby. Never let this happen. Recognise the warning signs and get to know when you have nearly reached the end of your tether. At this time seek help. It does not matter who it is from: it can be a partner, a friend, another young mum or even a sympathetic neighbour. If you are fortunate enough to have relatives living close by, they can often be called upon to come and lend a hand, but sometimes they live far away and this is not always possible. If no one else is available, call your health visitor, your midwife, your GP or the local child clinic. It is always helpful just to talk to somebody and obtain fresh ideas and advice. Not seeking help only makes matters worse.

If all else fails, put your baby down gently in his cot and simply close the door. He may well scream fit to bust, but provided he is not unwell he will come to no harm whatsoever in the short term. Walk away to a place where you cannot hear the noise, close your eyes and have a rest. Go back in ten to fifteen minutes and check that all is well. With any luck he will have fallen asleep or settled. If not, take another short break and go back again later. This may seem rather harsh on the baby but it is better than ending up harming him in any way. Anyone who reads the daily papers will know that, tragically, this does occasionally happen.

Professional Help

Often your health visitor will be able to give you the address and phone number of a local support group for parents of babies who cry all the time. The national organisation CRY-SIS has numerous branches throughout the country and is well worth contacting (see page 466).

Sleeping

When a baby does not sleep well at night, it is much more of a problem for the parents than for the child. Even moderate sleep deprivation is frustrating and exhausting and makes all the other tasks of the following day that much more difficult and time-consuming. Babies are as individual in their sleep requirements as adults are. Some will sleep contentedly without stirring right through the night from day one whereas others will be wide awake until late at night, restless and demanding. Some babies sleep for short periods at a time, waking frequently and wishing to play whereas others will go long periods without stirring. But eventually most babies establish a regular sleep pattern, the only problem being that although it may well suit the baby, it will not necessarily suit you.

Most babies in the first year of their life will require about fifteen hours sleep a day. This reduces to about twelve hours between the ages of one and three and then something in the region of ten hours between the ages of three and six. All children are different, however, and some will sleep more than average and others much less. What you do not need to worry about is whether they are getting enough sleep. The body's sleep regulating mechanism will ensure that, on the whole, babies get what they need. Perhaps the best news is that by the age of one and a half, three-quarters of all babies are sleeping right through the night. This is a fact to hang on to during your baby's first year when you are dragging your-self out of bed for the umpteenth time and wondering how on earth you are going to cope tomorrow. It will never be easy to manage sleeping problems, but there are certain tricks of the trade worth knowing.

Tricks You Can Try

It is sometimes possible to come to an agreement with your partner whereby you take it in turns to get up at night. When you are only getting up on alternate nights it is only half as bad, and you can look forward to three or four nights of uninterrupted sleep a week. Stimulate your baby as much as you can during the day by taking him out for walks, talking to him, playing music and changing his environment as often as you can. The more exhausted you can make him during the day, the more likely that he will sleep well at night. When your baby sleeps during the day, take a break yourself and a catnap if possible. Never allow your baby to sleep with a bottle still in his mouth as this can cause choking and is not good for any emerging teeth as they will be in constant contact with the sugar in the milk. As the child gets older you can try to cut down on his daytime sleep in order to encourage more sleep at night.

Ideally, the baby should be given a room of his own. This not only cuts down on the possibility of the baby being disturbed, but also reduces the chances of the baby disturbing others. Even if the baby merely breathes noisily or makes a single sound, a conscientious mother tuned in to her baby's noises may be woken unnecessarily. Co-sleeping experiments in which doctors have monitored the interaction between mother and baby when the baby is in the parental bed have proved this.

Provide a comfortable environment for your baby with soft music (such as a musical toy), low-level light and interesting things to look at like a shiny mobile over the cot. Establish a bedtime routine as early as possible and make sure that the child has a quiet time before being settled in his cot. If he is excited or stimulated there is less likelihood of his falling asleep quickly. When you wake in the night because your baby is not asleep, do not be tempted to go in to him immediately. It may well be that he will settle on his own within a few minutes. If this does not happen, check to see if his nappy needs changing or if he is hungry. A feed at this time, just like a feed before the normal bedtime, will often bring on sleep naturally and swiftly. The last thing you should do is to show your frustration and irritation, however difficult it may be to control it. Even a small baby will pick up on a parent's mood and if he is anxious he is less likely to settle down quietly.

Whether to have your baby in your bed with you is open to debate. Some parents feel that this is the only way to consistently get a baby to sleep at night and is something which they can all enjoy as part of the bonding process. Others feel it is important that the baby gets used to sleeping independently at night so that the parents can get some rest themselves. Relationships can suffer when the baby sleeps in the parents' bed ('something's come between us') and it can sometimes be very difficult indeed to get a child back into his own cot once the habit is established.

Help

The first two or three years with a young child are always tiring. Dealing with a constantly waking infant is perhaps one of the most harrowing tasks that any parent faces, and a great deal of effort and time has to be devoted to it. When you feel you can no longer cope it is important to seek help from any available source. Often this is a partner, but if a partner is not present, is working shifts or is simply unable to help then a relative may be called upon for assistance. It is also worth talking to your health visitor for help and advice, or get in touch with CRY-SIS, the national organisation devoted to parents with these types of difficulties (see page 466).

Very occasionally a doctor may consider prescribing a mild sedative for your child as a last resort. Where a family lives in cramped accommodation, where the father does shift work or where there is a great deal of street noise or other social irritations, this may be the only practical course of action. Sleep deprivation in these circumstances can have dire consequences for all concerned. If a mild sedative is used it should be for a short period only to re-establish a regular sleeping pattern. It should be used only in the stated dosage and the prescription should not be renewed. If the medication is used for more than two or three days at a time it can cause rebound insomnia when it is discontinued, which merely serves to make the problem worse. Rebound insomnia means that the infant's brain starts to become accustomed to the medication and then the child cannot sleep without it. Doctors who prescribe such medication do so knowing that they are really treating the parent rather than the child, but that sometimes this is a necessary, if temporary, measure.

Cot Death

Childhood is naturally and logically seen as the beginning of life rather than the end. When a child dies the shock for the parents is therefore profound and bewildering. Initially, there is complete numbness, then after a variable length of time, as the reality sinks in, this gives way to deep sadness and terrible grief. Later, anger may emerge as the parents struggle to make sense of what has happened and they yearn to know why it has happened to them. Often guilt features as well, the parents somehow, and quite unnecessarily, blaming themselves for the events which have taken place. After a cot death, these phases of bereavement may be particularly hard to bear. In cot death, also known as sudden infant death syndrome (SIDS), there is no explanation or reason for the loss of the baby. It is defined as the sudden death of a child which remains unexplained and in which a post-mortem examination fails to demonstrate any obvious cause of death.

Cot death, thankfully, is relatively rare, something like only one in seven hundred children being affected. To put it in perspective, a GP like myself will only see one case of cot death every ten years in a normal general practice, and the rate continues to decline. Having said that, it remains the commonest cause of death in babies from the age of one week to one year with a peak incidence at about three to four months. The usual tragic story is that the parents simply find their previously healthy baby dead in their cot. There will have been no warning signs and nothing to account for what has happened.

Although post-mortem findings reveal no abnormality, the cause of cot death is likely to prove multifactorial. Babies dying in this way may have a particularly immature respiratory drive centre within the brain, which means that they stop breathing when exposed to certain environmental conditions. Cot death is also more common in the winter months so it may yet be shown to be associated with a virus of some kind. We know that it is commoner in boys and in low birth weight or premature babies. We also know, despite recent media scares, that there is no evidence that certain types of modern cot mattresses or bedding are responsible. But what we do not know is the most likely cause of cot death. However, in the light of current information, there are four basic guidelines which, when adopted, will reduce the risks of a baby suffering a cot death. These are:

1 Lay your baby on his back or his side unless there is a particular medical reason for not doing so. If the baby lays on his back or side with the lower arm outstretched he cannot then roll forwards onto his tummy. Once a baby is able to roll over on his own, either from his back onto his tummy or vice versa, there is no need to keep readjusting his position as he will now be strong enough to do so on his own, should he need to.

2 Do not allow your baby to overheat. The ideal room temperature for the baby to sleep in is 18°C, a temperature which any lightly clothed adult would find comfortable. A baby placed in a centrally heated room and covered by thick bedding or wrapped in excess nightclothes cannot lose heat efficiently and may be more vulnerable to cot death.

3 Do not smoke, either during pregnancy or anywhere near the baby at all. It is best to give up cigarettes altogether if you can because there is a wealth of evidence to suggest that, not only cot death, but also many childhood diseases such as bronchitis, asthma, eczema and even abdominal complaints are more prevalent in children whose parents smoke. If both parents smoke the risk of cot death is five times higher than if neither parent smokes.

4 Have your baby checked over by the doctor if he is ill or unwell in any way. If your child has a slight temperature, is off his feeds or just not himself, it is better to be safe than sorry. Be extra vigilant and if you are worried ask your doctor for help.

In addition to these important recommendations, there are a number of questions which all parents concerned about cot death would like answered. These are some of the commonest ones with the most accurate and broadly agreed responses to them.

What Type of Mattress Should I Use?

Recent television programme claims that cot deaths were caused by toxic gases have not stood up to scientific research scrutiny and many parents have been alarmed unnecessarily. Some parents actually exposed their babies to increased peril by attempting to cover mattresses with dangerous materials like plastic sheeting and pillows. A mattress should be firm rather than soft. It should be kept in good condition, dry and well ventilated to avoid any possible contamination and micro-organisms.

What About Breast Feeding?

Research findings are unclear as to whether breast feeding reduces the risk of cot death, but since this is the natural and best way to feed your baby, and since it reduces the risk of infection in the baby, it should be encouraged.

Should my Baby be Immunized?

Babies should definitely be immunized as there is no evidence that vaccination is a factor in cot death. In fact cot death babies are less likely to have been immunized than babies who survive.

Is a Second Baby More Vulnerable if a Previous Child Died of Cot Death?

The risk is very slightly increased, and the amount of anxiety in the parents is naturally multiplied. For this reason the Foundation for the Study of Infant Deaths has set up a programme called CONI (Care of the Next Infant) to offer advice, practical help and support to every family affected in this way.

Can Baby Clinics Help?

The regular check ups and monitoring of growth and development are all useful ways of keeping an eye on your child's health.

What is the "Feet to Foot" Recommendation?

FSIDS encourages parents to lay their baby in his cot with his feet at the foot of the cot, not with his head at the top end of the cot as has previously been the norm. The cot should then be made up so that the baby cannot wriggle down under the covers which could then make the baby too hot. This is because over heating is a major risk factor in cot death, and there is no doubt that a proportion of victims have been discovered with bedding over their heads.

Should I Have My Baby In My Bed With Me, Or Just In The Same Room?

FSIDS advise parents to sleep their babies in the parental bedroom in a separate cot, not in the same bed. This should continue for at least the first 6 months of life. This advice has very recently been re-inforced by the latest research from New Zealand which took all other factors into consideration including whether sharing a room with another child made a difference. It did not seem to; so it is the presence of the adult which appears important.

Child-rearing practices differ amongst ethnic groups, and the rate of cot death is lower in UK Asian infants than in others. Perhaps their tendency to always have their children in the parental bedroom partly explains this. There has been a recent fashion for having the baby sleep in the same bed as the parent, but there are inherent risks in this practice. Over heating is the main concern, and there is always the potential risk of a parent rolling over in their sleep on top of the baby especially if alcohol or drugs of any kind, including medicinal ones, are being taken.

The Six Week Check

At the same time that mum is having her six week check-up after the birth, the baby should be having his first follow-up examination by the health visitor or doctor. This is certainly a convenient time to see the baby and to check on how he is getting on, but any parent who is worried about their child's health, growth or development can contact the healthcare team at any time. Mum will be asked some general questions to assess how she is feeling and whether she is coping generally. Any queries she might have about feeding the baby can be answered, and any worries about the baby's weight gain can be addressed too. The baby's mother may wish to know to what extent the baby should be watching her, whether he turns towards sound and light and whether he should be smiling by now. Some babies smile at six weeks, some take a little longer. More generally, the six week check is a good opportunity for mum to talk about any problems that she may have encountered looking after the baby and to discuss any ideas or pieces of advice she may have come across, however bizarre. It is amazing the things some people hear or read which bother them.

Next, the standard examination takes place, during which the baby's weight and length will be measured to check on his growth since birth. In general the six week review is reassuring for parents and a great opportunity to discuss any concerns or worries which they face. Occasionally some unexpected finding will require further observation, investigation or treatment. Difficult though this may be for the parents to accept, it will nevertheless mean that the routine six week check will have done the job it was designed to do – to identify any problem early and then to correct it.

Head Size and Shape

Head circumference is measured routinely to assess brain growth, and it provides an opportunity to discuss any asymmetry of the head which has been noticed. In fact, many babies are born with a degree of asymmetry of the head and it is usually of no great significance. Commonly, the baby's head is flat on one side from constantly lying on that side in his cot or pram. As the child grows older the head naturally becomes more symmetrical and no treatment is required. In very rare instances severe asymmetry can be due to craniostenosis which is caused by the premature closure of the sutures or gaps between the various bones which make up the baby's skull. This can be corrected surgically.

The size of a baby's head is closely related to the size of the brain within it. If the brain does not grow normally the head is likely to remain small. On the other hand, if the head is large and the fontanelle (the soft membrane at the top and front of the head) is bulging, increased fluid pressure within the skull, or hydrocephalus, is a possibility. Serial measurements of the head circumference in this instance would show that it is increasing abnormally fast.

There are a number of other rare causes of an abnormally small or large head, but by and large most variations are within normal limits. Small babies will obviously have relatively small heads and larger babies larger heads. Sometimes a baby's head is bigger or smaller than average because this feature runs in the family, and meeting both parents together may well reassure the doctor that this is indeed the case. In very rare instances there will be other underlying problems which require medical or surgical treatment.

The Physical Examination

After the head circumference has been measured, a full physical examination is usually carried out, looking particularly at the fontanelles, checking the eyes for cataracts, feeling the palate at the top of the mouth, looking at the inside of the mouth generally, listening to the heart and lungs, checking the areas where herniae occur and checking the hip joints and nappy area. Any problems with the stump of the umbilical cord should long since have settled down, but it is not unusual to see the first signs of a small umbilical hernia at the six week check.

Vision

At six weeks the baby is beginning to follow objects with his eyes. The eyes are checked for any signs of conjunctivitis or sticky eye and both eyes should move in the same direction together most of the time. The doctor may look at the back of the eye using a special torch called an ophthalmoscope to check that all is well there too.

Hearing

Tell the doctor if you have any suspicions at all that your baby is not hearing properly. Most parents are reassured if loud noises appear to startle the baby. Most babies will quieten and appear to concentrate when they hear certain noises and some will be soothed off to sleep if you play gentle music to them next to their cot. If the doctor is in any doubt about the baby's hearing a special test using an acoustic cradle or oto-acoustic emission (OAE) test can be arranged.

Movement

The doctor or health visitor will look at the way the baby moves his arms and legs and how strongly he can hold up his head when he is held with it unsupported. There should be good posture and muscular development and the baby should certainly not be unduly floppy or limp.

Social Behaviour

If you are lucky your baby will have smiled at you by the age of six weeks. However, this is not written in stone and some babies take a while longer to return your smiles. The six week check is a good time to talk about how much or how little your baby cries and how much sleep you and the baby are getting. Any major discrepancies from normal will be recorded and reassessed at a future date.

CHAPTER TWO

KEEPING YOUR CHILD HEALTHY

Immunisation

Immunisation protects both individual children and the community at large from infectious diseases that may cause serious handicap or even kill. Many people still consider the common childhood diseases such as measles and mumps to be fairly trivial conditions. The sad truth is that although this is usually so, in a small proportion of cases there will be damaging complications such as blindness, deafness, paralysis, brain damage or even death. In the case of measles, inflammation of the brain (encephalitis), pneumonia, bronchitis and deafness may all occur. With whooping cough there may be long, distressing bouts of coughing and choking. In a small infant this is terrible for the parents to encounter, let alone for the child to suffer, and convulsions, brain damage or death can even occur.

Not so very long ago many young children died of these illnesses because vaccination was not possible. Over the last half of this century, however, vaccines have become increasingly effective, simple and safe and are now available in either injectable form, or drops that are placed in the child's mouth. Vaccines work by preparing the body so that it can fight a specific virus or bacteria. The vaccine resembles the micro-organism, but is either a dead version or a live but drastically weakened version of it. In either case it causes the child's own defence system to produce antibodies against the real micro-organism so that active immunity is achieved. Here is a list of serious, preventable illnesses against which children can be immunised effectively.

IMMUNISATION PROTECTS AGAINST:

* Measles

* Mumps

* Rubella (German measles)

* Whooping Cough

* Polio

* Tetanus

* Diphtheria

* *Haemophilus Influenzae* Type B (HIB)

* Tuberculosis

* Hepatitis A and B.

When Should my Child be Vaccinated?

The Department of Health has a nationally agreed immunisation schedule which is believed to provide the best possible protection for children of all ages. At the appropriate time, parents will receive an appointment card automatically in the post inviting them to bring their child for vaccination. A full immunisation record should be kept in the personal child health record, which is provided to each child by the health visitor shortly after birth. The immunisation schedule is as follows:

CHILD'S AGE	IMMUNISATION
2 months	First triple vaccine (diphtheria, tetanus, whooping cough), polio and HIB
3 months	Second triple vaccine, polio and HIB
4 months	Third triple vaccine, polio and HIB
12–18 months	MMR (measles, mumps and rubella)
4–5 years	Diphtheria, tetanus, polio, MMR (unless previously given)
10–14 years	Rubella (unless previously given, girls only), HEAF test and BCG (if necessary) for tuberculosis
15–18 years	Tetanus and polio

Tetanus and polio boosters should be given every ten years throughout adulthood.

HIB

Haemophilus influenzae Type B is a relatively new vaccination protecting against life-threatening illnesses in young children. These diseases include meningitis and epiglottitis which resembles a serious form of croup. The new vaccine will prevent about sixty or seventy children dying each year in Britain from HIB infections, and it is very safe.

BCG and HEAF test

The HEAF test is carried out to discover whether a child is vulnerable to tuberculosis, a serious infection in children and adults alike which predominantly affects the lungs. This was once a leading cause of death in Britain until antibiotics were developed to treat it, but there has been a recent resurgence of the disease in inner cities where overcrowding and poor social conditions exist. Vaccination using BCG is normally given between ten and fourteen years of age, but where there is a family history of tuberculosis the BCG may be given in the newborn period.

Common Side-effects

The vast majority of children suffer no ill-effects whatsoever after vaccination. A few develop a small, tender red lump at the site of the injection which may last a day or two. A very few children spike a slight temperature and become a little irritable. If in doubt consult your doctor, although usually a small dose of paracetamol is sufficient to overcome the problem. There may also be a faint rash appearing on the skin after a baby has had the MMR immunisation, and occasionally the mumps component can produce a mild and short-lived swelling of the parotid salivary gland just below and in front of the ear. Neither reaction is serious.

Serious Side-effects

Although often quoted by a scare-mongering media, side-effects such as convulsions and encephalitis secondary to vaccination are incredibly rare. So rare, in fact, that a busy GP like myself would have to remain in practice for some 1,500 years before seeing a single case. Even then it is difficult to determine whether such symptoms would have occurred naturally anyway or are really a result of the reaction to the vaccination. The risks associated with immunisation are far smaller than the risks of any of the complications of the diseases themselves, including brain damage and death. There is universal agreement amongst scientists and doctors about this, and I personally know of no doctor who does not vaccinate his or her own children, myself included.

When Should A Child Not Be Immunised?

Even today there is confusion in some parents' minds about when a child should and should not receive an immunisation. A small minority of health visitors and doctors themselves may be a little uncertain, perhaps even basing their advice on ideas that are now out of date. If they are in any doubt whatsoever they should defer vaccination and refer the child to a paediatrician. All children should be carefully considered as individuals prior to immunisation procedures.

Always be guided by your GP or paediatrician, but in general all children should receive the vaccinations except for a tiny few who fall into the following categories:

1 Children who are feverish and unwell when the immunisation is due. In this case the vaccination should be postponed until the child has fully recovered.

2 Children who have had a *SEVERE* reaction to a previous jab.

3 Children who have a serious illness or who are taking medication such as oral steroid tablets. These could interfere with the child's capacity to fight infection. Children using steroid creams and inhalers, however, should still be immunised.

Because of the various myths that have abounded, many children who should have been immunised have missed out. Here is a list of children with conditions thought at one time to indicate that they should not receive immunisation. In fact, **they should all still be immunised.**

* Children who suffer from fits or convulsions.

* Children who have close relatives who suffer from fits or convulsions.

* Children who are snuffly or chesty on the day their jabs are due but who have no fever.

* Children on antibiotics.

* Children on steroid creams or steroid inhalers.

* Children who were premature or of low birth weight.

* Children with asthma, eczema or allergies.

* Children with a family history of asthma, eczema or allergies.

* Children with Down's syndrome or other chromosomal disorders.

* Children with cerebral palsy or other neurological conditions.

* Children who are breast-fed.

* Children whose mothers are pregnant.

If this information seems complicated and difficult to take in all at once, do not worry. Your doctor, health visitor or practice nurse are all able to advise you on which immunisations are due and at what time, as well as checking your child over to see that he is in a fit enough condition to be given the vaccine.

There have been fantastic medical advances through immunisation in recent years, notably the hundreds of thousands of lives saved by preventing whooping cough, measles, polio and so on. Smallpox, a serious, life-threatening disease, has been eradicated world-wide since 1971 as a result of vaccination procedures. Provided parents continue to have their children vaccinated, fewer and fewer children will be exposed to the risk of contracting these serious infectious diseases, and as the natural reservoir of the germs that cause them falls, their total eradication becomes ever more likely. It is the express intention of the Department of Health's vaccination campaign to put a stop to all such infectious diseases in Britain by the year 2000.

Hygiene

Babies, infants and children are particularly vulnerable to all kinds of infections, not least gastroenteritis which can lead to severe diarrhoea and vomiting, leading to the rapid onset of dehydration with all its attendant risks and consequences. It is vital, therefore, that parents teach their children thorough personal hygiene at all times and, of course, practice it themselves, particularly when preparing food for their children in the kitchen. You should also be constantly aware of the need to reduce any risk of infection spreading throughout the family, especially conditions such as coughs and colds, sticky eye, skin infections, worms and others. Here are some basic tips:

Personal Hygiene

* Wash your hands frequently to get rid of bacteria which can lead to food-poisoning.

* Always wash your hands after going to the toilet because germs can pass right through toilet paper onto the fingers and because bacteria can be picked up from moist areas around the groin.

* Wash your hands again if you have touched any raw foods such as vegetables, poultry, meat or fish. These too are likely to harbour bacteria.

* Wash your hands if you have been emptying the rubbish, wiping down kitchen surfaces or emptying the cat litter tray which can contain the germs responsible for an infection known as toxoplasmosis, affecting both adults and children alike.

* If you can, use a different sink for washing your hands from the one that you use for food preparation to prevent bacteria spreading from one to the other.

* Dry your hands with a towel reserved for that purpose and don't use a tea-towel which can allow bacteria to be transferred from your hands back to kitchen equipment.

* Change your hand-towels frequently to reduce any accumulation of bugs and moisture.

* Try to remember not to rub your nose or mouth with your

fingers or touch your hair as this also can transfer germs to food and kitchen equipment.

* Never cook if you are suffering from diarrhoea due to food-poisoning. With diarrhoea, it is always difficult to eradicate all germs and the risk of passing them on to other members of the family is high.

* In the kitchen, always try to keep raw food well away from cooked food to prevent bacteria being transferred. Use different parts of the kitchen for the preparation of raw and cooked foods. If you have a pet, keep its food in a separate part of the kitchen or in the fridge, and never dish up pet food with utensils which the family use. Keep pets well away from your family's food.

* Fill in any deep grooves or cracks around the sink and if the chopping board is deeply marked, throw it away because the crevices can allow germs to accumulate.

* Try to keep the kitchen clear of flies and other insects at all times, and empty rubbish bins frequently to prevent rats, mice, insects and pets from causing trouble.

* Keep any food left out covered at all times, and at any rate never leave food out of the fridge for longer than ninety minutes or so.

The above measures are really the very basic ones which anybody should adopt in maintaining good hygiene and preventing food-poisoning. But good hygiene is important in other areas too. These are outlined below.

Skin Care

Although some children may not like having their hair washed or their faces scrubbed, clean skin is important in reducing the growth of bacteria and preventing boils, abscesses and other infections such as impetigo. Bacteria thrive on sweaty skin and on babies where the moist nappy area is not cleaned properly. Thorough wiping is important to remove the ammonia-type products which come from urine and stools and which cling to the skin, making it red and sore. Most nappy rashes can be avoided by scrupulous skin care and by keeping the nappy area as dry as possible. With determination and patience, even thrush, which is due to a fungus, can be eradicated without medication.

Sterilising Baby's Bottles

One of the disadvantages of bottle-feeding your baby with formula milks compared with breast-feeding is that the risk of contamination of the milk is more likely. Bottles and teats must be cleaned thoroughly of any milk residues using ordinary washing-up liquid before being rinsed and sterilised thoroughly by one of a variety of methods (see pages 20–21).

Eggs

Eggs should really be excluded from an infant's diet until the age of one because of the risk of allergy or intolerance. Eggs are also a common reservoir for salmonella infection, a form of food-poisoning. The yolk is the part most likely to contain these germs, and the part least likely to cook well, but after the age of one, provided they are thoroughly cooked through, eggs are a perfectly healthy part of any child's diet.

Pets

Most children derive enormous pleasure from having pets around the house. Unfortunately, not all are as innocuous as goldfish. Cats and dogs can shed fur, skin scales and, in the summer, pollen, leading to a risk of allergic reactions such as eczema, asthma and hay fever. Shampooing the animals and vaccum cleaning thoroughly around the house can reduce this risk. Also, fleas can leap off animals onto children and produce itchy, infected bites. Pets, particularly cats and dogs, may also harbour parasites in their intestines which are passed in their faeces and can contaminate gardens and litter trays. Children do not think twice about what they pick up with their fingers in public parks, gardens and elsewhere, so worming the animals regularly and being cautious about where your children play is important.

Sticky Eye

Infectious conjunctivitis or sticky eye is common in children and highly contagious. The eye is red at first but within a day or two produces a yellow-green discharge which at night can sometimes stick the eyelids together by morning. Children rub their eyes and often transfer the infection from one eye to the other, and it is common for siblings and other members of the household to pick the infection up. Parents should wash the child's eyes thoroughly with boiled, cooled salted water on the end of a cotton bud to make the child more comfortable, using a fresh cotton bud for each wipe. Antibiotic drops or ointment will need to be prescribed by the doctor to eradicate the germs entirely. Ideally, a separate dispenser should be used for each eye and for each child, and care should be taken to provide each child with his own towel and flannel. Treatment needs to be continued for a good few days after the discharge has apparently cleared up to ensure that any germs left do not start multiplying all over again, producing a recurrence of the symptoms.

Coughs and Sneezes

Most coughs are infectious although the cough associated with asthma is an exception. Coughs and colds and other respiratory ailments are generally passed on through droplet infection which can be minimised simply by putting a hand over the mouth and using a handkerchief. Children can be taught to cover their mouths in this way from about the age of three and should be encouraged to do so.

Fingernails

Children's fingernails should be kept short at all times for several reasons. First, children are naturally clumsy and might easily scratch another member of the family accidentally while playing. Second, the space underneath a long nail is an ideal breeding ground for bacteria and this is an infamous source of contamination in food-poisoning cases. Third, intestinal worms depend on children with long, dirty fingernails for their continued survival. Although they are harmless, children with worms have an intensely itchy bottom where the worms are active, and so they scratch. Eggs of the worm are deposited under the nail and will then contaminate any food which the child touches. Whoever eats this food will in turn become infected as the eggs hatch out in their intestine. In this way, the lifecycle of the intestinal worm goes on.

Taking Your Child's Temperature

A child's normal temperature is between 36 and 37°C (degrees centigrade), or 96.8 and 98.6°F (degrees Fahrenheit). If your child has a fever his temperature will be over 37.7°C, and if your child is hypothermic, his temperature will have fallen below 35°C. What most parents will already know is that children's temperatures can fluctuate dramatically. It is not at all unusual for a child with a normal temperature to develop a fever of 40°C within a few hours, only for the temperature to subside again after simple treatment. In adults, a fever tends to take longer to rise and longer to settle down again. The reason for this is that the central temperature regulating mechanism in the brain is still immature in children, and control is less smooth and gradual. This is one of the main reasons that doctors are so often called by worried parents describing their children as 'burning up' or suffering with a raging temperature. Alarming though this is, it is not true to say that a high temperature always means a very ill child, or conversely that if the temperature is relatively normal, the child is perfectly well. A high temperature is merely a sign or a symptom of what is going on in the rest of the body, and as such it is well worth knowing how to measure a child's temperature accurately so that his progress can be monitored.

If a child has a higher than normal temperature, his skin, especially over the forehead, will seem hot to the touch. Often the back of the hand is used to assess roughly how hot a child seems, but to be accurate, and especially when reporting the symptoms to a doctor, a thermometer should be used.

Types of Thermometer

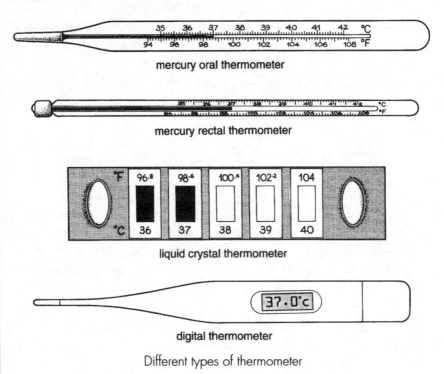

mercury oral thermometer

mercury rectal thermometer

liquid crystal thermometer

digital thermometer

Different types of thermometer

There are three types of thermometer that are commonly used. These are described below.

Traditional mercury thermometers are the most accurate. They consist of a glass tube with a reservoir (bulb) at the end holding mercury. An oral one is fine once your child is over the age of about seven, as by about this time he is unlikely to bite the thermometer and break the glass. When used with younger children, the temperature can be taken in the armpit with the arm held down firmly against the body, over the thermometer. Ideally, for a baby up to about eighteen months a rectal thermometer should be used, as this gives a much more accurate reading of the inner body temperature. This is important in this age group since any persistent fever is potentially more serious than in older children.

Digital thermometers have a plastic shell which is generally unbreakable, therefore they are safe and straightforward to use with children of all age groups. They are, however, slightly more expensive than mercury thermometers, and you may need to replace the batteries in the course of time.

Liquid crystal thermometers are plastic strips which are held against a child's forehead. They contain panels of heat-sensitive crystals which change colour at certain temperatures. They are safe and easy to use, although not quite as accurate as the other two types of thermometer. The heat-sensitive panel which illuminates corresponds to a digital temperature read-out above and below it.

Using a Liquid Crystal Thermometer

Read the manufacturer's instructions before using this type of thermometer as each may be slightly different. The important thing to do is to make sure the strip is held firmly against the child's forehead to maintain contact with the skin. The strip should be held there for about fifteen seconds during which time the heat-sensitive panels and their corresponding numbers will illuminate in turn before settling at your child's temperature.

Using a Mercury Thermometer

Whichever type of thermometer you are using, whether it is rectal or oral, it is important to return the column of mercury as far down into the bulb of the thermometer as possible before use. To do this, simply hold the thermometer at the top end and shake it vigorously downwards. Remember to wash the thermometer after use in cold water only, as hot water may break the glass.

Oral use: Place the thermometer under the child's tongue, asking him to keep it in place by pushing the tip of his tongue against his lower teeth. His lips should be closed to prevent air being breathed in and out of the mouth, which would reduce the temperature reading considerably. Remind him not to grip the thermometer too tightly in his teeth or to bite it. The thermometer should ideally be left in place for up to two minutes.

Armpit use: Lift your child's arm away from the body and place the bulb of the thermometer in the centre of the armpit. Lower the arm over the thermometer until the arm is fixed tightly against the side of the chest. Again, hold the arm in position for a minimum of two minutes. Remember that an armpit temperature will be about 0.5°C (or 1°F) lower than the child's inner body temperature.

Rectal use: Just as if you were changing his nappy, put your baby on his back and, holding both feet in one hand, lift the legs up and out of the way. Then gently insert the thermometer (lubricated with a little Vaseline or oil) to about one inch and hold it in place for a minimum of two minutes.

What Does Having a Fever Really Mean?

First of all, remember that in many ways a fever is a good sign. It means that the body is mounting resistance to the underlying disorder which has caused it in the first place. Also, whilst the symptoms of the fever are obviously unpleasant for the child, a raised temperature is highly unfavourable for the micro-organisms responsible for producing the infection.

Any child with a high temperature will be miserable. He will be floppy, flushed and lethargic. If the temperature has been high for any length of time, the child will be thirsty, will have a dry mouth and lips, and the parent may notice a sweet or acidic smell to the breath if the child is not eating. Older children may complain of a headache. At times he may feel shivery, as the fever leads to excessive sweating and heat loss from the skin which then cools, causing the child to feel cold and have goose-bumps. Because of this shivering, many parents in the past made the mistake of smothering their children in several layers of clothing and even greater numbers of sheets and blankets in an attempt to 'sweat out the infection'. This, unfortunately, only serves to make the child even more uncomfortable and miserable. It also increases the risk of dehydration and, most importantly, of producing a febrile convulsion, or fit, as a direct result of the fever, something which is particularly common in children under the age of seven. Because of these last two possibilities it is therefore important to take certain steps to treat the temperature rise and to keep it under control (see pages 244 to 246).

Children's Medicines

Drugs of any kind should only ever be taken when appropriate. If a particular drug is suggested by the doctor or nurse, make sure you know exactly why it is being proposed, for how long it should be taken and how it will help. Ask whether there are any more suitable alternatives and find out also about any possible side-effects. Some commonly used medications can make a child feel sleepy or irritable. Some may cause a rash or diarrhoea. If you know what possibilities exist, you will be less alarmed if they actually arise. Should your child get a reaction to the medication, remember to tell the doctor, not only for his or her immediate advice but also so that the problem can be recorded in your child's medical notes to ensure he will not be prescribed the same medication next time.

Make sure you know how much of the medicine should be given and how often. If this is not on the label, which it should be, write it down. Make sure that you finish the course that is prescribed, especially in the case of antibiotics. Not doing so encourages the emergence of resistant bacteria which can produce a worse infection than the original one.

When buying a medicine over the counter at a chemist, tell the pharmacist the age of the child who will be taking it. Make sure you read the label fully. Look at the expiry date as well because out-of-date medicine can do more harm than good. When any drugs in your medicine cabinet have passed their expiry date, hand them back to the chemist for proper disposal – too many unwanted chemical compounds entering our water supplies is bad news. Never accept medication from other people since you cannot be sure what has happened to it, and wherever possible use sugar-free preparations to save your child's teeth. Never give a child under the age of twelve aspirin as this has been associated with the very rare Reye's syndrome, which is characterised by brain and liver damage following a simple virus infection. Always keep the medicine cabinet locked and medicines well out of children's reach. Finally, make sure you have measuring equipment for liquid medicines in the form of droppers, syringes and specially designed measuring spoons. This is the best way of ensuring that your child obtains the correct dose.

Giving Medicine – A Spoonful of Sugar?

It is easy for the doctor to say, 'Here, take this medicine and give it to your child'. As we all know, when a child is unwell he is very likely to refuse anything unfamiliar or strange. This is perhaps one situation where a little bribery with a favourite food or drink is acceptable, but if this fails you may have to be forceful because if the medicine has been prescribed it should be taken. It will also, in many instances, make the child feel much better very quickly.

Giving Babies Medicine

Babies squirm and wriggle. They also cry a lot when they are sick. It is a good idea to get somebody else to help you, or else try wrapping a towel around your baby's body so that you can hold him steady. Prop him up in the crook of your arm and open your baby's mouth by gently pulling down on the chin if necessary. Syringes are generally used now to feed in the medicine, but if you are using a spoon make sure it is properly sterilised and that it contains the correct dose. Allow the medicine to run into your baby's mouth a little at a time. It is almost inevitable that some will spill out but try to get most of it to the back of his mouth and, having done so, close his mouth and allow him to swallow. If he will take some water from a bottle afterwards to wash it all down, so much the better.

Toddlers and Older Children

These days most medicines are available in liquid form and are attractively flavoured and palatable. The days of medicines which tasted and smelt disgusting have long gone. Even the few that remain can be disguised with sweet things like jam and honey. Tempting though it may be, do not add liquid medicines to drinks or bottles as the full dose will not be taken if all of the drink is not swallowed. It is all right to use drinks to wash away the taste, however, afterwards. To make tablets easier to take, they can be crushed up and mixed with something nice. Many preparations contain sugar or substances used to disguise nasty tastes, so it is always best to encourage your child to clean his teeth after taking a medicine.

Giving Drops

Drops may be used to treat eye, ear or nose infections. These are best given in the following ways:

Eye-drops: Lie the child flat and if necessary ask somebody else to hold his head and arms still. Gently pull down the lower eyelid of the affected eye and allow the drops to fall onto the eyeball just above the lower lid. Another way of doing this is to apply the drops to the corner of the eye with the eyelids closed. They will then run into the eye when the eye is opened.

Nose-drops: The child's head needs to be tilted slightly backwards. This prevents the drops running back down the nose after they have been dispensed. Three drops in each nostril are normally sufficient; any more will run down the throat and cause coughing.

Ear-drops: Put the child on his side with the bad ear uppermost. Allow two or three drops to fall into the ear canal and wait a few moments whilst they find their way downwards. Ear-drops are best given warmed slightly to body temperature to prevent the unpleasant sensation when cold drops are used.

The Medicine Cabinet

All households should have a properly stocked medicine cabinet, as few parents are lucky enough to have a 24-hour chemist open nearby every day of the year, and since it is very handy to have an immediate source of basic medication at all times. The medicine cabinet should be kept in a clean, dry, dark place and the first-aid kit within it should preferably be within an airtight box. Never mix different pills in one bottle and never hoard out-of-date medicines. Keep the medicine cabinet locked at all times and well beyond the reach of children. Essential items should include the following:

∗ Paracetamol in junior tablet or syrup form for babies. This is the classic pain reliever for children.

∗ Antihistamine. Older children can take non-sedating antihistamine tablets for allergies and travel sickness, and in combination with paracetamol for stings, sunburn, earache, sore throat, other pains and temperatures. Babies can take antihistamine syrup for similar conditions.

∗ Calamine lotion to apply directly to itchy, burnt or irritated skin.

The first-aid kit should contain at least the following:

∗ A thermometer, either mercury or liquid crystal (see page 54).

∗ Plasters of various sizes.

∗ Cotton wool.

∗ Gauze squares.

∗ Antiseptic cream.

∗ Paraffin-coated gauze dressings.

∗ A roll of surgical tape.

∗ A triangular bandage for shoulder and arm injuries to act as a sling.

* A roll or two of crêpe bandage.

* Scissors, tweezers and safety-pins.

* A simple plastic eyebath.

Your Child's Diet

Feeding your children is never easy at the best of times. Infants can make a terrific mess, young children waste food and most children are particularly fussy and choosy. Different children may want different food at the same meal, and the kind of diet that you want to give your children may be a million miles from the kind of food they have in mind themselves. It is also very common for children to go through a spell when they will only eat a particular type of meal, and all too often their choice is not terribly satisfactory. Buying healthy food that children enjoy is often not possible on a low budget, and shopping for recommended food which they will find tasty and tempting may not easily be accomplished in the time available.

Another problem is food refusal. At a very early age children soon learn to use food as a weapon. They know that the more they push their food around on the plate and refuse to eat it, the more attention they will receive from their parents. Parents can quickly get very worked up and frustrated about this, and many feel that the extra hassle involved in dishing up healthy food is just not worth it. But it is all too easy to give in to children's wishes and fill them up with fatty, processed 'fast' foods or bribe them with sweets in return for good behaviour. Difficult though it is, it is well worth persevering in these early years to ensure that your child eats healthily in the future.

Why bother?

The eating habits which an individual takes through life are learnt at an extremely early age, and bad habits are difficult to shed. Children who have got used to eating fatty, highly processed foods with lots of added sugar and salt will crave these for the rest of their lives. The delicate flavours inherent in vegetables and fruit will never be sufficient for them and they will prefer a diet rich in saturated fats unless drastic and painful action is taken. The problem is that this kind of diet begins a slow process leading to heart disease in later life. Doctors know that the deposits of cholesterol which form in the blood vessels start as young as two or three years of age, and the more saturated fat eaten throughout childhood the quicker coronary heart disease will develop in later life. This is perhaps the most pressing reason why it is worth bothering with your child's diet, and is particularly important if you have a family history of heart disease or obesity.

There are, of course many other reasons why children should have a healthy diet. Fresh fruit and vegetables not only contain healthy starches, vitamins, minerals and antioxidants (substances which help to prevent the harmful effects of toxins in the body), but they also contain plenty of fibre which maintains a healthy bowel and helps prevent the common problem of constipation. Reducing the amount of sugary foods in the diet and banning added sugar in cooking and drinks drastically reduces the amount of tooth decay your child is likely to suffer, and also helps to prevent obesity. Finally, being selective about what you give your child to eat and reading food labels carefully can reduce the possibility of allergy and other reactions to the components of his daily menu.

What Do Children Need?

Basically, children require a good variety of foods. This ensures that they get all the nutrients they require for normal growth and development. The essential building blocks of any food are protein, carbohydrate and fat, with vitamins and minerals thrown in too. Some foods, such as whole milk, contain almost all of these in a good balance, so dairy products are generally good news for children when given after the age of one. Carbohydrate is required to supply energy, and this comes best in the form of bread, rice, pasta, potatoes and fruit rather than in immensely sugary things like jam, honey, cakes, biscuits, chocolate and sweets. A certain amount of fat is essential in a child's diet as well, but too much fat is a bad thing. Unfortunately many of the foods which children like to eat, particularly fast foods and processed foods which are convenient for parents to buy, contain very high levels of saturated fat. Finally, children require adequate amounts of fibre which can be derived from a wide selection of fruit and vegetables. Children may not always go overboard about these, but there are clever ways of disguising vegetables in other foods or presenting fruit in an attractive and 'fun' way.

Helpful Tips for Reducing Fat

* Choose cooking oils which are low in saturated fat such as sunflower, safflower, rapeseed or olive oil.

* Avoid frying foods; grill or bake instead.

* Cut off as much visible fat as you can from red meat.

* When cooking dishes with fatty meat such as minced beef or lamb, skim off as much fat as possible during cooking.

* Get rid of the skin from poultry or fish as this is the fattiest bit.

* Go for low-fat spreads or polyunsaturated margarine rather than butter or hard margarine.

* When you buy cheese, buy lower fat ones like Edam, cottage cheese or low-fat Cheddar.

How to Cut Down on Sugar

Since high-energy carbohydrate calories can come from healthier foods, sugar is best left out. Once the habit of eating sweet foods is established, tooth decay and obesity can become a problem, and all too often a permanent one. Here are ways to prevent your child having too much sugar:

* When peckish, give your child healthy snacks from weaning onwards. These could consist of raw vegetables such as celery and carrots, unsweetened breakfast cereals, bread with

margarine or low-fat spread, unsweetened biscuits, fresh fruit or natural yoghurt sweetened with bananas, sultanas or other dried fruits.

* When it comes to drinks, avoid highly sweetened fizzy drinks and squash and use water, milk or unsweetened fruit juice instead. Remember, 'natural' products, such as orange juice, are also high in simple sugars.

* Keep stodgy things like cakes, puddings and chocolate biscuits to a minimum. They do not need to be banned altogether but they should be kept for special treats.

* Buy breakfast cereals which are not sugar-coated. These are cheaper as well as healthier.

* Try to avoid buying any sugar when you go shopping. If you have no sugar to put in your tea or coffee, none to sprinkle on cereals and none to add to your cooking, you will find you will get on quite happily without it.

* Reduce the amount of sugar you use in your recipes. Try using an artificial sweetener instead if you have to, although using these tends to maintain the sweet tooth habit.

* Get into the habit of reading the food labels on tins and packets carefully to see how much sugar has been included. If you must buy tinned fruit, buy those containing natural juice rather than syrup. Forget meaningless terms like 'low in sugar'. Read the label to find out just how low. And remember that the simple sugar in food may have a different name such as maltose, sucrose, glucose, fructose or dextrose.

How to Increase Carbohydrate and Fibre

Carbohydrate in the form of starch is an excellent source of slow-release energy, and fibre is important in the functioning of a healthy bowel and to avoid constipation. Starchy foods are high in carbohydrate and are also filling and satisfying. Vegetables and fruit, jacket potatoes, wholegrain cereals, pasta, rice, wholemeal bread and pulses such as lentils, beans and peas are all good examples. Beans and peas contain quite a bit of protein as well and are often quite popular with children. Dried beans need to be soaked overnight and then boiled for a minimum of ten to fifteen minutes. This destroys certain substances present in the beans which can cause tummy ache and diarrhoea. The recent trend of adding extra bran to everything is not really necessary if this type of diet is adopted. See the table on page 200 which lists foods which are particularly high in fibre.

Protein Intake

All children need protein to help them grow but, contrary to popular belief, meat is by no means the only available source of protein. It may be the most concentrated source, but children do not require huge amounts of protein anyway, and for many the texture of meat is unappealing. There is also a growing trend for older children to avoid meat on the grounds of vegetarianism, but again this is a problem which can be dealt with by including other protein-rich foods in the diet. Most dairy products, including milk, eggs and cheese, are good sources of protein and so is fish, although fish again is not all that popular with children unless it comes in the form of fish fingers, which can often be their staple diet. Luckily, cereals, peas and beans are also good sources of protein and if a child eats nothing else but these in addition to milk, he will almost certainly be perfectly well nourished.

Salt, Vitamins and Minerals

Although vitamins and minerals are absolutely essential in a child's diet there will be no need to add extra provided what he eats is varied and healthy. But children who are particularly faddy and difficult could still benefit from continuing with their vitamin drops until the age of five, though in most cases they can be discontinued by two. Iron is particularly important to a growing child, and this is present naturally in meat, dark green vegetables, bread, eggs, pulses and nuts. Infant formula milk and breakfast cereals are also fortified with extra iron.

Salt should not be added during cooking or to prepared food for a child since it is present in adequate amounts in food anyway.

Additives

There is continued controversy about the role of additives and preservatives in food intolerance, allergy and hyperactivity. The addition of any additives to food must be notified by law through food labelling, and many are recorded as an E number. Most of these are entirely safe and absolutely necessary as preservatives to prevent the growth of germs which can otherwise lead to food-poisoning. Continued research will determine just how important an influence additives are in food intolerance, although the consensus of current opinion is that only a tiny proportion of children are detrimentally affected by them.

Convenience Food

It's all very well suggesting a perfect diet for your children, but of course no such diet really exists. Mums are stressed and busy at the best of times and it is sometimes entirely reasonable to go for convenience foods to save time and trouble, especially when many children are gathered together at a party. Having said that, it is always possible to choose healthier options and go for wholemeal bread or toast, baked beans, baked potatoes, plain yoghurt, cooked eggs, wholegrain breakfast cereals, fish fingers, tinned fish and tinned tomatoes.

Any experienced parent knows that they will often see their child's worst behaviour at meal times. It is very tempting to give the child exactly what he wants in an 'anything for a quiet life' frame of mind. Provided that weak moments like these are the exception rather than the rule, a healthy and varied diet will set your child up well for the future, not only in terms of his growth and development but also in learning satisfactory eating habits.

Listening and Talking To Your Children

It is an outrageous but enduring fallacy that children in our society should be seen and not heard. But how easy it is to pretend that we are listening to the anguished attempts of our child to communicate with us as we are dressing in the morning, answering the telephone, laying out the breakfast, placing him in front of the television or kicking a ball around the garden. How easy it is for parents to talk over their child's head when he is trying to express his feelings about something because we do not really believe that what he is trying to say is important. But in fact the way we answer our children's questions is vital. By encouraging them to enquire, to be curious, to ask questions and to talk we can prepare them for two-way interactive discussion and the sharing of ideas about all sorts of things. If we listen as well as talk, we can help them think for themselves.

Talking to children should start when they are still babies. Of course they will not be able to understand what their parents are saying but they will pick up on visual cues and expressions and will derive reassurance from the familiar voices which can both soothe and stimulate them. Most children who have been chattered to in this way learn to talk earlier than children who have been brought up entombed within a wall of silence. It's also good for parents to get into the habit of chatting to their offspring as this fosters a spirit of free communication. As children grow up either we can ram our own values and ideas of acceptable human behaviour down their throats, or we can try to give them opportunities to form their own opinions. The trouble is that far too few parents feel that children are really capable people. They are seen all too often as helpless individuals totally unable to deal with the problems that life throws at them. It is natural to want to protect them from the harsh realities of life, but if we continually put ourselves forward as being omnipotent and all-controlling, the only message they will pick up is that only adults are capable of decisions and that they themselves are not.

Think back to your own childhood. Can you remember what it was like not to be believed when you told the truth about something? Can you remember how angry you felt when you were blamed for something somebody else had done? Can you recall how embarrassed, hurt or humiliated you sometimes felt? In many of these instances your own parents probably never gave you the opportunity to tell them exactly how you felt or what the actual circumstances were. You, like many children today, were probably given very little voice, either at home or at school, and nobody really listened to how you felt or what you wanted. Little wonder that so many children grow up totally unconvinced that they will ever get a fair hearing about anything. When this happens, children will withdraw and lose confidence. They will be reluctant to talk openly and express their feelings and parents will learn less and see less of their children's true potential. What parents have to do is try to become better listeners.

Listening

Listening to our children, or anyone else for that matter, is a hugely underrated social skill. Even when we think we are listening to what our child is saying, it is terribly easy to interrupt and impose our own ideas. Just as the child is telling you what is really wrong we jump in with reassurances, soothing words or judgements. Sometimes we totally contradict what he says if we do not like it. We either blame him or criticise him, which only makes the child feel worse, or we play the expert, robbing him of the ability to find his own solutions to a problem. Sometimes we divert the subject away from the real issue and reassure the child so that we, as parents, end up feeling better although he, unfortunately, does not.

Sometimes it is just a question of giving the child our full and undivided attention. Sometimes we need to take the phone off the hook, turn off the television or radio, put our work to one side and sit down face to face with our child and really listen. Set aside a minimum of 15 minutes every day to practise this one-to-one interaction. And strange as it may seem, we have to practise listening. Most of us are not very good at it so it takes time, but the longer you persevere the easier it will become for both of you.

Listening Tips

Because we are parents and because we want to share with our children our experiences and values, it is extremely hard to remain completely detached when they are talking to us, especially if they are expressing strong feelings or discussing problems. Try to let them say everything they want before butting in and giving advice. It is quite a good idea to repeat what they have just said in our own words as this not only tells them that we have listened and heard what they had to say, but it also gives them an opportunity to continue. It also tells them that we have accepted how they feel about something. The longer you can remain silent, just listening, the better. It is hard, but in many ways it is less risky than jumping in with questions which will distract them, or trying to diagnose the problem which prevents them from working it out for themselves. If we reassure them about any difficulties, this may make us feel better but it hardly ever helps them.

If we can also reflect back a child's feelings in our own words, this is helpful too. If a child, for example, tells his mother that he is cross with daddy, she has a number of options. She could simply say, 'Who isn't?', in which case the child is perplexed, or she could say, 'That's because daddy told you to stop playing football because supper was ready.', in which case the child is slapped down and rebuked. Alternatively, the mother could choose to probe further. She could ask, 'Something daddy has said has upset you?'. Then the child can continue his line of thought and express his feelings further. Mum can then go on to listen to the child's own views of where any injustice lies and to encourage him to find his own way of solving it which is acceptable to all. It is always good to allow your child to express feelings without judging them as over the top, trivial, silly or destructive.

Harsh Realities

Parents naturally want to protect their children from the harsh realities of this turbulent world. The most loving and caring parents of all make the mistake of trying to wrap them in cotton wool and protect them from the outside world. But in many ways, it is difficult to shelter children from reality, and they will come across violence, crime, war, bullying, cruelty, injustice and pollution whichever way they turn. They see newspapers, they hear conversations and they watch television. Our real duty as parents is to try to make sense of it all by discussing the issues with them and perhaps encouraging them to become involved in some small way in trying to make it a better world.

We cannot expect to bring up our children in a society which will remain identical to the one in which we ourselves were brought up. They, and us, will need to be versatile and show flexibility to change. They will need to be courageous and possess strong personal values so that they can find their own solutions, either alone or in association with others. Children respond best to openness and honesty, even if that means at times exposing our own inadequacies, personal conflicts and failures. By sharing everything with our children, not only do they grow and develop, we do too.

When To Call The Doctor

It is very difficult for parents to decide exactly when to call the doctor when they are worried about their child. Much depends on how experienced the parents are, and it is well known that most parents show much more caution and concern for their first child than for their subsequent children. Every little cry or whimper and even a small regurgitation of milk in the first-born can lead to anxiety, whereas in the case of the second or third child it is simply met with an 'Oh yes, the first one did that as well.' You may be reassured to know that doctors and nurses, with all their medical knowledge and skills, are no better. They still tend to panic when it is their own child that is suffering, so non-qualified parents need not feel guilty about worrying unduly.

Children are somewhat different from adults in that their symptoms can change quite dramatically from one hour to the next. A child can be listless and pale with a high temperature and lying flat out on the sofa one minute, and then running around again full of energy the next. In general, if a child seems unwell one moment and well the next, this is less likely to be serious than if a child is constantly unwell and is deteriorating. Not only do children's temperatures fluctuate very quickly (see page 244) but pain can come and go rapidly as well. Children are also not very good, quite understandably, at telling us exactly what is wrong. They may be too young to understand concepts such as 'headache' or 'sore throat', and even when they do they may experience pain at a different site from the one where the problem really lies. For example, tonsillitis may be felt by the child as ear pain and a hip problem may be felt as knee pain. Often it is some vague, general symptoms which the parent notices rather than a specific ailment. The child who is off his feeds, for example, who is clingy or particularly whingey may be behaving so out of character that the parent simply knows that something is wrong. Sometimes the symptoms are even less obvious than this, but the parent, out of sheer instinct, is convinced that something is going on.

In my opinion, a parent who is in any doubt should ask the advice of the doctor. A good and conscientious doctor will never mind being consulted about a conscientious parent's anxiety, and if the parents cannot take reasonable steps to ensure their child's health and welfare, who can? It is surely better to be an overworried parent who likes to play safe than a parent who neglects their offspring's symptoms and allows his condition to deteriorate before it is appropriately treated. Sometimes parents will need to ask for advice more than once. This is not to say they are dissatisfied with the first diagnosis, nor that they are making a nuisance of themselves. All doctors know that symptoms change and develop over time, especially in children, and an update as to the child's condition every few hours is often very helpful indeed. Provided the doctor is given all the relevant information, a plan of action can be established with the parents, and the doctor can then decide whether a child should be visited at home rather than the parents demanding it. Part of the GP's role is to medically educate his or her patients, and this includes giving parents some guidance about when and why to call the doctor about a sick child. All doctors have different styles of practice, however, so it is useful to ask your own GP exactly how he or she likes things to be done.

Urgent Conditions

It is impossible to be specific about which symptoms and conditions should be referred to the doctor. There are too many variations and too much symptom overlap to make this possible. If it were feasible, we would not need GPs at all, merely hospital departments to which children with any given symptoms would automatically be referred by their parents. But luckily we have highly trained GPs to make sense of sometimes bewildering symptoms, to diagnose and to treat or refer where appropriate. But even then, the GP may need to see a child on more than one occasion to remain confident about the nature of the condition and its treatment.

Particular Concerns

Certain emergencies can arise which necessitate immediate help. Any kind of breathing difficulty, especially where there is blueness of the lips or distress, is one example. Loss of consciousness, head injury, heavy bleeding, serious burns and suspected fractures are others. Most of these probably require immediate admission to hospital and are dealt with later. But there are a number of other common conditions for which a call to your GP is generally warranted. A high temperature present for more than an hour or two and which is associated with other symptoms may not always have an obvious cause, and may require examination by a doctor. If the child has suffered from convulsions in the past, in association with fever, or if he has symptoms such as a stiff neck, headache and vomiting, the matter is particularly urgent; meningitis needs to be eliminated, particularly in infants. Diarrhoea of more than a few hours duration, especially if associated with pain and temperature, requires immediate help. Dehydration is dangerous. Vomiting is another worry, particularly if it has been going on for more than a few hours, is violent or, in an older child, is associated with pain in the lower right-hand side of the abdomen. This could be the result of acute appendicitis. Any unexplained pain, discomfort or loss of appetite in a listless, apathetic child also requires proper and urgent evaluation. There is such a huge variety of symptoms and possible conditions that they cannot all be listed here, nor can any comprehensive or concrete guidelines be provided. The bottom line is – if in doubt, shout.

The Doctor's Role

Doctors know that one of their major roles is to reassure parents that their child is not seriously unwell. Family doctors are the filtering system for all sorts of conditions, and they know that in a small proportion of the cases they see they will unearth a more significant condition than the usual sore throats and earaches which form the largest portion of their work. Through a series of careful questions aimed at the parents about the timing, severity and nature of the symptoms, the doctor will start to form an idea about the likely diagnosis. A full physical examination will, in almost all cases, confirm the doctor's suspicions and allow him or her to treat the illness appropriately. Sometimes, however, things are not so clear-cut and further tests and investigations will need to be carried out before any conclusions are reached.

Ultimately, the diagnosis needs to be made so that the correct medication can be prescribed. The GP's role, however, does not stop there. He or she should be available to answer any questions that the parents may have and to explain how the medication will work, what its side-effects may be and how long the condition is likely to last. Each consultation with the child and parents should be viewed as part of the continuous development of the doctor–patient relationship.

The Doctor–Patient Relationship

As I have already said, conscientious parents should play safe and seek the doctor's help if they are in any doubt at all about their child's health. As well as seeking the doctor's help as regards diagnosis and treatment, they should ask for advice on nursing the child at home. They also need to know what to do in the case of recurrent conditions such as asthma, eczema and colic. Leaflets and other publications containing advice on specific conditions may be available from the doctor's surgery. The practice nurse may run health promotion clinics which the child could attend regularly. Finally, information about the spread of infectious diseases has implications for the rest of the family and, for that matter, anybody with whom the child has come into contact. Holiday travel arrangements may need to be discussed as well.

Regrettably, the doctor–patient relationship has evolved in recent years to a position where the chances of a child's parents being able to talk directly with the doctor who knows him, keeps his medical records and may even have delivered him as a baby, have diminished considerably. This is especially so when the parents make an emergency call during the night and weekends. At the end of the day, however, the GP with whom your child is registered is responsible for his care 24 hours a day, no matter which deputy or medical partner is on call in his or her absence.

Your Child In Hospital

Every year in Britain almost one million children will be admitted to hospital for one reason or another. Half of them are under the age of five so this is a worrying and emotional time for the entire family. But parents who remember hospitals from their own childhood as frightening, bewildering places will be reassured to know that things have changed dramatically in the last few years. Organisations such as the National Association for the Welfare of Children in Hospital (NAWCH) have been working at both a local and national level to increase awareness of the emotional needs of children and to make their stay in hospital less fraught.

Although the provision of specialised care for children may still vary a great deal between hospitals, it is true to say that separate children's wards are now taken for granted and the nurses working within them are specially trained to understand children's needs. Most children's wards are now friendly, happy places to visit with bright murals and plenty of toys and activities on display. Many hospitals allow for pre-admission visits whereby parents can take their child into the hospital ward in advance so that the child can familiarise himself with it and see that it is a 'fun' place. Most children in hospital are looked after by a dedicated, named nurse who becomes their friend as much as their carer, and parents are also encouraged to become as involved as possible to allay any anxieties the child may have.

How to Prepare Your Child for Hospital

Many children will still regard hospitals as unfamiliar, frightening places where some awful fate awaits them. It helps if you can talk to your child about their admission, say two to three days before being admitted. To try to do so any earlier than that may provoke more anxiety than it allays. It is worth encouraging children to play doctors and nurses, to play with a toy medical kit, and to read children's stories about going into hospital. There are many suitable ones which should be available from your local library. There are even special toys which can be purchased resembling miniature hospital words, ambulances, etc. together with the associated staff and equipment. These provide an excellent opportunity for the child to learn about the sorts of things he will encounter in hospital, and I have seen many children actually look forward to going in as a result. Failing this, the child's favourite cuddly toy can be used as a model patient, having bandages applied and so on, so that the child learns that patients are well cared for when poorly.

If a child asks you directly whether he will have injections or whether something will hurt, it is best to be honest if economical with the truth. If you reassure him that it will not hurt he will get a nasty shock if it does and may never trust you again. On the other hand, if you agree that it will be uncomfortable but that it will not last long and that it will help to make him better, he will probably accept this fairly readily.

Your Child in Hospital

Most hospitals allow parents to stay overnight when children under six are in hospital. In the past, separating children from their parents when they were ill only made things worse, not only for the child but also for the parents as well. It also meant that the job of the nurse was made that much more difficult and that doctors had to cope with a fretful child rather than a cooperative one. Research has also shown that the presence of a child's parent can lead to a reduction in the amount of anaesthetic and other drugs used prior to, and after, the operation.

The child's routine whilst in hospital should be kept much as it is at home. So a parent can help to wash, change, feed and put their child to bed in the way that is familiar to him. Some parents even get involved in the actual nursing care once they have gained confidence and been shown what to do by the nursing staff. Children who are in for a relatively long spell may continue their education in the ward with a specially trained teacher, or alternatively his normal school work can be brought in by the parent for the child to get on with.

It is not always possible, of course, for one parent to stay all the time and a rota should be organised to include the other parent or another relative. Remember to tell the ward sister when you come in and when you leave, and those parents who, for whatever reason, are unable to arrange for anybody to be there at all, can still communicate by telephone or by letter. In these situations, the hospital social worker and the social services generally can be of great assistance. It is important for single mothers, for example, not to ignore the rest of her family, and there will be times when the single parent just has to be at home, leaving the professionals to care for the child.

What To Take In With You

The standard items that your child will need are as follows:

* His favourite toy, muslin, blanket or comforter.

* Two sets of nightwear.

* Toiletries.

* Comfortable day clothes.

* Favourite books, games and toys.

* Drawing paper, crayons and pens.

✱ Favourite cup, dummy or bottle.

The parent will need the following:

✱ Cool, comfortable clothes.

✱ Alarm clock.

✱ Toiletries and towel.

✱ Nightwear, dressing gown and slippers.

✱ Small coins for the telephone.

✱ Books or magazines.

✱ Simple snacks and drinks.

✱ Sleeping bag if needed.

Note: Mobile phones are best left at home. They can interfere with some of the monitoring equipment in intensive care areas and payphones are always available on the wards.

The Day of the Operation

Some children like to know more than others about what will happen on the day of the operation. If your child needs to have a bath then there is no reason at all why the parent cannot give it to him. Next, the child will generally be expected to wear a special gown which does up down the back. He is normally allowed to wear some underpants and will almost always have to miss a meal so that the stomach is completely empty prior to the anaesthetic. This helps prevent nausea and sickness after the operation. Often, the child will be given some special medicine an hour before the operation called a pre-med. This is to make him sleepy, to dry up secretions in the nose and mouth and to make the anaesthetist's job that bit easier. A special 'magic' cream called Emla cream may be applied to the back of his hand to numb the skin there. This is to prevent the needle, used later for the anaesthetic, from hurting.

Increasingly, anaesthetists are willing to allow parents to accompany their child to the room where the anaesthetic is given. Special masks are now available which, unlike the dreadful black rubber ones of days gone by, actually smell of bubble-gum or chocolate, although even now these are not placed over a child's face until he is unconscious. After the operation your child will be nursed in the recovery area of the operating theatre and will be brought back to the ward as soon as his condition is stable and he is coming round from the anaesthetic. Of course, it is comforting for the child to have one or other parent there when he begins to wake up and the ward sister should inform you when it is all right for your child to have his first drink.

Home Again

It's important for parents to know who they may contact if they have any queries after their child has come home. Your GP should certainly have been informed as to what has happened in hospital, and both the children's community nurse and the children's ward itself are on hand to assist if any problems arise. Do not be surprised if your child reverts to slightly babyish behaviour for a while and becomes more clingy than usual. It is understandable that he needs reassurance that no further periods of separation from his home and family are about to happen, and he may well have enjoyed the extra attention his stay in hospital afforded. Beware of any jealousy from the poorly child's brothers and sisters who will have missed you whilst you stayed in hospital with him, and may well have resented the extra care he received.

Further Help

There are many helpful publications available concerning children being admitted to hospital, and many of these come in the form of leaflets available not only in English but also in Urdu, Somali, Bengali and Cantonese. For further information, advice and support contact Action for Sick Children, Argyle House, 29/31 Euston Road, London NW1 2SD.

CHAPTER THREE

GROWTH AND DEVELOPMENT

Growth

The way in which your baby grows is a simple but accurate gauge of his general health and progress. After your baby is measured at birth, regular measurements will be repeated at frequent intervals to ensure all is well. These checks are usually carried out by the midwife and health visitor to start with, and later at the doctor's well baby clinic. Various aspects of your baby's growth will be recorded, in particular weight, length and head circumference. The measurements are plotted on special graphs called centile charts. The chart below is a typical example. It is for a girl born prematurely at thirty-four weeks in order to check her weight gain over a period of time.

The middle one of the horizontal lines is known as the fiftieth centile. It means that fifty per cent of children of a certain age will be heavier than this weight and fifty per cent will be lighter. The fiftieth centile is therefore merely the average. The outermost continuous lines are the second and ninety-eighth centiles which means that only two per cent of babies fall outside each of these lines, because they are either very small or very large. Since this little girl was born prematurely at thirty-four weeks, the first recorded weight is to the left of the vertical black line which represents the date when a full-term baby is born, that is, at forty weeks. When this little girl reaches the twenty-week point on the chart she will actually be twenty-six weeks old. In fact, as premature babies grow older the difference becomes negligible and is generally gone after the second year.

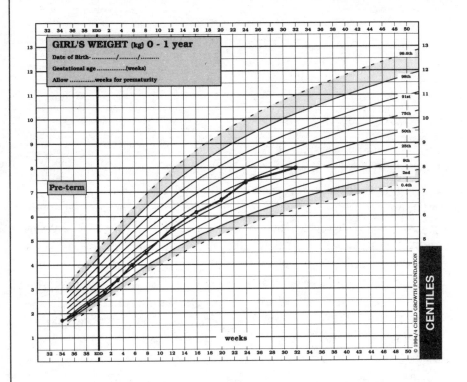

Centile weight chart for a girl born at 34 weeks

Understanding the Charts

Many parents are confused by centile charts and become worried if their child is above or below the fiftieth centile. The thing to remember is that 'average' does not mean the same as 'normal'. Children with small parents will probably be smaller than average children of the same age but will still be entirely normal. There are also variations between ethnic groups, and since the centile charts

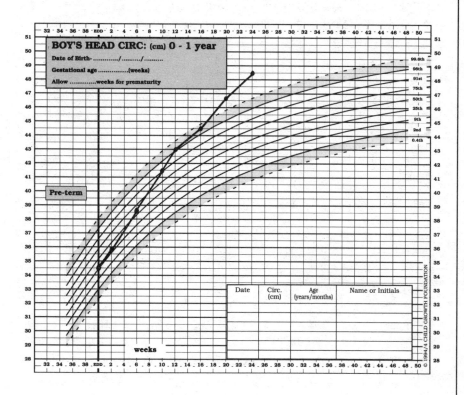

A crossing centile chart showing an abnormal increase in head circumference (size when measured around the outside)

were drawn up using data from a white, British population, there will be racial variation also. In addition, girls have slightly different shaped growth charts from boys because they have a pubertal growth spurt earlier.

The overall pattern of growth is more important than individual measurements. For example, an infant can have a bad week now and again as a result of illness and his growth may temporarily slow down. Healthy babies quickly catch up again, however, and the line of growth which your baby follows will usually be a gradual, smooth, steady slope parallel to one of the centiles. If your child's centile chart for height, weight or head circumference does not follow a steady curve, but crosses the centile lines suddenly, it can alert the doctor that something may be wrong. Generally speaking, a normal pattern of weight gain is for a baby to double his birth weight by six months and triple it by one year. Many babies lose a little bit of weight straight after their delivery although they should have recovered their birth weight by about ten days. After that the usual weight gain is somewhere between four and eight ounces per week.

Development

All children develop new abilities and skills at different rates, simply because everyone is different. But having said that, what they do, what they achieve and their pattern of behaviour normally evolve within acceptable age ranges. Physical, mental, social and emotional development is a complex process, with new capabilities appearing as existing patterns of behaviour develop into new ones. Much depends on genetic factors but environmental influences can also be important. One the whole, the more time and energy that parents can devote to teaching and stimulating their child the better. If brothers and sisters are around too and the child is exposed generally to other children, his development can be accelerated even more.

Learning and Playing

Children love to play as part of the learning process and it is through creative action that they learn about the world around them, about other individuals and about themselves. The trouble is, most small children will not play alone for very long. This puts demands on the parents' time and attention which have to be divided amongst all the other things that life throws at them. But the more time you can devote to filling your child's day and to stimulating him, the more his curiosity will be satisfied and the more you will be aiding his development. Try to make this as much fun as possible for both of you. Talking to your child about anything and everything from a very early age is vital. It does not matter that he may not understand much of what you say, he will gradually pick up intonations of speech, nuances, moods and finally the meaning itself. Children like to feel included. They need to learn that communication should go on all the time. They need to know that expressing themselves through speech is important.

Here are just a few of the kinds of useful activities you can encourage your child to enjoy during the course of a day:

* Provide toys which allow various methods of construction such as Playdoh, Plasticine, clay, building bricks, Lego, Meccano, sand and water, etc.

* Tell stories to the child and listen to the stories which he tells you, embellishing them as you go on.

* Provide noisy musical instruments which make different kinds of sounds. Allow them to bang, ring, blow, buzz, pluck and hammer.

* Play games like hide-and-seek and matching shapes and colours.

* Experiment with language using 'silly' talk, funny noises, pretend words, rhyming words and other kinds of word games.

* Encourage physical activity in the form of climbing, jumping, bouncing, dancing, riding on your back, swinging, kicking or catching a ball.

* Provide toys and books which encourage role play, for example model houses, books about doctors and nurses, farmers, etc., dressing-up outfits.

* Be prepared to get messy. Buy waterproof mats or polythene sheets, plastic aprons, paint pots and brushes.

* Act out little plays using dolls, or make puppets out of gloves or socks. A play can incorporate all sorts of important concepts

such as right and wrong, cruelty, kindness, anger, love and compassion.

* Get on the floor yourself and join in your child's games. Make lines of cars, mimicking the noises they make. Tell a story to describe what is happening as you move the vehicles about.

* Play with water in the sink, bath or paddling-pool. Provide plastic bottles and cups, funnels and straws for the child to experiment with.

* Let your child dress up in masks, hats, scarves, blankets or any items which you have little further use for.

* Encourage simple cookery using manageable quantities of real ingredients such as rice, flour, sugar and eggs.

* Keep television and videos to a minimum, although most children over three will follow cartoons and animal programmes quite well for a few minutes at least, giving the parents a bit of a break. Ensure that you know exactly what your child is watching at all times, and watch television with your child when you can so that you can discuss and if necessary explain what is going on.

Playing in Groups
Children like to play in the company of other children. When they are very young, children in groups will tend to play on their own, but they do at least get used to other children being around. Parent and toddler groups are super for children from about eighteen months of age, and they give harassed parents a decent break as well as providing them with an opportunity to relax and mix with other adults. From about three, your child can go to a playgroup or nursery school offering organised play with new and exciting toys and equipment. To find out about local playgroups, ask your health visitor or local social services department and get into the habit of looking on notice boards in the newsagent's, at the doctor's clinic or at the health centre. Libraries often contain addresses and contact numbers and the Pre-school Playgroups Association can give you local addresses too.

Infant school starts at around the age of five and by law all children have to start by the beginning of the school term following their fifth birthday. It is of course possible, if the child is ready, for him to start slightly earlier. Some schools are more popular than others so it is wise to visit local schools well before your child is due to start to see which ones you like and to get your child's name down at the earliest opportunity. Lists of local infant schools are available from your local education department.

Choosing Where Your Child Goes
When thinking about a playgroup, nursery or infant school for your child, you need to be absolutely sure that you choose the right one. First of all, check that the nursery or playgroup is registered. Go and take a look at it and talk to the people who work there. Find out how many children attend and what the staff/child ratio is like. The more staff per child the more stimulation and supervision your child is likely to receive. Find out about the qualifications of the staff, what equipment and facilities are provided, what kind of discipline is imposed and how your child's day is likely to be structured. Talk to other parents whose children go there to see whether they are really happy with it. Ask how the playgroup or school would help to settle your child in and what their policy is in the event of illness or injury. You should soon get a feel for a place and know instinctively whether it is the sort of environment which would be good for your child to grow and develop in.

The Developing Child

Since all children are different it is inevitable that they will develop certain skills at different times. A child who learns to stand and walk fairly late may well have compensated for this by learning to talk earlier than is average. The important thing is to distinguish this sort of child from the one whose development is delayed in almost all areas. In the latter case, the child may well have a specific disability such as a hearing or visual impairment which when treated will enable him to catch up. Children who have generalised developmental delay may simply have inadequate stimulation at

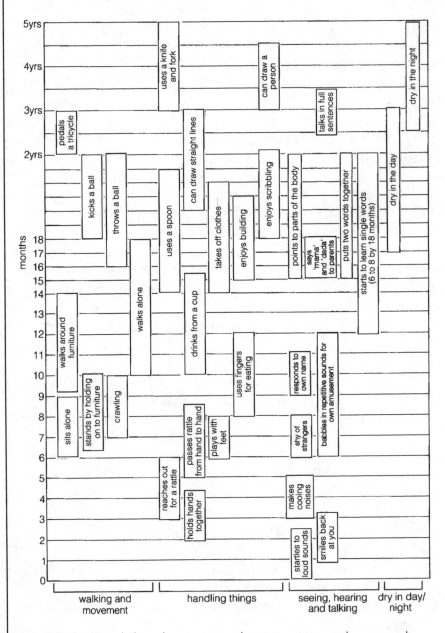

Developmental chart showing normal variation in time taken to reach milestones

home or perhaps are just a little slower than expected because of restricted intellectual capability or because of illness or disability. Important examples of specific developmental skills are described below and are summarised in the developmental chart.

Walking and Movement

A baby of about three months will have begun to lift up his head when lying on the floor. Later, somewhere between six and eight months, the child will generally sit when supported and by the age of nine months most children can do this without assistance. Crawling usually begins at about seven or eight months but does not always follow the same pattern. Sometimes the child starts off by crawling backwards, and some children miss out the crawling stage altogether, a child perhaps shuffling along on his bottom before learning to stand holding onto furniture and then later beginning to walk. Bottom shuffling and creeping along on the tummy appear to be features which run in families.

When it comes to walking itself there is tremendous variation in the age when children achieve this. Most are able to stand holding onto the furniture or their parents' legs at about eight months and walk at about thirteen months, but walking can start as young as nine months or as late as fifteen months. With children who are late in walking, no significant cause is usually found. A child who is quite happy with crawling, and can do so particularly speedily, may have less incentive to learn to walk and may therefore walk later than usual. It may be an inherited feature, and just like delayed control of the bladder, appears to be due to slow maturation of certain aspects of the nervous system. Most children will learn to kick or throw a ball from about one and a half to two years of age. Parents might like to know that the first really big present they can give their child, the tricycle, can be pedalled by most children at about the age of two and a half to three. In rare instances, delayed walking and other movement abilities is due to weakness of the leg or other muscles as a result of nerve or muscle conditions such as spina bifida or muscular dystrophy. Cerebral palsy may affect all areas of movement, first manifesting itself as slowness in developing head control and later as delayed sitting and walking.

Using the Hands

One of the features which distinguishes humans from other animals is advanced hand–eye coordination which allows fine finger movements and complex manipulative skills. The development of these abilities requires practice and experience, and children can be stimulated and encouraged in this by giving them small objects as well as large toys to play with and sitting them up as much as possible rather than leaving them lying down all the time.

Most children will be able to reach out for objects which take their fancy at about four months. Within another two months they can lift a plaything and bring it to their mouths to suck. They can also start to pass an object from one hand to the other, sometimes via their mouths. At ten months they can start to feed themselves with solid foods and at around fourteen months can even shovel food messily from a spoon. The ability to stack bricks will usually start just before a year and a half, as will drawing with a crayon on anything put in front of them. By the age of about three it may become apparent whether a child is right- or left-handed and somewhere between the ages of three and four he is likely to draw for you his first anatomically correct person.

Hearing and Speech

Right from day one most babies will jump at, or be startled by, loud sounds. At three months they are babbling and cooing in their cots and by about sixteen to eighteen months most children are managing single, simple words like 'daddy' and 'mummy'. Two or three months after this they know who daddy and mummy actually are and restrict these words to their parents. At a year and a half most children have learnt about half a dozen or so words and by three years of age most children are talking in full sentences.

The most significant cause of speech delay is a hearing problem, but lack of stimulation and genetic factors are also worth considering. Funnily enough, twins often begin to talk rather later than other children, either because they receive less individual attention from their parents or because they have developed a private language between themselves which gives them less incentive to learn true speech. Offspring of bilingual parents may also learn to talk slightly later than others, but learning more than one language at a time more than compensates for this.

Sight

Normal vision is essential for normal development. Children can only learn the names of objects once they have recognised them by sight, and they learn about sounds by observing which objects make which sounds. Their motivation to crawl, sit and walk also stems from their curiosity and their wish to explore the environment which they observe around them.

Although newborn babies appear not to be able to see or focus on anything, they do in fact see all kinds of things and are able to focus on objects that are very close to their faces. Anything further away is just a blur of light, and it takes a while before a baby's brain can make sense of the images relayed to it through his eyes. Many babies squint for the first few weeks of their life, or appear to, and if this is still noticeable after the age of three or four months, the doctor should take a look (see pages 366–369). They begin to recognise their parents' faces at two weeks or so and start to smile at about six weeks. At six weeks a child can also begin to follow a colourful and slowly moving toy at a distance of about eighteen inches from his face. It takes about six months before an infant can see things on the other side of a room.

Potty Training

Children learn to control their bowels and bladders at vastly different ages. Bowel function is usually mastered first, delay in bladder control being much more common. By and large, about fifty per cent of two-year-old children are dry during the daytime and in another year, at the age of three, ninety per cent are dry. Staying dry at night usually takes longer and it is not until the age of five that most children are dry at night as well. Having said that, twenty per cent of normal five year olds will still wet the bed at least twice a week, and even the two per cent of twelve year olds who wet at night can still be considered normal as they too will grow out of it in time.

For practical reasons, it is always advisable for parents to start potty training during the summer months when it is easier and more economical to get the washing dry outdoors and there are fewer clothes to take off in the first place. The first stage is for the child to become aware of when his nappy is dirty or wet, and the second is for him to realise when his bladder or bowels are actually working. Finally, the child will come to recognise when he needs to empty his bladder or bowels and will actually instruct his parents accordingly. There is a lot to be said for allowing a child to develop these skills at his own pace, although using nappies can be both costly and time-consuming and parents may well wish to do away with them as quickly as possible. The best developmental stage to start potty training is probably when the child has learnt to recognise when he actually needs to 'go'. Attempts to potty train too early are frustrating for the parents and can exert undue pressure on the child which merely makes the situation worse.

Developmental Checks

Developmental checks are carried out routinely at certain ages, though the timing varies slightly between different regions. The first one is at about six weeks, the second at about eight months, the third anywhere between eighteen months and two and a half, with the final one being pre-school, when the child is aged between three and three and three months. Obviously, if a parent is concerned about any aspect of their child's development in the meantime, the child can be checked over by the doctor or health visitor at any time.

The purpose of routine development checks is to spot any problems as early as possible so that any weak areas can be corrected. Any special educational needs can be identified and notified to the local education authority. Many of the skills described earlier will be tested to make sure that your child is developing at the correct rate for his age. It is not a question of passing or failing such assessments, because some areas of development will be slower than others. It is the overall progress and maturation of the child which are important. Often it will be the parents themselves who are the first to observe that something may be wrong. When this occurs, the child should be examined thoroughly by the doctor, in particular to test hearing and vision. Referral to a paediatrician, speech therapist, physiotherapist or psychologist may then be in order. The priority is to diagnose the cause of the developmental delay, and then to instigate appropriate treatment. Usually no significant problem is discovered, and the parents can be reassured and advised as to which toys and other forms of stimulation to choose for the correction of certain weaknesses. Depending on the nature of the developmental delay, therapy might well include a number of health professionals, such as occupational therapists, speech therapists, physiotherapists, clinical psychologists as well as the provision of hearing aids or glasses. Occasionally, a long-term problem or handicap is discovered and children affected by these physical or intellectual difficulties will require special consideration.

Children with Special Needs

Many health authorities and trusts have set up child development teams consisting of doctors, health visitors, social workers, paediatricians and therapists who are there to support children with special needs and their families. They can provide much needed information, support and advice, though this is also available from a large number of voluntary organisations. Other sources of help include speech therapists, physiotherapists, occupational therapists, playgroups, nurseries, nursery schools and home learning schemes. Educational advisors for special needs can be contacted at your local education department, and your health visitor or social worker can tell you exactly what has been set up in your particular part of the country.

Children over the age of two who may have special needs have to be fully assessed, and even children under two can be formally assessed if the parents request it. The parents can take part in the assessment themselves, and the Advisory Centre for Education provides information on the implications of the assessment for the child's future learning. It is tough, to say the least, when parents are informed that their child has some kind of learning disability. But with the help available from all the various healthcare professionals and voluntary organisations, combined with the love and support of families and friends, the seemingly insurmountable hurdle which may be perceived at the outset can become a good deal more manageable in time.

CHAPTER FOUR

ACCIDENTS AND EMERGENCIES

Prevention

Although *all* children are accident-prone in most situations the majority of unforeseen injuries in children occur in the home and more than half of them involve the under-fives. These account for half a million admissions to hospital, representing one child in six, every year in Britain. Believe it or not, such accidents are the commonest cause of death in all children aged between one and five years.

There is a great deal that parents can do to prevent such injuries, though it is never possible to remove the risks altogether. As well as being vigilant and observant, there are two major contributions parents can make to reduce the chances of accidents happening in the home. First they can have a good scout round every room in the house to identify and remove potential hazards. Second, parents can start to teach their children an awareness of dangers and risks at the earliest possible age, reinforcing the message at every turn. Very young children learn by experience but it still takes several falls before they learn to watch more carefully and become more nimble. The same applies to road safety – children need to develop the infallible habit of having their seat belts attached whenever they are passengers in a car.

There are a number of areas where parents need to be particularly careful. These are described below.

Suffocation and Choking

A child's windpipe is narrow and easily blocked. Make sure that your young child does not play with objects small enough to be put inside his mouth and then accidentally inhaled. Beads, hard sweets, dolls' eyes, marbles and peanuts are common culprits. Peanuts and hard sweets should ideally not be given to any child younger than seven. Also make sure that your child does not play with lengths of ribbon or string which he can accidentally wrap around his neck and choke himself with. Regrettably, doctors still see far too many tragedies every year from children who have suffocated after putting polythene bags over their heads, despite the warnings printed on the bags which, of course, children themselves are unable to read. Make sure that *all* bags of this type are stored well out of children's reach.

Falls

Do not allow your child to run about in socks or tights if you have any slippery, non-carpeted floors. This is a very common cause of sometimes quite serious head injuries as a child's feet skid forward bringing the back of his head hard down on a tiled or wooden surface. Make sure all upstairs windows are safely secured and that there is no furniture positioned close by on which children can climb in order to reach them. Check that banisters are strong and that the gap between them is narrow enough to prevent a small infant from wriggling through. Do the same for any balcony in your house. Stairgates are a must to prevent small children from tumbling down the stairs. Place babies in bouncy chairs or safety chairs only on the floor, not on tables or kitchen worktops. Baby walkers are fine provided they are kept away from the top of ungated steps or stairs, ledges on which they can turn over or hot radiators against which they can become wedged.

Cuts

One of the commonest causes of cuts in children is from broken glass. Make sure that any low-level glass, for example in windows or French doors, is safety glass or is coated with safety film. This prevents shards and splinters from forming, which can cause nasty lacerations, should the window be broken. Do not allow your child to play with any glass objects such as milk bottles or ornaments. Go round the house removing anything with sharp edges or points, especially those which can be put in a child's mouth like pencils or ballpoint pens, as these can cause severe injuries if the child falls. Finally, keep scissors and knives well away from children as they are not only fascinated by them but experiment with them from a very young age.

Burns and Scalds

Always keep hot drinks out of children's reach at all times and, however fussy it may seem, ask any visitors who are unfamiliar with children to do the same. Make sure that tablecloths cannot be pulled off tables which have hot food or drink on them. Kitchens are dangerous places for children, and if you cannot put a safety gate across the kitchen door to keep children out, there are various other precautions you should take. Make sure your cooker has a safety guard and ensure that any pan handles are pointing towards the back. Never sit children on worktops where they can touch a hot kettle or stove. Beware of the kettle flex hanging down over the worktop which children might be tempted to pull on – coiled flex is much safer. Teach your children how dangerous hot radiators and towel rails can be and always keep a fireguard around an open or electric fire. When it comes to the bath, obviously check the temperature of the water before your child gets in, and never leave him alone in the water for a moment.

Accidental Poisoning

All medicines should ideally be kept in child-resistant containers in a locked medicine cabinet well out of reach of any children. Similarly, parents need to lock up, or keep out of reach, any household chemicals such as bleach or methylated spirits which children might be tempted to swallow. This can result in extremely nasty burns to the mouth, gullet and stomach. Special child-proof locks fitted to kitchen cupboards are particularly useful here. If you have a garden, take the same precautions with any garden chemicals such as weedkiller or creosote and check around for any potentially poisonous plants, berries or seeds which your child, in his innocent curiosity, could chew on and swallow.

Accidental Electrocution

Children love poking their little fingers into unused electrical sockets, which are often within their reach. Buy enough plastic safety covers to block these sockets or at least hide any exposed sockets behind furniture. Any worn or split flexes should be replaced.

Drowning

Tragically, young children still die in the bath every year. It only takes a few inches of water for a child to drown in so never leave your child alone in the bath, even for a moment. If the phone rings or there is somebody at the door, either take your child with you to answer it or ignore it altogether. If you have a garden pond, fence it off so that children cannot fall in, and when you take your child to the seaside, to the swimming-pool or to any open stretch of water never leave him out of your sight for a second. Teach your child to swim as early as possible but also teach him respect for the water. Many strong swimmers are lost every year purely because they have no experience of currents and tides.

Dangers Outside the Home

Although children are vulnerable both inside and outside the house, there are probably fewer safety measures you can take outdoors. There are inherent hazards in many public places, including parks and roads, and on stairs and escalators. In playgrounds, for example, it is a good idea to carefully watch your child at play and to be there to help him if he attempts anything you consider too dangerous. You do not want to stifle his adventurous nature but nor on the other hand do you want him to run any unnecessary risks. Hold his hand in public places or use reins if this is easier, and teach him sound road safety drill as soon as this is practically possible.

You can certainly make it safer for your child to travel in cars. When it comes to seat belts, make sure your child is strapped in for every journey. If it becomes a habit from day one, children are more likely not to rebel against it. Never be tempted to hold your baby in your arms, even if he is screaming. It is particularly dangerous and foolish, as well as illegal, to do this in the front of a vehicle, and is very dangerous even in the back. In an accident the baby or child becomes a tiny projectile which will rocket through the windscreen with great force if not restrained by a seat belt. Babies are safest in a special baby seat which is facing backwards, strapped onto the car seat by the existing adult seat belt. An alternative is a carry cot secured to the back seat of the car with a special safety harness. Some areas run loan schemes which provide baby seats free of charge. Check with your midwife, health visitor or road safety officer for more information on these.

When your child is older he should really sit in the back seat, again secured into a child safety seat or on a booster cushion strapped in with a child safety harness or adult seat belt. However much your children may pester you, do not let them play in the rear luggage compartment of a car unless the manufacturer has provided special seats with harnesses designed for the purpose, and do remember that you are committing an offence if you travel in the back seat of a car without wearing a seat belt.

Finally, Be Prepared

However well prepared you may be, accidents will still happen. Keep emergency numbers such as the doctor, the casualty department of your local hospital and even a neighbour by your telephone, and if you can book up one of the many locally organised courses set up by St John Ambulance or the Red Cross to learn some basic first aid (see page 99). Remember that however safe you have made your own house, you and your children will no doubt visit relatives and friends whose houses may not just be unsafe, they may be potential death traps.

Emergency Resuscitation

In an emergency, when your child is unconscious or has stopped breathing, it is easy to panic. Everybody realises that seconds count and yet they may not have the first clue as to what to do. Probably the first thing to do is to scream for help because a second pair of hands is better than just one and, if nothing else, can be used to dial 999 and summon an ambulance. Knowing that you need to keep calm is one thing, but actually doing it is enormously difficult.

It is certainly possible to resuscitate a child by following the instructions given here. I know of many cases where parents have followed similar instructions to the letter with a successful

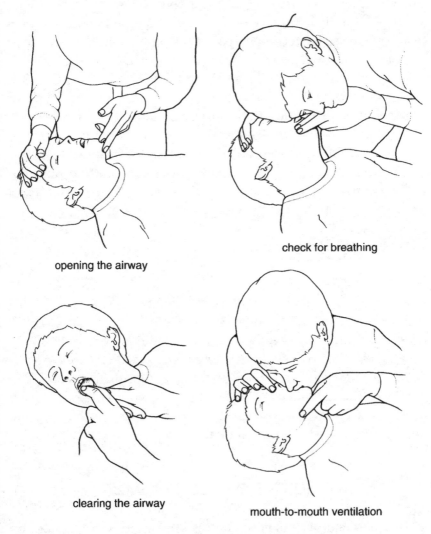

opening the airway

check for breathing

clearing the airway

mouth-to-mouth ventilation

Initial steps in emergency resuscitation

outcome. Confidence, however, is the key. It is difficult to put into practice instructions read from a page in a state of shock, and there is no substitute for going on a first-aid course and learning sound practical techniques through hands-on experience. On the St John Ambulance (St Andrew's Ambulance Association in Scotland) and the British Red Cross courses you will be allowed to practice on an artificial dummy as well as on fellow students in order to really get to grips with the resuscitation procedure. Once learned it is never forgotten and may one day save a life.

Step One: Mouth-to-Mouth Resuscitation

When a child has stopped breathing you may need to give mouth-to-mouth resuscitation.

Before you start
1 Lay the child down on a flat, hard surface on his back and tilt his head backwards. Do this by bringing the forehead back with one hand and pushing the underside of the chin upwards with the other hand. This brings the tongue away from the back of the throat where it may be obstructing breathing in an unconscious child. Sometimes this manoeuvre alone will allow the child to start breathing again naturally.

2 If you cannot hear the child's breathing start up again, put your ear right up against his mouth and listen again. Quickly feel with the back of your hand for air going in and out of the mouth and take a glance at the front of the chest to see if it is moving up and down. If it is not, and you cannot hear or feel breathing, mouth-to-mouth resuscitation will need to be carried out quickly.

What to do
1 Clear the airway by using your finger to hook out anything which may be in the child's mouth such as food, mud, dirt or vomit.

2 Remembering to keep the child's head tilted right back with the chin up, squeeze the nose with the fingers of one hand whilst covering the child's mouth completely with your mouth, and blow gently into the child's chest.

* For a baby it is easier to cover the baby's nose as well as his mouth with your mouth, and it is safest only to blow as much air into his lungs as is held within your cheeks as over-inflation can damage a baby's lungs.

3 Once you have breathed into the child's chest, take your mouth away and let the air flow out of the child's chest on its own.

4 Repeat this mouth-to-mouth breathing twenty times every minute and continue until help comes or the child starts to breath again on his own.

5 Once the child is breathing again, put him gently in the recovery position (see step three below).

Step Two: Heart Massage

If the child remains ashen or even blue in colour and you cannot feel a pulse, heart massage will be necessary as well as mouth-to-mouth resuscitation.

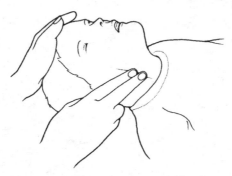

Checking for the carotid pulse

Before you start
Place the child on his back on a hard surface and kneel or stand by his side. Check for the presence of a pulse either in the neck, as shown above, or on the inside of the upper arm.

What to do
1 To start heart massage, press downwards over the lower part of

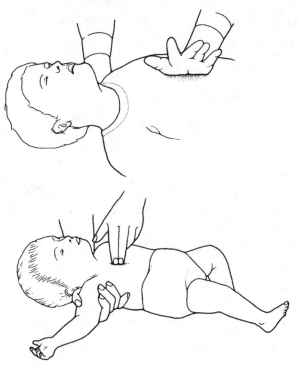

Heart massage in children of different ages

the breastbone using the hard under-surface of the hand and wrist. Aim to depress the breastbone about an inch and a half.

✱ *For a baby* use only the tips of two fingers and aim to depress the breastbone between half and one inch.

Pushing down on the breastbone squeezes the heart and artificially pumps a small amount of blood around the body.

2 You will need to repeat this manoeuvre about a hundred times a minute, so there is no time to slacken.

3 Mouth-to-mouth resuscitation will need to be carried out at the same time – give one breath after every five presses on the chest. This ratio of five heart compressions to one breath should be continued indefinitely until help arrives or until the heart gets going again. Even when the heart does start up, you will need to continue the mouth-to-mouth breathing.

4 When both the heart has started up again and breathing has recovered, place the child in the recovery position (see step three below).

Step Three: The Recovery Position

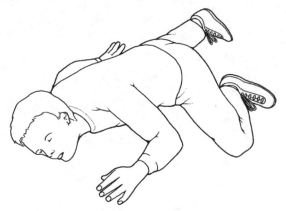

The recovery position

Before you start
If the child is breathing and his heart is beating but he still remains unconscious, place him safely in the recovery position. An unconscious child lying on his back is in great danger because the airway can easily become blocked by the tongue falling backwards into the back of the throat or by the presence of collected fluid or vomit.

What to do
1 Position the child half-way over onto his front with the lowermost arm behind the body and the uppermost arm bent at the elbow in front.
2 Put the uppermost leg with the knee bent at a right-angle so that the body cannot roll forwards or backwards.

3 Tilt the head right back so that there is no danger of the tongue blocking the airway again.

Poisoning

What to do

1 If you suspect that your child has swallowed something he should not have done, whether it be medicines or household or garden chemicals, try to discover exactly what it is and how much has been consumed.

2 If you think that he has swallowed something poisonous, take a sample of whatever it is, or the label from the appropriate container (preferably both), and go directly to your GP or local casualty department, whichever is quickest. *Do not under any circumstances give the child large amounts of salt water to drink in an attempt to make him sick as this in itself can be dangerous.*

3 If you suspect that any corrosive substance has been swallowed, such as bleach then take a careful look at the child's lips and mouth. Corrosives will cause redness, inflammation, soreness and blistering in these areas.

4 If this is the case, encourage the child to drink milk which as an alkali will help to neutralise any corrosive acid which may still be active. *Do not try to make a child sick in this situation as any corrosive present in the vomit will cause further burning.*

5 In the case of a child who has lost consciousness, shout for help and then embark upon the usual resuscitation manoeuvres described on pages 97–102.

Burns and Scalds

These are common injuries in and around the house and when they occur the sooner treatment is begun the better.

What to do

1 Right away put any burned skin under running cold water to take away the excess heat from the skin. Do this for ten to fifteen minutes. The cold water also has a numbing effect which will help to alleviate pain.

2 Afterwards, cover the burn or scald with a clean, soft, non-fluffy material such as cotton or lint which has been soaked in cold water. Cling film is a suitable alternative if nothing else is available. This will reduce the risk of infection and keep the area cool.

✳ *Do not try to remove any clothes which are stuck to the skin.*

✳ *Do not apply butter or any other oily or fatty substance as this only serves to cook scalded or burned skin even further.*

✳ *Do not burst any blisters that are present as they act as a natural covering for the burn, preventing fluid loss and keeping out germs.*

3 For anything larger than a very small burn or scald, the child should be taken to the casualty department for assessment to see how deep, extensive and serious it might be. Even if the burn is trivial, pain relief in the form of paracetamol and an antihistamine preparation can be very helpful.

Cuts and Bleeding

Children are forever falling and grazing their knees, elbows and hands. Cuts and lacerations are not uncommon either.

Treating Minor Cuts

What to do
1 Clean the surrounding skin with soap and water if available, taking care to wipe away from the open wound. Leave any blood clots which have already formed – nature's methods of stemming bleeding should not be interfered with.

2 If any bleeding continues, apply direct pressure with your hands, cover any small wound with a first-aid dressing and then raise and support the injured part. This helps to reduce the circulation within it and prevents further bleeding.

Treating Larger Cuts or Wounds

What to do

1 Where there is a lot of bleeding, first expose the wound and look for any foreign material which may be lodged in it. Anything sharp or dirty must be removed at once.

2 Apply direct pressure using your fingers or the palm of your hand over a pad of clean cloth or sterile dressing. If nothing else is available, use an article of clothing or your bare hands. *Take care not to tie a tourniquet or any article of clothing around the wound so tightly that it impedes the circulation completely.*

3 Raise and support the wound if it is on an arm or leg. This helps to stop the bleeding. Obviously this cannot be carried out if there is any likelihood of a broken bone being present.

4 Place sterile pads or dressings over the wound, pressing down firmly and fixing with a roll of bandage. If bleeding continues through the bandaging, do not under any circumstances remove it but add further layers of dressing on top of the original ones, applying them even more firmly.

5 Finally, take the child to hospital directly or call an ambulance. ***Do not give your child anything to drink, not even a sip of water, just in case an anaesthetic will be required on arrival in hospital.*** Remember to check with the casualty officer whether your child will require a tetanus injection in case the wound has been contaminated.

Fractures

There are a number of general symptoms and signs common to all broken bones:

* Sometimes the snap of a bone may have been felt or heard the moment it happens.

* There will be pain which is made worse by movement.

* The child may find it difficult or even impossible to move the injured area without help.

* There will be tenderness over the site of the fracture when even gentle pressure is applied.

* Gradually, swelling and bruising will occur.

* In many instances there is a deformity present where the fracture has taken place due to shortening, angulation or twisting of an arm or leg.

* With a fracture of a large bone such as the thigh bone or femur, the child may go into shock – he will be pale and feel faint and shivery.

In the case of any fracture, do not give the child anything to eat or drink in case an anaesthetic may be required later.

Treating Arm Fractures

What to do
1 Sit the child down with the fractured arm bent at a right-angle at the elbow and supported as it lies across the chest. The whole arm can then be supported in a sling or triangular bandage (every first-aid kit should contain one of these).

2 Secure the arm to the chest with a broad-fold bandage applied over the sling near the elbow, but obviously avoiding the site of the break. Any knot should be tied in front of the uninjured side.

This type of bandaging is applicable for breaks in the clavicle, the collarbone, the wrist and all three large bones in the arm.

Treating Leg Fractures

What to do
1 Lay the child down with the broken leg held steady and supported by holding it above and below the site of the injury.

2 Put some padding between the legs to fill in the natural hollows.

3 Tie the injured leg gently but firmly to the uninjured leg using

broad-fold bandages or articles of clothing, taking especial care to avoid placing bandages anywhere near the site of the suspected fracture. This acts to immobilise the injured leg as much as possible, reduce pain and minimise risk of further damage to nerves and blood vessels which may be in contact with the sharp ends of any broken bones.

4 Arrange for the child to be taken to hospital in an ambulance.

Neck and Spinal Injuries

If you even suspect a child of having injured his neck or spine, resist moving him at all but get immediate and expert help. Any movement of a broken neck or spine can seriously damage the sensitive spinal cord, potentially leading to paralysis. Trained paramedics or doctors will need to supervise the child's removal to hospital using special equipment to immobilise the neck and achieve this safely.

Choking

Children are at particular risk of choking because they love putting small, hard objects inside their mouths. If they then become excited or if they fall, the object may be inhaled, partially or totally obstructing the airway. It is essential that the obstruction is removed as soon as possible and initially it is worth encouraging the child to try to cough the object out. If it is lodged firmly this may not work, in which case first-aid treatment must commence (see below).

Signs of Choking

* When choking occurs, the child will probably be unable to speak or breathe and may be holding his throat.

* He may well not be able to make any noise at all.

* The face will gradually become red at first and then blue as the blood vessels become congested.

* If the obstruction is not totally removed, loss of consciousness will eventually take place.

Treating Choking in Older Children

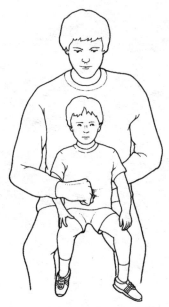

Heimlich manoeuvre used in the treatment of choking

What to do

1 Sit in a chair and lay the child over your lap with his head downwards. Alternatively, kneel on the floor on one knee and lay the child over your other knee.

2 Support the child's chest with one hand underneath and slap the child vigorously between the shoulder blades up to four times with the other hand.

3 If this does not work after the fourth attempt, go on to carry out the abdominal thrust, or Heimlich manoeuvre, described below.

Treating Choking in Infants

What to do
1 Sit in a chair or kneel on the floor on one knee. Lay the infant over your lap or knee with his head downwards and his chest and tummy lying along your outstretched forearm using your hand to support his face and chest.

2 Slap him firmly between the shoulders up to four times. Remember that the pressure required in infants is much less than for older children or adults.

3 If the cause of the obstruction appears to move, be very careful indeed when putting a finger into the infant's mouth in an attempt to remove it since there is always the risk of pushing the obstruction further back down his throat.

4 If the back-slapping technique does not work, go on to perform the abdominal thrust described below.

The Abdominal Thrust (Heimlich manoeuvre)

What to do for older children:
1 Sit the child on your lap with one arm in front of his tummy. Clench your fist and position it with your thumb pointing inwards right in the centre of the upper part of the child's tummy. Support the child's back with your other hand.

2 Using a quick, sharp inward and upward movement, press your clenched fist into the child's abdomen. The thrust should be strong enough to dislodge the obstruction. If the first thrust is not sufficient, repeat the manoeuvre up to four times.

For infants:
1 Lie the infant down on his back on a hard surface with the head tilted back and the chin lifted upwards.

2 Put two fingers of one hand on the upper part of the tummy, between the bellybutton and the breastbone, and press quickly and sharply inwards and upwards. Again, the thrust should be hard enough to remove the obstruction. Should the first thrust fail, repeat it up to four times.

Unconsciousness

What to do
1 If a choking child becomes unconscious despite your best efforts to remove the obstruction, lie the child on his back, tilt the head backwards to open the airway as much as possible and begin mouth-to-mouth resuscitation (see pages 97–102).

2 If it is impossible to blow air into the child's chest, repeat back slaps and abdominal thrusts, reposition the child's head and try again.

3 Carry on until help arrives or until the obstruction is dislodged.

4 If the cause of the obstruction is coughed up, remove it from the mouth carefully and position the child in the recovery position (see page 102).

Drowning

Drowning occurs through either water entering the lungs causing asphyxia or the throat muscles going into spasm so strongly that the airway is completely closed off, again leading to asphyxia (dry drowning). The aim of treatment is to get air into the child's lungs as quickly as possible, if necessary while the child is still in the water. Admission to hospital after the event is essential as the lungs can continue to become congested long after the accident occurred, and because cold water can lead to hypothermia if the child is not kept warm.

What to do
1 As soon as you can, make sure there is nothing in the mouth obstructing breathing.

2 Open the airway by tilting the child's head right back. If you have to, do this while the child is still in the water.

3 As soon as the child is back on dry land, check his breathing and check for a pulse. Carry out mouth-to-mouth resuscitation and heart massage if necessary (see pages 97–102).

4 As soon as breathing starts again, place the child in the recovery position (see page 102). Keep him warm and arrange for his urgent transportation to hospital.

Shock

Shock occurs in a child when the circulation fails. Usually, because of blood loss, there is insufficient blood flowing to the vital organs to keep them supplied with oxygen. It is a serious condition which, if left untreated, can prove fatal.

Signs of Shock

* A child who is in shock looks ashen in colour or even blue around the face and lips.

* The skin is clammy, cold and sweaty.

* If the child is still conscious, he will feel faint and weak.

* Breathing is rapid but shallow and the pulse, if you can feel it, is also rapid but weak.

* The child may feel thirsty or sick.

* He will often be agitated or may vomit.

* If the condition deteriorates the child will eventually lose consciousness.

What to do
1 If there is any obvious source of external bleeding, try to stem the flow using direct pressure.

2 Lay the child down flat on his back and turn his head to one side in case he is sick. Do not let him sit up or move as this will affect his blood pressure. Instead, raise his feet on a chair or bundles of clothes or pillows and loosen any tight clothing around the neck, chest or waist.

3 Do not allow the child to become excessively cold but do not be tempted to overheat him either in too many blankets or coats. This will merely bring precious blood to the surface of the skin, taking it away from more important internal organs.

4 Never leave the child alone and check his state of consciousness at regular intervals. If necessary, place him in the recovery position (see page 102) and use emergency resuscitation techniques (see pages 97–102) should they become necessary.

5 Obviously the child should be admitted to hospital as soon as possible.

Head Injury

Head injuries must always be taken seriously in children as they can result in concussion or even a fracture of the skull with possible brain damage. Severe head injuries are the ones which cause loss of consciousness – unless this happens, it is most unusual for a child to suffer any lasting harm. Occasionally, however, a child who is briefly knocked out may recover consciousness and feel fine for a short spell before once again becoming drowsy and losing consciousness. Because of the possibility of these delayed effects, it is important for every child who has been knocked out by an injury to be admitted to hospital for a period of investigation and observation.

What to do
1 If a head injury has taken place and the child is still conscious or has recovered from loss of consciousness, he should always be assessed by a doctor. Further investigations and observation will then be arranged if appropriate.

2 If the child is unconscious as a result of a head injury then the general treatment for such cases, using the recovery position or emergency resuscitation (see pages 97–102), should be applied and the child admitted to hospital as soon as possible.

3 If the child is conscious, check for the following vital symptoms:

* Noisy or laboured breathing.

* Drowsiness or confusion.

* A strong but very slow pulse.

Any of these might suggest brain swelling or damage.

CHAPTER FIVE

RASHES AND SPOTS

People mean different things when they talk about 'rashes' and 'spots'. Individual spots, or a small group of them in a localised area, are seldom referred to by doctors as a rash, although patients themselves may describe them as such. Because they are distinct from one another, 'spots' and 'rashes' are dealt with in separate sections.

There are hundreds of different types of rashes, ranging from a small group of spots in a localised area of the skin to a widespread, generalised area of red, inflamed skin. Rashes may be similar in colour to the surrounding skin, or bright red. They may be flat with discoloration visible beneath the surface of the skin, or they may be raised above it, appearing irregular and lumpy. Sometimes a rash forms blisters, which can be large or small, on the surface of the skin.

Most rashes are relatively trivial and rarely represent any sign of serious underlying disease. Most are also fairly short-lived. Some, however, are longer lasting, such as the rash of eczema, and a few may very occasionally be associated with more significant internal disorders.

Infective Rashes (usually non-itchy)

Perhaps one of the most important aspects of any rash is the symptoms which accompany it. Rashes generally occur as a result of infection or allergy. In these instances there will often be a fever or an itching of the skin respectively. In other cases the cause may not be so obvious and a little more detective work may need to be done.

CAUSES OF INFECTIVE RASHES

* Chickenpox

* Measles

* Rubella (German measles)

* Roseola infantum

* Meningitis

* Scarlet fever

* Rheumatic fever

* Slapped cheek syndrome (erythema infectiosum)

When a child has a skin rash as well as a temperature of 38°C or above, the most likely cause is one of the childhood infectious diseases. The common ones are listed here, and although the appearance alone can often suggest the diagnosis, there is a great deal of visual similarity and overlap between them. Often, even a doctor is unable to make a precise diagnosis by the appearance of the rash alone. To be absolutely accurate in every case, blood tests, throat swabs and other tests would have to be carried out, but this is time-consuming, unpleasant for the children concerned and, in most instances, unnecessary. It is always useful, however, to try to achieve as accurate a diagnosis as possible since it is valuable for people to know which infections they have and have not had. A woman planning to start a family, for example, should always know whether she is immune to rubella which could otherwise harm her developing baby, so knowing that she had the infection

in childhood is reassuring. The ideal policy for any woman planning a pregnancy is to have a blood test in advance to confirm that
she is immune. If not, she should have a rubella vaccination,
although a gap of at least three months between the jab and
becoming pregnant is required. Rubella vaccination has significantly reduced the incident of maternal rubella, but unfortunately
a few women still slip through the immunisation net.

Whilst on the subject of immunisation, it is worth pointing out
that a short-lived rash with a fever may occasionally appear in a
child about a week after having the MMR vaccination (measles,
mumps, rubella). The rash is fine and indistinct, does not mean
that the child is infectious and will clear up of its own accord within
a few days. A mild temperature may occur at the same time and
the only treatment necessary is symptomatic treatment of the
temperature itself by means of sponging with tepid water and the
use of paracetamol.

Chickenpox

Chickenpox is now one of the more common childhood infectious
diseases in Britain because it is one of the few not immunised
against. Some countries use an effective chickenpox vaccine
routinely, however. The illness is classified here for convenience,
along with the other infective rashes, although it is the one
example which does produce itching and irritation. The disease
has an incubation period of 11–21 days and it generally causes
only minor symptoms. Some children develop a slight temperature
or a headache and the crops of fluid-filled blisters, which are characteristic of chickenpox, can irritate and itch, especially in sensitive
areas like the inside of the eyelids, the mouth and vagina. The rash
can occur over all areas of the body, with spots coming along in
clusters every few days. Little fluid-filled blisters form which then
burst leaving a reddened, itchy scab. Theoretically your child is
infectious until the last of the blisters have scabbed over and dried
out. Some of the larger blisters may occasionally cause permanent
scarring, but this usually only happens where the child has
scratched and secondary bacterial infection has occurred.

WHAT CAN YOU DO?

A raised temperature can be treated with paracetamol and sponging with tepid water if necessary. The main problem is usually the itching, and this can be reduced by using oily calamine lotion on the skin or by giving your child a warm bath containing some bicarbonate of soda. Intense itching in the eyes, mouth, ears or vagina is more difficult to alleviate and in these instances anti-histamines in syrup or tablet form are ideal. Cutting the child's fingernails and tying on mitts can help to prevent harmful scratching. If the spots become weepy or are particularly deep and on the face then ask your doctor to see what can be done. An antibiotic may well be needed. Your child should remain isolated from other children until the scabs have all dried out.

Finally, for young children still in nappies, there is a greater risk of the blisters becoming infected. If possible, leave the nappy off for as long as you can and ask your doctor or health visitor about the use of water-resistant barrier creams.

IF YOU REMEMBER NOTHING ELSE, REMEMBER THESE THREE THINGS

1   The chickenpox rash consists of a number of small, fluid-filled blisters.

2   The worst symptom is irritation and itching in sensitive areas.

3   Should the blisters become red and weepy, an antibiotic may be necessary to deal with secondary infection.

WHAT CAN THE DOCTOR DO?

Again, confirmation of the diagnosis is useful. If any of the spots are oozing a nasty milky or yellowish substance, then secondary infection is likely to have occurred and antibiotics may be required. Also, if other symptoms which seem unusual are reported such as neck stiffness or very high temperature, then the doctor would be wary of the possibility of rare complications.

Measles

Since the MMR vaccination programme began, measles has become relatively rare. It is caused by a very contagious virus and starts with the symptoms of a common cold. The child then develops a fever with a temperature that can rise as high as 40°C (104°F), and if you look inside the child's mouth on the insides of the cheeks, you may sometimes see tiny white spots which resemble grains of salt (Koplik's spots). The child's nose will stream, the eyes will become red and sore and the child is generally very miserable. Within two to three days of the onset of fever, blotchy red spots begin to appear on the face and trunk, gradually fusing to form a generalised red rash.

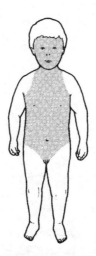

The typical distribution of the measles rash

WHAT CAN YOU DO?

Measles infection is extremely uncomfortable for the child, who will undoubtedly be miserable and unhappy. Try to reduce his temperature if you can using the usual methods of sponging with tepid water and giving paracetamol. Encourage your child to drink plenty of fluids, even if it is only a sip at a time. Close the curtains in the child's bedroom since bright light will irritate his sore eyes. Bathe his eyes if you wish with cool water and administer regularly any eye-drops which your doctor may prescribe.

Bear in mind that any other children in the house will be likely to pick up the measles infection unless they are already immune, either through having had the infection previously or through immunisation. Your child is infectious for about a week after the symptoms begin, so do not be tempted to send your child back to school too soon. Any other children living in the house should be immunised, if they have not been already, and the usual schedule is to have the MMR vaccine (measles, mumps and rubella at the same time) at the age of about thirteen months. Babies under the age of about eight months very rarely develop measles as they are still protected by their mother's antibodies in their blood.

WHAT CAN THE DOCTOR DO?

Although measles is less common than it used to be thanks to vaccination, and it is considered by many to be a trivial childhood illness, it is in fact potentially a very serious condition. Complications include ear infection, pneumonia and inflammation of the brain or encephalitis. World-wide, deafness, brain damage and even death is still seen occasionally. The doctor should always confirm the diagnosis of measles and, because of the risk of a secondary bacterial infection which may complicate the viral infection, he or she may well decide to prescribe antibiotics at the outset. The doctor will certainly do so if your child complains of earache or has signs of a chest infection. He or she may or may not also prescribe antibiotic eye-drops or ointment to treat the sore eyes. You will be advised to keep the child in bed whilst the temperature remains and to confirm that all is well within a few days.

IF YOU REMEMBER NOTHING ELSE, REMEMBER THESE THREE THINGS

A child with measles:

1   has a high temperature;

2   has a streaming nose, red eyes and is miserable;

3   has a rash which is blotchy and red and affects mainly the face and trunk.

Rubella

Rubella, or German measles, is such a trivial disease in children that many show no symptoms of it whatsoever. Occasionally there may be a slightly raised temperature, and the spots, if any, tend to begin just behind the ears before they move onto the face and the rest of the body. One characteristic feature, however, is slightly tender, enlarged lymph glands behind the ears and at the back of the neck, which when you feel them are pea-sized, mobile and rubbery. Occasionally, aching or swelling in the joints can also occur. The incubation period is between two and three weeks and any rash generally lasts only a day or two.

The main thing to remember about rubella is that although it is not serious in children, it is potentially very serious in early pregnancy (see page 116). Rubella contracted by a developing baby in the first three months of its life can result in severe congenital defects.

WHAT CAN YOU DO?

Usually there is little you need to do because your child will probably be unaware of any problem. If, however, he feels unwell, as some older children do, then paracetamol may be used to reduce any fever and a day in bed would do no harm. Certainly, he needs to be kept away from any pregnant women and any other children in the house who have not been vaccinated. These children should, of course, be vaccinated in due course.

WHAT CAN THE DOCTOR DO?

Ideally the doctor should try to identify the infectious agent responsible for the rash, but this may not always be possible. Should the child become unwell in other ways, for example

---

IF YOU REMEMBER NOTHING ELSE, REMEMBER THESE THREE THINGS

1   Rubella is usually an extremely mild childhood illness.

2   A characteristic feature is enlarged glands at the back of the neck.

3   The rash is a faint, pink, flat rash, usually beginning behind the ears.

---

increasing drowsiness or persistent vomiting, the doctor should certainly examine him to rule out any of the possible rare complications of rubella.

Roseola Infantum (3-day fever)

This is a common infectious disease caused by a herpes virus which usually affects children of between six months and two years of age. The infected child suddenly becomes irritable and feverish, often with a sore throat and enlarge lymph glands in the neck. The temperature can go as high as 40°C, falling back after three days to normal. The rash starts on the body as the fever begins to subside and then spreads to the face, arms and legs.

WHAT CAN YOU DO?

The most important thing to do is to reduce the child's temperature and prevent the possibility of a febrile convulsion. Plenty of fluids, sponging with tepid water and giving paracetamol are the traditional methods. The condition is infectious so other children should be kept away from the sufferer as much as possible.

WHAT CAN THE DOCTOR DO?

The characteristic symptoms of roseola infantum are that the illness takes a dramatic turn for the better as the child's temperature drops, and the rash appears after about the fourth or fifth day. On this basis alone, the doctor may be able to confirm the diagnosis. Advice about reducing the temperature is important, but antibiotics are usually not necessary.

IF YOU REMEMBER NOTHING ELSE,
REMEMBER THESE THREE THINGS

1   This illness is common, especially in younger
     children.

2   The rash begins as the fever subsides and
     affects mainly the trunk and face.

3   The child is usually remarkably well in spite
     of the high temperature.

Meningitis

There are many different types of meningitis depending upon the type of micro-organism responsible, and the rash, when it occurs, is uncommon. The bacteria that does cause a skin rash is a particularly nasty one called meningococcus and when this produces blood-poisoning (septicaemia) in association with the meningitis, a purply-red rash visible below the surface of the skin may appear. This rash is caused by bleeding from small blood vessels and is an alarming sign that the bacteria causing the meningitis are already present in large numbers. If the other signs and symptoms of meningitis are also present, namely:

* stiff neck

* high temperature

* persistent vomiting

* increasing drowsiness

✳ discomfort when looking at bright lights

emergency medical treatment is needed. The best thing to do in this situation is to **get your child to hospital as fast as possible.** If your doctor is able to attend promptly then an intravenous injection of penicillin could well be life-saving.

SIGNS OF THE MENINGITIS RASH

✳ The rash is purply-red and flat.

✳ Unlike most rashes, the redness in the skin cannot be 'squeezed out' by pressing a clear piece of glass against the skin to flatten swollen blood vessels.

✳ Typical meningitis symptoms may or may not be present and the child may not always look ill.

WHAT CAN YOU DO?

There is only one thing for a parent to do in this situation and that is to arrange urgent medical help as a matter of emergency.

WHAT CAN THE DOCTOR DO?

Children with meningococcal meningitis or septicaemia need the most urgent hospital admission and treatment. Immediate administration of intravenous penicillin is required and control of fluid balance and steroid administration in Intensive Care will quite possibly also be needed. It is a condition with a high mortality so prompt and appropriate medical treatment is the key to a happy outcome.

IF YOU REMEMBER NOTHING ELSE, REMEMBER THESE THREE THINGS

1 Any child with symptoms of meningitis and a rash requires urgent hospital admission and treatment.

2 The rash is purply-red and flat.

3 Prompt treatment with antibiotics, fluids and/or steroids may mean the difference between life or death.

Scarlet Fever

Scarlet fever typically begins with a sore throat and there may be an accompanying temperature. This is followed by a rash, starting with an appearance of tiny red spots on the neck and upper body and soon spreading to the face which then becomes scarlet in appearance (hence the name 'scarlet fever'). Only a circular area around the mouth remains pale. The redness is caused by a toxin produced by the infecting streptococcus bacteria. On the tongue there is a characteristic white coating interspersed with little red spots, descriptively referred to by doctors as a 'white strawberry tongue'. This can progress to a 'red strawberry tongue' as the disease evolves. As the temperature drops and the rash disappears, it is not unusual to see a little peeling of the skin, especially on the hands and feet.

WHAT CAN YOU DO?

Your child should rest in bed and drink plenty of fluids to replace those lost as a result of his temperature. Paracetamol can be used to both reduce the fever and ease the sore throat. Again, as with any infectious disease, other children should be kept away as much as possible and the doctor notified so that confirmation of the diagnosis and appropriate treatment can be carried out.

WHAT CAN THE DOCTOR DO?

Since the infection is caused by a bacteria, treatment consists of antibiotics, usually penicillin or, if the child is allergic to penicillin, *erythromycin*, and a short course is usually sufficient to result in full and rapid recovery. It can be difficult to distinguish a sore throat caused by a more usual viral infection from that caused by the streptococcus. If in doubt, the doctor will treat the child with an antibiotic.

IF YOU REMEMBER NOTHING ELSE, REMEMBER THESE THREE THINGS

1 Scarlet fever produces a sore throat, a temperature and a bright red facial rash.

2 There is often a pale area around the mouth.

3 Treatment is usually with penicillin.

Rheumatic Fever

Rheumatic fever, thankfully, is now rare in the West but is still fairly common in the developing countries of Asia and Africa where it remains a significant cause of heart disease. Children between the ages of five and fifteen are most at risk. It always begins after a throat infection caused by a certain type of streptococcal bacteria, and indeed a simple sore throat is often the first sign of this potentially serious condition. For some reason, the infection sets up some form of autoimmune reaction in which the body's immune system is stimulated to attack its own tissues. As a result, a temperature develops, the joints become painful and swollen, there may be general malaise and fatigue, the child loses his appetite and there may also be a blotchy, red, circular rash on the body, arms and legs.

WHAT CAN YOU DO?

If your child has had a sore throat or ear infection recently, and later complains that his joints are painful or swollen, then you should contact your doctor to rule out the possibility of rheumatic fever. It is obviously worth checking all the joints to see if there is any tenderness or swelling. You should be even more suspicious if a circular rash starts to appear on the child's trunk and limbs. It is worth remembering that although rheumatic fever is rare now in Britain, prompt treatment can reduce the risk of developing heart disease in later life.

WHAT CAN THE DOCTOR DO?

If there is any likelihood of rheumatic fever, a firm diagnosis needs to be made. This may be done clinically purely by weighing up all the symptoms, but blood tests should be performed to confirm the diagnosis. These tests rely on the detection of antibodies in the blood specific to the particular type of bacteria responsible for the infection. Penicillin is then used to eradicate the bacteria and aspirin is used to reduce pain in the joints and inflammation generally. Sometimes steroids are used to prevent the possibility of any long-term heart damage.

IF YOU REMEMBER NOTHING ELSE, REMEMBER THESE THREE THINGS

1   Rheumatic fever produces a blotchy, red, circular rash on the trunk, arms and legs.

2   It produces inflammation of the joints and the heart.

3   Early treatment with antibiotics can prevent long-term ill-health.

Slapped Cheek Syndrome (erythema infectiosum)

This infectious childhood disease, also known as erythema infectiosum, causes a widespread and distinctive rash. It is the least well known of the common childhood infections. It is caused by a parvovirus and often occurs in minor epidemics during the spring. The rash starts as individual, raised, pink spots on the cheeks which gradually merge together. Over the next few days the rash spreads over the arms and legs but only to a minor degree on the rest of the body. A very mild temperature may occasionally be present too.

WHAT CAN YOU DO?

The only treatment required is plenty of fluids and paracetamol to reduce any discomfort or temperature.

WHAT CAN THE DOCTOR DO?

The doctor should confirm the diagnosis, thus reducing the parents' anxiety concerning other more serious conditions. He or she should explain that the rash usually settles down after about a week and a half, although occasionally it can return over a period of some weeks. The doctor should warn parents that, very occasionally, adults who pick it up can develop swelling and tenderness in their joints.

IF YOU REMEMBER NOTHING ELSE, REMEMBER THESE THREE THINGS

1   Slapped cheek syndrome is caused by a virus infection.

2   There may be a mild fever.

3   Treatment consists of symptomatic relief for temperature or discomfort.

Allergic Rashes

Apart from the widespread, itchy rash of chickenpox, which is dealt with on pages 117–119, the commonest cause of a temporary, widespread, itchy rash is allergy.

This type of rash tends to affect all areas of the body although it is often worse where there is any friction on the skin from tight clothes, belts or the tops of elasticated socks, for example. It is usually a reddy-pink, blotchy rash, often raised off the surface of the skin, and the natural temptation is to scratch the rash which, unfortunately, only tends to make it worse. Even where the skin is not visibly affected by the blotches, there is an increased sensitivity to any kind of irritant, and where any scratching has occurred, swollen red lines of reaction in the skin (weals) can be seen. This is known as urticaria.

In general, allergic rashes are caused either by something which comes into contact with the skin and which irritates it, or by something which the child has eaten or swallowed. There are an infinite number of possible culprits (allergens) and indentifying the exact cause of the rash usually proves impossible, even after a reasonable amount of detective work. Of the irritants which affect the skin directly, many of the low-temperature, biological washing powders often prove to be responsible, the active enzymes in the products having a direct digestive action on the skin. Natural fibres like wool and some synthetic ones can also irritate the skin, as can metals such as nickel used in buttons, zips and fasteners on clothes. Children who run around the garden in their swimming clothes in the summer and roll around in the grass may develop an allergic rash and certain household and garden plants are notorious for producing reactions. Of the dietary factors commonly incriminated in allergy, shellfish, strawberries, nuts and tomatoes are usually to blame, though the additives, colourings and preservatives in food may also have a lot to answer for. Medicines can also cause rashes, and ten per cent of the population, are, for example, allergic to penicillin, still the most commonly used antibiotic of all.

One important feature which distinguishes an allergic rash from other rashes is that the child is not otherwise generally unwell. He may be irritable as a result of the itching, but he is not lethargic and listless, or off his food, and there is certainly no fever. If, however, the rash is severe and accompanied by swelling around the eyes and lips, then great caution needs to be exercised. These could be the early symptoms of a severe and potentially life-threatening condition known as angioneurotic oedema. This may cause the tongue to swell and the respiratory passages to narrow and inflame, causing breathing difficulties. It is a medical emergency and requires urgent treatment with adrenaline, steroids and antihistamines.

WHAT CAN YOU DO?

If you suspect that your child has an allergic rash, check to make sure that he has no temperature and that he is not unwell generally. If this is the case, and the rash is very itchy, you are probably right in assuming that it is allergic in origin.

Consider where the rash is distributed over the skin. Is it in a line, where the elasticated waist of the child's trousers or pants, for example, touch the skin? If so, this suggests that something the clothes have been washed in may be responsible, because this is where the clothes are tightly applied to the skin and rub against it. Do you use a low-temperature, biological washing powder, or have you begun to do so lately? Is there anything else unusual that your child may have been in contact with? You can also ask yourself whether he may have eaten anything different or slightly unusual. Has he had any shellfish or fruit in the last few hours which he may not have had before? Is he taking any medication, especially aspirin or antibiotics? Aspirin is a common cause of allergy in people of all ages and should, in fact, never be given to children under the age of twelve because of a rare condition called Reye's syndrome which has occasionally been reported after taking aspirin. You should also ask yourself when the rash came on as this can also give useful clues as to what has caused it.

Often a child just has particularly sensitive skin capable of reacting to a number of environmental irritants, making it impossible to identify and avoid any specific cause of the rash. It helps in these cases to minimise the number of synthetic chemicals coming into contact with your child's skin, so any kind of detergent including perfumed soaps, bubble baths and anything but the mildest shampoos should be avoided. *Simple* soap or aqueous cream, which are inert on the skin, can be purchased over the counter at the chemist, and emulsifying ointment can be used in the bath water to moisturise and protect dry, sensitive skin.

If, despite all your efforts, the skin rash recurs frequently and causes problems, symptomatic relief in the form of oral antihistamines, which again can be purchased at the chemist, will usually relieve itching and irritation. Antihistamine creams, on the other hand, are not effective and can, themselves, sometimes irritate the skin.

WHAT CAN THE DOCTOR DO?

The doctor's most important role is to exclude other causes of a sudden rash including those of an infectious nature. Once the rash has been identified as allergic in origin, he or she may be able to pinpoint the most likely cause. In up to ninety per cent of cases, however, the rash is a one-off, requires no treatment and never happens again. On the other hand, if the rash recurs frequently, certain tests can be performed to try and discover the cause. Skin prick tests are amongst the commonest used and involve pricking the skin through a droplet of the suspect agent being tested. Possible agents would include common item such as grass, pollen, wool, animal fur and mould. When the skin is inspected a few hours later, a positive test is recorded if the area of skin around the scratch has become reddened, inflamed and itchy. Classic food allergies, on the other hand, are more difficult to diagnose. A RAST test, in which antibodies in the child's bloodstream can be demonstrated to react with certain components of his diet, can be performed, but the results are frequently disappointing in practice. A small blood sample is required from the child in order to carry out this test.

The doctor can advise as to how to avoid certain factors that might cause an allergic reaction, and can certainly prescribe non-sedating antihistamine tablets or syrups to take away any itching and the tendency to scratch. In the worst cases, he or she can provide special mitts for the child's hands and encourage the parents to make sure that his fingernails are cut short to avoid further scratching, which can only make the allergic rash worse. The doctor can advise about using soap substitutes such as aqueous cream and emulsifying ointment in the bath water and, occasionally, he or she may sanction the short-term use of mild steroid creams such as hydrocortisone for the worst types of skin irritation.

In the very serious condition of angioneurotic oedema, an injection of adrenaline may prove life-saving as any accompanying swelling of the lips, tongue and respiratory passages can seriously interfere with normal breathing. This is a medical emergency and requires the most urgent treatment.

IF YOU REMEMBER NOTHING ELSE, REMEMBER THESE THREE THINGS

1   Allergic skin rash is usually due to something which irritates the skin directly or something that is swallowed.

2   The child is not generally unwell and does not have a temperature.

3   If breathing difficulties occur, get medical help urgently.

Other Short-lived Rashes

There are a number of short-lived rashes which do not fit into the main two categories above but which are nevertheless common and important. Three of them, which all parents should be familiar with, are nappy rash, heat rash and a little known but nevertheless very important rash called purpura. All of them may produce a fairly widespread rash and all of them have different causes and treatments.

CAUSES OF NON-ALLERGIC SHORT-LIVED RASHES

* Nappy rash

* Heat rash

* Purpura

Nappy Rash

Nappy rash is common and usually unmistakable and occurs whatever type of nappies you use – disposable or reusable fabric ones. Although it is always confined to the nappy area, its appearance and severity can vary enormously. In mild cases there are merely a few red spots around the genital region. In the most severe cases, however, the whole of the skin underneath the nappy is bright red and inflamed with oozing, infected blisters or ulcers present.

The underlying problem in this condition is that the sensitive baby's skin is constantly exposed to moisture and to the chemical irritants contained in the baby's urine and stools. The bacteria normally present in the motions begin to act immediately on the urine to produce ammonia which attacks the skin. Bottle-fed babies are particularly susceptible as their stools are more alkaline and provide a more favourable environment for the bacteria to flourish in.

Patterns of Nappy rash
1 Around the genital region. This is the commonest type of nappy rash. A number of red, inflamed spots are seen at the tip of the baby boy's penis or around the vaginal lips in a girl and the

surrounding skin may become bright and shiny. There may be a strong ammonia-type smell and the baby may suddenly cry when passing urine or when placed in a warm bath.

2 In the skin creases. When the rash is confined to the creases at the top of the thighs and lower tummy, it may merely be excess moisture that is causing the problem. Fluid becomes trapped in these skin creases and if this can be avoided the rash will often settle down without treatment.

3 Around the anus and buttocks. This type of nappy rash suggests that a thrush infection may be responsible. Thrush, or candida, is an organism which normally lives in the bowel but which can occasionally produce inflammation of the skin. When it is seen in the nappy area it is well worth looking in the baby's mouth to see if there are any white spots adhering to the tongue or cheeks, as thrush here will pass down through the baby's intestine and be excreted in his stools. Make sure not to confuse these white spots with curds from any milk your baby may have been drinking recently and which, in contrast, can easily be scraped off. Thrush is more likely to be a problem if the child has recently had treatment with antibiotics.

4 An all-over rash. This more severe type of rash often suggests that it is caused by some kind of general allergy or skin inflammation (dermatitis). It may be an early sign of atopic eczema in a child where there is a strong family history of it, and often a biological washing powder or fabric conditioner in which reusable nappies have been washed are to blame. In this situation there are two factors responsible for the rash – extra sensitive skin plus chemical attack from ammonia-like substances.

WHAT CAN YOU DO?

The first thing to do with nappy rash is to make sure that the baby's skin is washed gently with warm water and a non-perfumed soap and then dried thoroughly. This removes any existing chemicals which may be irritating the skin, and all traces of moisture. Baby wipes, which are usually both effective and convenient, may sting if used on sore skin, and possibly make the rash worse. A suitable barrier cream (there are many to choose from) should then be applied to prevent the skin from coming into further contact with the baby's urine and stools. The baby should be changed as soon as the nappy is dirty and the skin washed thoroughly each time. If possible, it is best to leave the nappy off for as long as possible in a warm, dry room to allow the skin to 'breathe'. Talc is probably best left off since it can cake and thus irritate the skin. Plastic pants should definitely not be used as they cause more moisture to be retained.

With generalised nappy rashes, where there is a possibility of allergy, it is imperative that reusable nappies are first sterilised, then washed, then thoroughly rinsed and dried before being used again. If this doesn't work and the rash remains defiant, it is always worth trying disposable as opposed to reusable nappies. Finally, check your baby's mouth to see if there are any white spots sticking to the inside of his cheeks or tongue. This could suggest a thrush infection which will require specific treatment.

WHAT CAN THE DOCTOR DO?

In any case where the nappy rash is bothering a child or where it has been present for more than a few days, the doctor or health visitor should certainly take a look. I have seen some terrible cases of very sore-looking nappy rash in babies whose mothers thought they were just making a fuss, and severe nappy rash can occur even in babies whose nappies are changed regularly. Your doctor may prescribe a cream that, in addition to acting as a barrier, may contain a mild steroid, antibacterial and antifungal agent all combined in one.

IF YOU REMEMBER NOTHING ELSE, REMEMBER THESE THREE THINGS

1   Nappy rash may have a number of different causes.

2   Change your baby's nappy frequently and leave the nappy off whenever you can.

3   See your doctor if the rash does not clear within a few days.

Heat Rash

Heat rash is very common in infants and consists of many tiny, itchy, red spots and blisters which converge to produce a faint, red rash in those areas of the body where there are most sweat glands. These include the face, neck, shoulders and chest and the skin creases in the elbows, the groin and behind the knees. Basically, the skin becomes inflamed by the presence of sweat and sometimes tiny white spots can be seen where sweat has built up below the skin surface.

WHAT CAN YOU DO?

Since the condition is caused directly by heat, cooling your child down is the key. Remove as many of his clothes as possible, give him a tepid bath and pat his skin dry thoroughly. Avoid dressing him in clothes made of synthetic fibres, choosing cotton clothing instead. Open a window and direct a fan onto him if you have one. For the itching, calamine lotion is quite effective. All these measures combined together usually result in the heat rash disappearing within a few hours.

WHAT CAN THE DOCTOR DO?

Obviously, the doctor needs to rule out other causes of a rash in these commonly affected areas, particularly intertrigo. This is caused by wet skin surfaces rubbing together and setting up an infected inflammation.

IF YOU REMEMBER NOTHING ELSE, REMEMBER THESE THREE THINGS

1   Heat rash is very common in infancy.

2   It is restricted to areas where there are numerous sweat glands.

3   Adequate cooling and drying of the skin solves the problem rapidly.

Purpura

This rash is different from almost all other rashes in that it can have a serious underlying cause and cannot be blanched by pressing a piece of clear plastic or glass down on the skin or when the over-lying skin is stretched. In contrast to other rashes, the purple/reddy-brown areas of discoloration are not only beneath the skin but also outside the blood vessels, the underlying cause being abnormal bleeding. In effect, the rash is caused by tiny bruises which may range in size from that of a pinhead to two to three centimetres in diameter.

The abnormal bleeding is due to a deficiency of either tiny particles in the blood called platelets or clotting factors, both of which help the blood to coagulate. In addition, it may be caused by inflammation and damage to the smallest blood vessels (capillaries) beneath the skin. There are a number of causes for this, which may be either short lived and trivial or long-lasting and serious. Platelets may be reduced temporarily by certain medications, allergies and viral infections. They may also be reduced in number in autoimmune disorders where, for some reason, the body produces antibodies to its own structures and tissues, including components of the blood itself. This phenomenon also occurs in the blood-poisoning associated with certain forms of meningitis (see pages 124–126). Another possible cause is in where damage to the bone marrow results in the platelets being reduced.

WHAT CAN YOU DO?

If a rash of this type occurs, check to see if you can blanch the rash by pressing down on it with a piece of clear plastic or glass. If you can't, it is probably purpura and you should take your child to see the doctor as soon as possible whether or not he is showing any other signs of illness.

WHAT CAN THE DOCTOR DO?

The doctor needs to carry out a full physical examination of the child and to take blood samples so that the blood clotting mechanism and the number of platelets present can be evaluated. Treatment will depend entirely on the cause of the condition, although to prevent further purpura occurring, blood clotting factors or platelets can be replaced through transfusion.

IF YOU REMEMBER NOTHING ELSE, REMEMBER THESE THREE THINGS

1   Purpura is more likely than other rashes to have a serious underlying cause.

2   The purpura rash cannot be blanched.

3   Treatment depends on the underlying condition.

LONG-TERM RASHES

The rashes which accompany childhood infections and allergy are normally gone within a few days. There are, however, a number of rashes commonly seen in children which may last very much longer than that. The commonest are eczema, psoriasis and fungal infection.

CAUSES OF LONG-TERM RASHES

* Eczema

* Psoriasis

* Fungal infection (ringworm)

Eczema

Eczema is extremely common. There are about five million sufferers in total throughout the UK. It is an inflammation of the skin producing severe itching, and the skin itself is reddened, dry and scaly. Where it has been present for some time, the skin is often thickened, cracked and chronically infected. Where scratching has occurred, bleeding and weeping may also be seen. Eczema often starts with a cluster of pearly coloured blisters just below the surface of the skin, which often triggers the itching in the first place.

There are many different types of eczema and because of this it is easy to become confused about the causes and treatment. The commonest types in children are atopic eczema (otherwise known as infantile eczema) and seborrhoeic eczema, both of which are treated in different ways. The good news about atopic eczema, which affects more than 12 per cent of all children, is that many children grow out of it by the age of three and ninety per cent will do so by the time they are eight.

Two other types of eczema are also commonly seen, namely contact eczema (contact dermatitis) and pompholyx eczema. Contact eczema occurs where a chemical irritant produces a local reaction in the skin, examples being certain glues, concentrated washing powder, metals in jewellery and certain plants. Pompholyx eczema is usually confined to the sides of the fingers and toes and is triggered by warm weather. Both are more common in adults.

Symptoms of atopic eczema
Atopic or infantile eczema is the most common type of childhood eczema and always begins in the first two years of a child's life. Often it begins at between two and three months when bottle-feeding is substituted for breast-feeding, or a little later, between four and five months, when the child is weaned. The distribution of the rash is very characteristic. It is seen on the face, scalp, neck and in the skin creases and nappy area. It is often worse where the joints flex, sometimes being known as flexural eczema, and is therefore usually most obvious at the front of the wrists and

elbows, at the back of the knees and around the ankles. It is also commonly seen on the fingers and hands. The skin appears very dry and scaly and it may be reddened, cracked and thickened. Where scratching has occurred, there may be bleeding and, if bacterial infection has taken place, weeping and oozing are typical complications.

Causes of atopic eczema

A strong, positive family history of allergy is almost always present, and if either parent or a brother or sister has suffered with a similar kind of eczema, the next child has a fifty per cent chance of suffering too. It is closely associated with hay fever, asthma, glue ear and migraine as well, and whereas some children have all of these conditions together, many escape with just the eczema alone.

The genetic component of atopic eczema makes a child much more vulnerable to a number of trigger factors, but why this should be is not fully understood. What is understood, however, is that if certain trigger factors can be avoided, the severity and duration of the eczema can be reduced drastically.

TRIGGER FACTORS FOR ATOPIC ECZEMA

* Wool

* Biological washing powders

* Pet fluff and pet dander

* Parental smoking

* Emotional factors

* Detergent

* House dust mite

* Foodstuffs, food additives and colourings

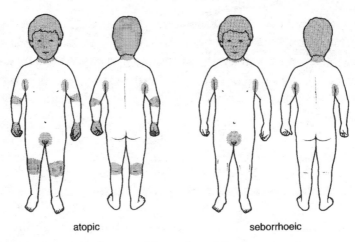

atopic   seborrhoeic

The typical distribution of the rash in different types of eczema

Seborrhoeic eczema

Although seborrhoeic eczema is seen in teenagers and adults, it is also commonly seen in babies as well. It affects areas of the skin where the sebaceous, or oil-producing, glands are in abundant supply and it produces a thick, yellow crust over the skin. Cradle cap is a good example of this and most babies, for several weeks at least in the first year of life, will develop the characteristic flakes on the top of their heads until the skin naturally becomes drier. It is also seen on the cheeks and on the neck at the level of the hairline, and is often prominent behind the ears. It may produce flaky scales on the eyelashes and crust formation at the outer part of the ear canal, and tends to favour greasy areas of skin such as around the nostrils, ears and groin. The best thing about seborrhoeic eczema is that it is not nearly as itchy as atopic eczema and responds very readily to simple treatment.

WHAT CAN YOU DO?

Although childhood eczema responds extremely well to treatment, the one thing that you cannot do is alter your child's genetic susceptibility to it. If he has inherited a tendency to eczema, hay fever or asthma, the best you can strive for is to avoid the environmental factors which make it worse and use whatever treatment is prescribed correctly and frequently. If you are breast-feeding your child, then it is to his advantage that this is continued for as long as possible. If it can be continued for up to six months, this will certainly delay the onset of symptoms and may reduce their severity as well. It is recommended that cow's milk, eggs, orange juice and wheat in the diet should be deferred until after the age of one. Exposure to these common causes of allergy (allergens) make the development of eczema all the more likely. It is well worth checking the labels on baby food to confirm that these products are not among the listed ingredients. When weaning your child, it is best to wean him onto vegetables, fruit, meat, cereals and a form of baby rice which is milk free. Finally, some children appear to react badly to additives and colourings in food, so again check the E numbers and ingredients on all food labels.

Allergies to the house dust mite contribute to eczema as well as to asthma (see page 449), so the same precautions to reduce exposure to this source should be taken for both. Plasters used on the skin for cuts and minor wounds should be hypo-allergenic. Wool in clothes is particularly irritant when worn in direct contact with the skin and, if it cannot be avoided altogether, it should certainly be worn only over cotton vests and undergarments. Unfortunately, the fur and dander (skin scales) shed from household pets is another potent source of skin irritation. It is extremely difficult, however, once a child has made an emotional attachment to a pet to separate them, so it is well worth thinking about the wisdom of providing such a pet in the first place. Sometimes a doctor may advise getting rid of a pet, but the distress caused can often do more harm than good. There is an enormous number of irritants capable of inflaming eczematous skin, some of the less obvious ones being biological washing powders, fabric conditioners, scented or perfumed soaps, bubble baths and shampoos. For most of these, more inert alternatives may be substituted.

If a child is scratching badly, particularly in bed at night when the skin is warm, cotton mittens may be worn over neatly trimmed fingernails. Finally it goes without saying that one of the most important jobs for a parent to do is to follow the doctor's advice to the letter, religiously applying any creams or ointments as directed.

Everyone wants their child to have clear, healthy, babysoft skin and it can be distressing to see a child with severe eczema. But it is important to remember that the child is extremely likely to grow out of the condition and that even if he does not, modern treatment is highly effective. In addition, anyone who does not know otherwise should be told, in no uncertain terms, that the condition is certainly not infectious or contagious and that the child does not need to be isolated or treated differently in any way.

WHAT CAN THE DOCTOR DO?

The first task of the doctor is to make an accurate diagnosis. There are many different types of eczema, and the doctor needs to be quite sure which type he or she is dealing with so that the appropriate treatment can be chosen. Usually there is little doubt, and even where it has occurred in the family before, a full explanation of the condition and its trigger factors is recommended for the parents. Avoiding the trigger factors can sometimes create real problems, and the doctor can certainly help with this. In terms of diet, for example, he or she can give specific advice about elimination diets which are designed to identify factors in the diet that trigger the eczema, and cow's milk alternatives such as soya milk can be provided on prescription.

If the eczema is weeping or oozing the doctor may prescribe antibiotics to eradicate any bacterial infection which is likely to be present, since until this is treated the eczema will certainly not improve. Some very recent research suggests that even where there is no obvious infection present, a specific bacterium called *Staphylococcus aureus* is usually found on the skin of eczema sufferers. This bug produces a toxin which itself irritates the skin and triggers further eczema. The eczema then encourages further infection and so a vicious circle is set up. Accordingly, the best treatment for eczema should consist of a cream or ointment combining antibiotic and steroid properties.

Where severe itching is a problem, the doctor can advise which antihistamine would be the best choice. He or she should then organise regular follow-ups to monitor the effect of the treatment chosen. In general, eczema treatment consists of a combination of emollients and steroids.

Emollients

An emollient is a mixture of oil, fat and water. It comes in the form of ointments, creams and lotions or in liquid form which can be added to bath water. Emollients are designed to be used every day in order to keep the skin moist and soft, and may be purchased directly over the counter at the chemist or can be obtained on NHS prescription. The advantage of emollients is that they avoid excessive drying of the skin which in itself can cause itching that in turn produces further inflammation. It also means that the total dose of any steroid used may be reduced, and this is of real benefit in cases of severe eczema where absorption of the steroid through the skin, with resulting side-effects, is always a possibility.

When an emollient cream is applied, it is important that the parent does not transmit any chemical that may be present on the hands, even in microscopic amounts, to the child's skin. You should therefore wash your hands before applying any cream, the ideal time to do this being after the child's bath, and the emollient should be massaged well into the skin. Some children respond better to one kind of emollient than another, and since there are so many it is well worth trying several out. If your child is sensitive to lanolin, a component of wool, avoid those that contain lanolin by checking the labelling on the container. Emollients need to be used as often as possible since they are not active drugs and are thoroughly safe however much is used. Sometimes, wrapping the skin with polythene sheeting or clingfilm (which is softer) after an emollient has been applied can allow more of it to be absorbed into the dry skin. It also prevents staining of the bedclothes.

Emollient bath liquids are particularly useful since children who bath in water alone, especially in hard water areas, will end up with even drier skin than before. Sometimes, cutting down on the number of baths helps, and is usually popular with children! A good soak for fifteen to thirty minutes is advisable and detergents of any kind, such as commercial soaps and shampoos, should be avoided as these merely remove any natural oil from the child's skin. Alternatives to soap are aqueous cream or emulsifying ointment which are totally inert but effective. These, like the emollients, however, will make the bath very slippery so take care when the child is getting in and out. The child should be patted dry with a soft towel rather than rubbed, and once dry any steroid cream prescribed should be applied.

Steroids

Steroid creams reduce the inflammation of the skin and prevent itching. Their effectiveness depends on the strength of the preparation and, as a general rule, the mildest steroid cream that is able to control the symptoms should be used. The more potent steroid creams may be partly absorbed through the skin into the bloodstream and, if used long term, might theoretically cause reduced skeletal growth and a moon-shaped face. Hydrocortisone one per cent cream and ointment is almost entirely safe, however, even if used all the time and on the face, and this may be purchased without prescription over the counter. Sometimes, more potent steroid creams are used when eczema flares up badly. These are used for a short period of time only to control the symptoms, and then later a milder steroid is substituted to maintain long-term treatment. Again, wrapping with clingfilm or polythene can improve and accelerate results. Occasionally, low-dose oral steroids such as predmisolone are used for severe cases and can be very effective and safe.

Antihistamines

Although antihistamines, which prevent itching, are available in skin cream form, these are best avoided as they are ineffective and may themselves contain additives to which the child may be sensitive or allergic. Non-sedating antihistamine tablets and syrups are now available which, if used just once a day, can control skin irritation.

Oil of evening primrose

Some medical studies have suggested that oil of evening primrose may, in a proportion of eczema sufferers, result in an improvement over the course of time. It should not be used in children under the age of one, nor in epileptics because of possible side-effects, but it is worth trying with other individuals since it is otherwise safe. It is available over-the-counter and also available on prescription in the form of Epogam (gamolenic acid) when it is taken in a dose of one to two capsules twice a day.

Chinese herbal medicine
There has been a great deal of interest shown lately in the beneficial effects of Chinese herbal medicine in the treatment of atopic eczema. In individuals with severe eczema, even those where the most potent steroids have failed to work, dramatic results have been reported in a proportion of cases. What's more, medically conducted trials by conventionally trained doctors at Great Ormond Street Hospital for Sick Children have been able to confirm the results scientifically. The active ingredient of the Chinese herbs used in the medicine has not yet been identified, the drink which the sufferer takes being concocted from a large number of different plants. On the safety side, there have been reports of certain side-effects including liver damage, but although

---

IF YOU REMEMBER NOTHING ELSE, REMEMBER THESE THREE THINGS

1 Eczema is extremely common in children, especially where there is a positive family history, although the majority of children grow out of it by the age of eight.

2 Avoidance of identified trigger factors is essential.

3 Emollients are the main form of treatment, with steroid creams and antibiotics being reserved for flare-ups.

no proven link with the Chinese medicine has been established, it seems appropriate that its use should be carried out under supervision in hospitals, with regular blood tests to check on the healthy functioning of the liver. This form of complementary therapy is not generally available as yet on the NHS.

Psoriasis

Psoriasis causes a patchy rash which can sometimes be mistaken for eczema although the sites of the body affected, as well as the cause and treatment, are totally different. Unlike eczema, it is rare under the age of two and becomes more common with increasing age. In adults, something like one per cent of the population may be affected at some stage in their lives.

There is often a family history of psoriasis and the rash may be triggered by a sore throat or some other common infection. In children, it often starts with a widespread crop of small, dry patches on the skin which are round or oval in shape and reddy-pink in colour. Overlying the redness there is a characteristic layer of silvery scales which heap up and flake off. The distribution of the

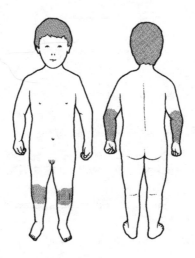

The typical distribution of the rash in psoriasis

rash is unique too, occurring particularly on the back of the elbows, the front of the knees and the scalp. Other areas commonly affected by psoriasis are the ears, chest and upper part of the cleft between the buttocks. In babies, psoriasis is occasionally the cause of a very severe and widespread nappy rash (napkin psoriasis). Luckily the rash of psoriasis is not nearly as itchy as that caused by eczema.

The underlying cause of psoriasis is an increased rate of cell formation in the skin, although quite what triggers it is not understood. The spotty form of the condition, guttate psoriasis, which is seen in young children, tends to last about three months before it spontaneously disappears. It is quite likely, however, to recur sometimes in the next five years and then possibly again in adult life.

WHAT CAN YOU DO?

One of the most important things which you should do if your child has psoriasis is to establish the diagnosis. It is easy to assume that the rash is due simply to patches of eczema or cradle cap, but the treatment for these common conditions is quite different. If in doubt, take your child to the doctor so that a proper examination can be carried out. Older children with larger patches, or plaques as they are known, need to be reassured that the condition will almost certainly clear up within a few weeks leaving no blemishes or scars. This is especially important if the rash affects the face or scalp as, even these days, tactless people who are ignorant of the condition are quick to attach some kind of stigma to it.

One natural remedy is to expose your child's skin as much as possible to mild-to-moderate ultraviolet light from sunshine, so it is well worth letting your child run around with no clothes on in the garden during the summer. Unaffected areas of the skin should still be protected against excess exposure to the sun by means of high SPF sunscreens. Finally, regular, careful application of the various treatments prescribed by the doctor is important in keeping the condition under control.

WHAT CAN THE DOCTOR DO?

The first job for the doctor is to establish the correct diagnosis. Psoriasis is quite distinct from seborrhoeic eczema or atopic eczema and needs to be dealt with differently. Initially, bland ointments should be tried as these moisturise the skin and prevent flaking. They also avoid any staining of the clothes or bedlinen. If these are not sufficient, the two other main types of treatment are mild cortisone creams and coal-tar preparations. Coal-tar preparations are particularly good for larger areas of psoriasis on the scalp or body, and they also come in shampoo form. Hydrocortisone creams suppress the inflammation and redness of the skin and in time reduce the amount of scales produced. It is worth using coal-tar solutions in the child's bath water too, and where there are widespread small spots, this is much easier than rubbing cream into each one.

In more resistant forms of psoriasis, dithranol is useful but since this can produce a slight burning sensation as well as some skin staining it is best used in a short-contact regime. In other words,

---

IF YOU REMEMBER NOTHING ELSE, REMEMBER THESE THREE THINGS

1   Psoriasis affects different areas of the body compared with eczema.

2   The elbows, knees and scalp are most commonly affected.

3   Hydrocortisone and coal-tar preparations are the two main treatments.

---

the cream is applied at night for say thirty minutes at a time, and then all excess cream is rubbed off again. This is probably the most effective treatment at the current time, but care should be taken that it is never applied to raw or blistered areas of skin.

Fungal Infection (ringworm)

Although a fungal infection may start as an individual spot, it usually enlarges to form a more widespread rash in certain moist areas of the body. A rather old-fashioned term for this type of infection is ringworm, although ironically the rash produced is not always in the shape of a ring and has absolutely nothing whatsoever to do with worms.

Areas most commonly affected are moist skin creases such as the groin, between the toes, under the arms and on the face. Occasionally, circular patches may also be seen on the limbs. On the scalp, distinct patches can show themselves as localised areas of hair loss. Between the toes, where it is known as athlete's foot, the infection can produce a soggy, white, swollen mess.

Fungal infections may be passed on through touch alone, and can also be picked up in bathrooms and shower rooms which provide a constantly warm and moist environment.

WHAT CAN YOU DO?

One of the most important things to do is to dry the child's skin thoroughly after showers and baths. The drier the skin, the less chance of a fungal infection developing. The feet really need to breathe in order to allow sweat and moisture to evaporate, so on the whole sandals and leather shoes are better than trainers. Various anti-fungal foot powders are useful if applied regularly, but once the infection has taken hold and the rash is spreading, more potent antifungal therapy is required.

WHAT CAN THE DOCTOR DO?

If there is any doubt at all about the nature of the rash, the doctor can take a sample of skin scrapings, using a sharp instrument, which can be examined under the microscope to identify the fungal elements. Once confirmed, an anti-fungal cream can be prescribed which, when applied regularly say two or three times a day, will eventually result in a straightforward cure. Treatment should certainly be continued for at least two weeks after the rash appears to have gone completely to prevent it from recurring, as not every single fungal element may have been eradicated.

IF YOU REMEMBER NOTHING ELSE, REMEMBER THESE THREE THINGS

1 Fungal infection is normally seen in the moist skin creases of the body.

2 On the body or face, the rash consists of a flat, pink circle with a slightly raised edge and a pale centre.

3 Treatment involves keeping the skin dry and using antifungal powders and creams.

ITCHY SPOTS

Children develop spots for any number of reasons, and they may or may not be itchy. Of the itchy variety, chickenpox is one of the commonest culprits. The characteristic blisters quickly become widespread to form an overall rash (see pages 117–119). The spots produced by insect bites may be particularly itchy too, although generally these are confined to one small area. Occasionally, cold sores, shingles or another viral infection known as hand, foot and mouth disease can produce itchy spots too.

CAUSES OF ITCHY SPOTS

* Chickenpox (see pages 117–119)

* Insect bites

* Viral infections:

   Cold sores

   Shingles

   Hand, foot and mouth disease

Insect Bites

Many insects can inflict bites as they puncture the skin in order to get to the blood on which they feed. Mosquitoes, gnats, bed bugs, fleas, lice, horseflies and midges are amongst the most common, but spiders, mites and ticks can all produce itchy spots too. The spots are usually short-lived, producing irritation for no more than a day or two, but some children develop an allergic reaction to the insect's saliva or faeces which can be rubbed into the skin through scratching. If this is the case, instead of small, red pimples there may be intensely itchy and painful lumps which soon become infected with bacteria and start to weep. In the worst cases, they can produce redness and discomfort in a whole limb. Depending upon the degree of allergic response, some children hardly seem to notice their spots, whereas others bitten by a similar insect can develop extremely severe reactions.

In warmer countries, mosquitoes are notorious for inflicting the most damage, and in the tropics they can transmit diseases such as malaria as well. In Britain, however, most insect bites come from cat or dog fleas which live not only on the pet but in certain parts of the house where the pet sleeps. These include animal sleeping baskets, settees, carpets and other soft furnishings, and fleas are often present in locations where the pet has been absent for some time. When fleas which have temporarily jumped off an animal are unable to jump back on because the animal has moved elsewhere, they may be forced to feed on humans instead.

Scabies infestations occur where the scabies mite burrows under the skin and lays its eggs. It produces a particularly itchy crop of spots which can look just like eczema. The spots are usually tiny, grey and pearly, often seen in the webs of the fingers, on the front surfaces of the wrists, in the armpits and around the genitals. The spots are most irritant at night when the skin is warm, and vigorous scratching often produces bleeding and infection. Scabies is spread relatively easily through close physical contact or from sharing contaminated bedding, so it is commonly seen in people living in institutions.

WHAT CAN YOU DO?

The first thing to do is to try to avoid insect bites in the first place. This is especially important for summer campers and people travelling abroad. Bites inflicted when children are out can be partially prevented by putting them in long socks, long-sleeved shirts and trousers, especially after dark. Insect repellents are also worth using, as are flea collars for cats and dogs. Indoors, various aerosols containing insecticides are helpful, and where mosquitoes are a real problem, screens over open windows and mosquito nets may be necessary.

Once a bite has been inflicted, it should be washed with ordinary soap and water before applying a soothing lotion such as calamine. Scratching should be avoided, as this will only take the top off the spot and lead to secondary infection with bacteria. Antihistamines can be taken to prevent itching, and these are much more effective in tablet or syrup form than in creams.

Scabies is treated by applying a special insecticide lotion to the whole of the skin from the neck downwards. The lotion is best applied after a tepid bath and left on for 24 hours before being rinsed off. The lotion kills the mites although the itching may persist for up to a fortnight. All other members of the family should be treated at the same time, and bedlinen and clothes should be washed thoroughly at high temperature and ironed.

If itching is restricted to the scalp, head lice are a possible cause, in which case special shampoos and lotions will be required (see page 289–291).

WHAT CAN THE DOCTOR DO?

The doctor needs to confirm the likely cause of the spots and examine them to determine whether any secondary infection has occurred. If it has, treatment with antibiotics either in topical cream form or, if more widespread, in oral form will be required, and the doctor can advise about which type of antihistamine it is best to use to relieve itching. Scabies and lice infestations are sometimes more difficult to diagnose in the early stages, but your doctor should be able to do this and to prescribe the necessary treatment.

> ## IF YOU REMEMBER NOTHING ELSE, REMEMBER THESE THREE THINGS
>
> ---
>
> 1   Insect bites in Britain are most commonly inflicted by fleas from cats and dogs.
>
> ---
>
> 2   The size of the spot depends on the extent of any allergy or infection and the extent of the child's reaction to the bite.
>
> ---
>
> 3   If prevention has not worked, calamine lotion, antihistamines and antibiotics are effective in treating the skin condition, whilst insecticide preparations can be used to eradicate the parasites themselves.

Viral Infections

There are three common viral infections which can produce localised, itchy spots.

Cold sores
Cold sores generally appear around the mouth, often between the ages of one and four. The infection is often accompanied by a temperature and little ulcers in the mouth, and the child may also complain of a sore throat. It usually settles over a period of a few days, but it may be precipitated in the future by exposure to sunlight, intense cold, dry wind or a fever.

Shingles

In this condition, a group of tiny blisters on a red background is seen in a small area on one side of the body. It starts with an itch and then often becomes very painful as the blisters erupt over a period of two to three weeks. As the blisters break, secondary infection with bacteria can occur, with crusty scabs forming on the surfaces.

Hand, foot and mouth disease

This is a relatively trivial condition which can occur in epidemics. It has nothing to do with foot-and-mouth seen in cattle. It is a very mild disorder lasting about a week or so, and consists of tiny, superficial blisters on the insides of the cheeks and on the tongue, with similar flat, empty blisters over the hands and feet. It is quite contagious, so other children and even adults in the family are often affected too.

WHAT CAN YOU DO?

With these viral infections, it is important to keep the skin clean to reduce the possibility of secondary bacterial infection. Salted water or soap and water are probably as good as anything since some antiseptic lotions may penetrate the blisters and sting.

WHAT CAN THE DOCTOR DO?

Antiviral therapy in the form of cream and ointment as well as in tablet form can reduce the duration and severity of both cold sores and shingles. This needs to be applied as soon as the character-istic tingling is experienced in the skin before the blisters appear, so ideally you should keep a supply of the appropriate treatment for a child who is prone to recurrent eruptions. If in the later stages the spots become weepy, antibiotics can prevent further spread. No treatment for hand, foot and mouth disease is required.

IF YOU REMEMBER NOTHING ELSE, REMEMBER THESE THREE THINGS

1   Recurrent itchy spots may be caused by viral infections.

2   Antiviral creams reduce the severity and duration of attacks.

3   Antibiotics may be required if secondary bacterial infection has occurred.

NON-ITCHY SPOTS

There are a number of different types of non-itchy spots which can occur in infants and young children. Sometimes the diagnosis is obvious, but this certainly is not always the case.

CAUSES OF NON-ITCHY SPOTS

* Milia

* Infantile acne

* Boils

* Warts

* Impetigo

Milia

Milia is a localised area of hundreds of tiny, white-headed spots on the nose and cheeks of a newborn baby. The spots are not itchy and do not bother the baby in any way. They are merely the result of immature sweat glands that are not yet able to discharge sweat properly, thus producing tiny collections of fluid. Milia is a normal condition and requires no treatment.

Infantile Acne

This condition appears at any time between the ages of four months and five years. There is hardly ever any glandular disorder responsible, but the typical white heads and cysts of adult acne may be seen. In most cases there is a spontaneous improvement within a few years, but in some of these children severe acne may develop in adolescence.

WHAT CAN YOU DO?

There is no immediate cure for infantile acne although the importance of general hygiene should not be overlooked. Frequent washing with soap or mild antiseptic lotions helps to prevent the secondary bacterial infection in the pores from spreading to other areas of the skin. Exposure to moderate degrees of natural sunlight is also helpful as this helps to dry out some of the skin's natural oiliness.

WHAT CAN THE DOCTOR DO?

The doctor may prescribe sulphur preparations in cream or paste form, although watery antibiotic lotions are now also available which are very effective. The tetracycline antibiotics, which are often used in the treatment of adult acne, should be avoided in children as they may cause a yellow-brown discoloration of the teeth.

IF YOU REMEMBER NOTHING ELSE, REMEMBER THESE THREE THINGS

1   Infantile acne may appear at almost any time before the age of 5.

---

2   Frequent use of soap and mild antiseptic helps.

---

3   Antibiotic lotions eradicate any troublesome bacteria.

Boils

A boil is simply a large, fluid-filled lump which occurs when a hair follicle becomes invaded by bacteria. There may also be a surrounding redness of the skin. The boil often has a white or yellow top which bursts onto the surface of the skin after a few days, oozing characteristic pus. Boils can spread easily to nearby areas of the skin as other hair follicles are readily infected. Areas where clothes rub are particularly vulnerable. Boils on fairly insensitive areas like the front of the thigh are not usually too troublesome, but those that occur over joints where the skin can become stretched or on the inside of the ear canal can be extremely tender.

WHAT CAN YOU DO?

If your child has a boil, it is important to prevent the infection from spreading to other nearby hair follicles. This can be done by applying antiseptic lotion or surgical spirit, and the boil should be covered with a sterile pad. Do not be tempted to squeeze the boil as this can further irritate the skin and help to spread the infection. Even when a boil has burst, it is still important to keep the area sterile and to cover it with a dressing to reduce the shedding of any further bacteria. The child should also use a separate towel and flannel to reduce the chances of other members of the family being infected.

WHAT CAN THE DOCTOR DO?

If the boil is in a particularly painful area of the body, your doctor will be more inclined to prescribe antibiotics at an early stage. He or she will also do this if, instead of discharging towards the surface of the skin, the boil remains deep-seated and the infection spreads sideways or downwards into neighbouring areas of skin. If this happens there may be tell-tale red streaks under the skin and enlarged lymph glands some distance from the boil itself. Larger boils of this type need to be lanced under local anaesthetic with a small, pointed scalpel. This can drain the pus quickly leading to a reduction in pain and quicker resolution of the

IF YOU REMEMBER NOTHING ELSE, REMEMBER THESE THREE THINGS

1   Boils cause large, painful, red lumps.

2   Deep-seated or painful boils may require surgical treatment.

3   Short- or long-term antibiotics and antiseptic scrubs will prevent recurrences.

problem. Finally, if the child is bothered by recurrent boils then a long-term course of low-dose antibiotics may be required to reduce the number of micro-organisms responsible for the infection on the skin's surface.

Warts

Warts produce small, hard lumps on the skin surface, either individually or in crops and clusters. They are caused by the human papillomavirus which invades cells in the outer layers of the skin where it multiplies, causing overgrowth of the skin itself. Warts are very common in children and young adults, and they are usually seen on the fingers, soles of the feet, knees and face. In nearly all children the warts disappear spontaneously within about three years, as this is how long it takes for the immune system to eradicate them. Many will find that their warts clear up within months rather than years.

Except on the sole of the foot where they are known as verrucae, warts are not usually painful, and if they are it usually means that secondary infection with bacteria has taken place in the surrounding skin. The virus is spread by direct contact with other warts, but children with verrucae do not need to be excluded from swimming or take any special precautions as they are nowhere near as infectious as was once thought.

WHAT CAN YOU DO?

If you suspect that your child has a wart, first look around the surface of the skin for others. If there is only one and it is small, probably the best course of action is to ignore it as it will almost certainly clear up on its own in time. However, if the child has numerous warts or a single very large one, or if they are on the face and are unsightly, treatment is certainly possible. There are many patent wart cures which you can buy over the counter at the chemist, although it is essential to follow the manufacturer's directions carefully to avoid damaging healthy skin. These treatments usually consist of acid solutions designed to burn away the horny, superficial layers of skin. They should be applied within a special corn-plaster which protects the adjacent healthy skin. They should never be used on the face or in the genital area as scarring can occur.

WHAT CAN THE DOCTOR DO?

If you are uncertain as to the cause of the skin lump, then the doctor should certainly be consulted so that a diagnosis can be made. He or she may well advise you to do absolutely nothing as the majority of warts will clear up in their own time. If the wart is single and large, treatment with special anti-wart solutions can be prescribed, which should generally be applied at night. The wart should be covered to keep the solution in contact with the wart only, and in the morning a pumice stone or mild abrasive can be used to remove the top layer of dead cells. Many GPs now run special wart clinics where warts can be removed using cauterisation (burning) or cryotherapy (freezing). For widespread multiple warts, especially unsightly ones, liquid nitrogen treatment (freezing) may be carried out in specialised dermatology clinics in hospital.

IF YOU REMEMBER NOTHING ELSE, REMEMBER THESE THREE THINGS

1   Warts and verrucae are caused by a virus.

2   The vast majority of warts clear up on their own within two to three years without treatment.

3   Large or multiple warts can be treated by acid solutions, burning or freezing.

Impetigo

This is a highly contagious infection of the skin which is common in children and usually occurs around the nose and mouth. It is caused by a bacteria which gets into a broken area of skin, often through a cut, a cold sore or a patch of eczema. Sometimes thumb-sucking, nail-biting or nose-picking, all of which break the skin, can trigger it off. The germs which cause the problem may be those which normally live on the skin and in the nose.

The first sign of impetigo is that the skin becomes red, after which small, fluid-filled blisters appear on the surface. The blisters then burst open leaving weeping areas underneath which dry out to form honey-coloured crusts on the skin. These look a little like brown sugar. The infected fluid may spread across the surface of the skin causing further patches of infection nearby. As the infection is drained through lymphatic channels, the lymph glands in the face or neck may swell and occasionally a slight fever may occur.

WHAT CAN YOU DO?

The first thing to do is to get your child to stop spreading the infection by scratching, picking or wiping the rash with his hand. It is best to clean away any crusts using warm, salty water and then to pat the skin dry with a towel or flannel which you keep separate from those used by the rest of the family. It is important to prevent the child from sucking his thumb, picking his nose or biting his nails.

WHAT CAN THE DOCTOR DO?

Since impetigo spreads so quickly, not only on the child but to other people in close contact with him, it is important for the doctor to prescribe an antibiotic cream or oral preparation as soon as possible. This will usually cure the condition within a matter of days. If the infection is recurrent, oral antibiotics are best to prevent the infection being spread further afield.

IF YOU REMEMBER NOTHING ELSE, REMEMBER THESE THREE THINGS

1   Impetigo is a weepy, crusty, yellow-coloured skin rash usually seen around the lips, mouth and nose;

2   Spreads rapidly to other skin sites and to other people;

3   Responds quickly to treatment with antibiotics.

CHAPTER SIX

A TO Z OF SYMPTOMS

Abdominal Lumps

The commonest lump on a child's tummy is an umbilical hernia.

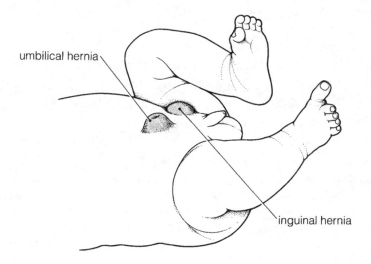

umbilical hernia

inguinal hernia

The typical position of a hernia

It is caused by a weakness in the muscular wall at the front of the abdomen where the umbilical cord passed to and from the baby. A small loop of intestine is able to push through this weakness, distending the skin on the surface of the tummy. Parents notice that the lump bulges out when the intestinal pressure increases, say when the child cries or strains. The lump feels extremely soft and soggy to the touch and, although it looks alarming, in almost all cases it is quite harmless. The general tendency is for the hernia to correct itself naturally by the age of about six months to a year. By this time the child has grown taller, the abdominal muscles have strengthened, the abdomen has enlarged and the intestine has been pulled up further inside the tummy.

The health visitor or doctor will be able to demonstrate that the hernia can easily be pushed back gently inside the abdomen causing a slight gurgling sound. This is normal. If, however, the very rare case of strangulation of the hernia occurs, the loop of the bowel is pinched by the muscular edges of the weakness, shutting off its blood supply and damaging it severely. In this situation, the lump becomes hard and tender, the child will be distressed and sick, and it is very difficult or impossible to push the lump back inside: If these symptoms occur, urgent medical attention should be sought. Parents should remember, however, that this virtually never happens to an umbilical hernia, although it commonly does to inguinal herniae (see page 256).

There are one or two other causes of abdominal lumps, notably constipation (see pages 196–202) which can produce a barely visible but palpable hard lump on the left-hand side of the tummy, and fatty lumps and cysts in the skin, although these are rare.

Generalised abdominal distension is commonly seen in children and usually has a trivial cause. Occasionally, however, it may be a sign of dietary malabsorption so if the symptom persists and the child is listless, medical help should be sought.

WHAT CAN YOU DO?

It is worthwhile taking a child with an abdominal lump to the doctor for reassurance if nothing else. The important thing to realise is that a strangulated umbilical hernia, though rare, is a surgical emergency, so if you cannot push the lump back gently inside the child's abdomen and it is hard and tender to touch, consult your doctor straightaway.

WHAT CAN THE DOCTOR DO?

Most umbilical hernias require no treatment whatsoever, the doctor's job being to merely observe and advise.

IF YOU REMEMBER NOTHING ELSE, REMEMBER THESE THREE THINGS

1　Most abdominal lumps are umbilical hernias, which are common and usually harmless.

2　They are characterised by a soft lump which comes and goes and gets bigger when the child cries.

3　Any abdominal lump should be examined by a doctor.

Bad Breath

In most cases, when children have bad breath it is a temporary problem. It is common in children with enlarged adenoids or who are nasally congested, as they continually mouth-breathe which dries up the saliva that washes away dead cells on the surface of the mouth and prevents them from decaying. Children with sore throats and colds will often have smelly breath for the same reason. Sometimes even a mild cough may be responsible. Other causes include lack of dental hygiene which results in food being trapped between the teeth, tooth decay and gum infection.

A simple explanation of bad breath but one which is often over-looked is the consumption of spicy foods such as curries or highly flavoured snacks such as crisps which may form a staple part of the child's diet. Really bad breath may occur in children who have a small, foreign body stuck up their nose. In this instance there is usually a watery, bloody discharge from one nostril as well.

WHAT CAN YOU DO?

The child's teeth should be brushed regularly using a fluoride toothpaste, if fluoride is not already added to the local water supply, and occasional antiseptic mouthwashes are helpful. Children who mouth-breathe, for whatever reason, should be supplied with drinks at night to solve the problem of dry lips, tongue and mouth.

WHAT CAN THE DOCTOR DO?

In cases of nasal congestion, decongestants and steroids in the form of paediatric nose-drops and nasal sprays together with oral antihistamines for allergy can be used. Serious adenoidal enlargement which produces snoring, mouth-breathing, speech problems and regular ear infections as well as the antisocial problem of bad breath, may require surgery to overcome the problem. Finally, removing a foreign body from a nostril in a child with bad breath can solve the problem almost overnight.

IF YOU REMEMBER NOTHING ELSE, REMEMBER THESE THREE THINGS

1   Bad breath in a child is usually short lived.

2   Enlarged adenoids and cold infections are usually responsible.

3   Decongestants for colds and adenoidectomy are usually the answer to persistent bad breath.

Bedwetting (nocturnal enuresis)

This is defined as the passing of urine at night by a child who is over the age of five and where there is no identifiable physical reason for it. But children differ enormously in the age at which they learn to control their bladders and stay dry. Most children will become dry by day somewhere between the ages of one and four, and the majority of children become dry at night anywhere between the ages of two and five. In fact about three-quarters of all children are dry at night by the age of four and a further ten per cent join them by the time they are five. This means that something like fifteen to twenty per cent of five year olds are still wetting the bed two or three times a week.

Secondary enuresis means that a child who was previously dry at night has started to wet the bed again. It usually points to some kind of anxiety or stress such as the arrival of a new brother or sister (who can be seen as a rival for his parent's affections), starting a new school, or simply 'fear of the unknown'. Occasionally there will be a physical cause, and bladder infection or even diabetes should not be ruled out until proper tests have been conducted.

CAUSES OF BEDWETTING

* Late control of bladder function

* Bladder infection

* Constipation

* Stress

* Diabetes

* Anatomical abnormality

Late Control of Bladder Function

Bedwetting is not only upsetting for the child concerned, but stressful for the parents as well. Parents who are constantly changing damp sheets, duvets and mattresses soon become tired, irritable and frustrated. If, in addition, the child is still wet by day, some nurseries and infant schools will be reluctant to take him. It may be some help to know that late control of bladder function tends to run in families, and that the children are certainly not lazy or dirty, and virtually all of them will become dry in time. If either parent continued to wet the bed until the age of eight or nine, then the children will have a much higher chance of doing likewise. Similarly, children within the same family will tend to control their bladders at a similar age, although boys tend to be a little later than girls. For some reason, firstborn children are more affected than later siblings, and certainly any child with learning difficulties, delayed development or any form of social deprivation may be more vulnerable to delayed bladder control.

There are many myths about bedwetting which need to be debunked. Many parents think that if they restrict the amount of fluid the child drinks during the evening this will reduce the possibility of bedwetting. This is simply not true. Many also believe that if they 'lift' the child from his bed and get him to empty his bladder when the parents go to bed, this will also cut down on wet bedding. Again, this is not the case and may actually train the child to pass urine whilst half-asleep. Nor is it true that children who wet the bed are just deep sleepers, have smaller bladders or are too lazy to get up.

Finally, allowing your frustration and anger to show will not help in any way. In fact, the last thing a child who wets the bed in his sleep needs is to be scolded, chastised or beaten. It is not his fault and he would certainly far rather be dry at night than wet. This is where your handling of the problem becomes so important.

WHAT CAN YOU DO?

The first thing is to remember how common bedwetting is. It is all too easy to listen to other mums of young children and think that your child is far behind in terms of bladder control. Eventually, however, all children learn to stay dry at night, although it requires a lot more patience on behalf of some parents than others.

On the practical side, before you put your child to bed it is obviously a good idea to get him to empty his bladder. Also, using a waterproof rubber or polythene sheet over the mattress is essential so that a top sheet which does become wet can be washed and dried each day if necessary. If the bathroom is a long, cold, shadowy corridor away, having a potty by the bedside may encourage your child to use it during the night, especially if a dim light is left on in the bedroom. Lastly, it is worth avoiding giving your child certain drinks as some contain caffeine which acts as a diuretic, making your child's kidneys produce more urine. Cola and chocolate drinks are particularly worth avoiding, but normal tea and coffee, which is drunk by some children, also contain significant amounts of caffeine.

A very important thing to remember is never to show how angry you feel when your child wets. It is far better to encourage and praise him when he has a dry night. This prevents the build up of any anxiety or fear, and increases his incentive to stay dry. A 'star chart' is an ideal way of helping your child over this problem. Help the child to draw up a weekly calendar and place it in a prominent position in the bedroom, such as at the foot of the bed. If he wets the bed in the night, nothing is indicated on the chart, but if he rises in the morning and is dry, he may stick a coloured star on the chart on the relevant day. When he manages, say, three stars in a row, he is awarded a special gold star which entitles him to a little present or treat. Usually the star chart kept like this for a month or two is sufficient to get a five- to seven-year-old child dry by night.

WHAT CAN THE DOCTOR DO?

The doctor needs to listen carefully to what the parents have to say about the child's bedwetting and to reassure them about the normal age range for achieving bladder control. Stress and anxiety in a child is one possible cause for bedwetting, so any sources of fear or worry should be discussed. More importantly, the doctor needs to exclude any of the physical reasons for bedwetting. Constipation is common in small children, and when the bowel becomes distended there may be pressure on the bladder which can lead to persistent bedwetting. Another possible cause is infection, which can creep into the bladder and kidneys from outside, especially in girls, producing 'frequency', the desire to pass urine all the time. Usually, however, this will produce problems during the day as well as during the night. If the child is unusually thirsty as well as producing excessive quantities of urine, diabetes mellitus might be the cause. Other symptoms to look out for in this case would be loss of weight and fatigue, and any child who potentially might be suffering from this serious condition needs urgent investigation and treatment. Finally, and rarely, there is a group of children who are born with an anatomical abnormality of the kidneys or bladder which can lead to problems.

Once the doctor has excluded these physical causes he or she can get on with the treatment of true nocturnal enuresis. Here, even if the star chart has been tried unsuccessfully, a child over the age of seven still has an eighty per cent chance of responding to an enuresis alarm. This alarm is designed to wake a child from his sleep as soon as he starts to wet the bed. The alarm is battery operated and is connected to a small, electronic sensor pad which fits snugly between two pairs of pants worn by the child. As the

WEEK	1	2	3	4
Monday	✳			
Tuesday				
Wednesday	✳			
Thursday				
Friday	✳			
Saturday	✳			
Sunday	✳			

star chart

battery operated alarm

sensor pad

The star chart and enuresis alarm used in the treatment of bedwetting first drops of moisture come into contact with the sensor, the alarm is immediately triggered, waking the child. The child can then stop himself from passing any more urine until he reaches the toilet or potty. The alarm usually needs to be used for a few weeks because it takes this length of time for the child's nervous system to link the sensations of a full bladder with starting to wet the bed and the buzzer going off. As soon as the link occurs, then the alarm becomes unnecessary, and the child wakes up in response to a full bladder rather than the sound of the buzzer. Often, for the first few weeks, the child's parents will need to sit by his bed to wake him up *immediately* the alarm goes off. It is very important that he is thoroughly woken, otherwise he will be conditioned to pass urine when still half-asleep. Various types of alarm are available, and your doctor may be able to arrange to have one lent to you from a local paediatric or hospital enuresis clinic.

Alternative treatment involves the use of medication. An anti-depressant known as imipramine (Tofranil) can be effective in the majority of bedwetting children, although a significant proportion of them will revert to bedwetting once the treatment is stopped. For reasons not fully understood, the drug seems to allow their nervous system to recognise the sensations of a full bladder and to react accordingly. Certainly, the fact that Tofranil is an antide-pressant has nothing to do with it, as there is no evidence whatsoever that such children are depressed. Since bedwetting symptoms may return when the imipramine regime is stopped, the therapy should not be discontinued abruptly but gradually tailed off over a period of a week or so. If this drug is used, it is vital to keep it away from younger children as an overdose can be dangerous. Nowadays, a second form of medical treatment is more likely to be used, namely desmopressin tablets taken at night. These contain a special hormone (desmopressin) which makes the kidneys produce less urine. About three-quarters of children using this regime respond very well and, if nothing else, it at least shows them that they can be dry and that control of their bladder func-tion is in sight. However, as with imipramine, some children will revert to bedwetting when therapy is discontinued, although when used in conjunction with the alarm system, it can be particularly effective.

IF YOU REMEMBER NOTHING ELSE, REMEMBER THESE THREE THINGS

1   There is enormous variation in the age at which children gain bladder control.

2   Physical reasons for persistent bedwetting need to be excluded.

3   Star charts and enuresis alarms are effective treatments which the parents themselves can supervise.

Behavioural Problems

Behavioural problems can come to light in several ways in children. Temper tantrums, food refusal, sleeping difficulties, excessive activity and aggressive acts such as biting, hitting, kicking and fighting are just a few. Parents will have different ideas about how to deal with these problems, and any established family rules will depend on the culture, ethnic background and social circumstances of the family itself. A lot, of course, will also depend on the parents' personalities and their own childhood experiences. Some parents believe in a highly disciplined and rigid approach to child rearing, whereas others are more liberal and laid-back in their attitude. In medical terms, there is no absolutely right or wrong way to bring up a child (provided there is no abuse of any kind), and at the end of the day, the most important thing is for parents to do what they feel happiest with.

A child who is brought up to observe a regular routine is usually less likely to become obstreperous and difficult to handle. In fact, there is much evidence to suggest that the imposition of a regular routine at a young age is the best way of dealing with children, even those who have short attention spans or a degree of hyperactivity.

Parents will tend to seek help for their child's behavioural problems when both feel that their child has become uncontrollable and that nothing they try to do seems to work. At this point they may have already consulted other parents, and they may well have talked to nursery nurses, teachers, health visitors and other members of local playgroups and schemes. Of course no child is perfect and there are as many little terrors as there are little angels – in a recent survey, 75 per cent of mothers when asked said their children were hyperactive, suggesting that in most cases this was a misconception. The question is whether behavioural problems are beginning to upset normal family life, and whether the difficulties are something that can be lived with or whether they need to be sorted out. Sometimes a lot of pressure can be relieved just by knowing that a problem can be solved if certain actions are taken. A lot also depends on who perceives there is a problem. What may be tolerable for parents may well be unacceptable to neighbours, grandparents, teachers or even the police. Overtly antisocial behaviour certainly needs to be corrected.

The child's underlying personality is probably the overriding factor in determining his behaviour. Some children are born shy and placid, others extrovert and aggressive. A child who tends to be anxious and fearful may be more prone to sleeping badly or having nightmares, accounting for disturbed sleep and tiredness the following day. A child who feels pressurised in any way, either from school, from brothers and sisters or from parental tensions, may well behave badly in an attempt to gain the attention and security which they need so much.

Often bad behaviour is the result of measures the parents have unwittingly taken in the past. For example, a child who will not settle at night and who has always then been taken into the parental bed will have learned that making a fuss pays dividends and is rewarded with cuddles and special treatment. A child who has thrown tantrums and who has been bribed with sweets or cakes will have picked up a similar message.

Sometimes bad behaviour occurs at certain critical times such as when the child is over-excited, thirsty, tired or hungry, and if this type of behavioural pattern exists then the obvious remedy will suggest itself before too long.

Occasionally there may be un underlying disorder such as undiagnosed autism, dyslexia, deafness or hyperactivity which produces such immense frustration in the child that naughty behaviour inevitably follows as a result.

WHAT CAN YOU DO?

There are different trains of thought on how to deal with aggressive behaviour such as biting, hitting, kicking and fighting, but it is best not to retaliate by, for example, taking a child who has bitten and biting him back, because although this shows that it hurts, it also serves to condone this type of behaviour. It must be explained to the child why such behaviour is not acceptable, and the message needs to be repeated as often as is necessary. In general, children respond to increased affection even if they do not apparently deserve it, as often their naughtiness is an attention-seeking device born out of insecurity. It is not a bad idea to allow particularly exuberant children who are also aggressive a certain period of time every day to let their hair down and go completely wild so that they burn up excess energy and do not feel restricted or physically confined.

By and large, parents should do what feels right, but often professional guidance is required. Sometimes the most loving and caring mothers and fathers can pamper their offspring, giving them far too much of a free rein to manipulate to their advantage. Spoiling is not in the best interests of any child and sometimes being cruel to be kind and taking a firm line is the best way. Saying 'no' must mean 'no', but reserve it for the things that you really don't want your child to do, for example, for reasons of health and safety.

There are different ways of achieving the results you wish to see, and the important step is to make a firm decision about what is to be done and to then give it a fair trial with the support of the rest of the family as well as perhaps the health visitor and doctor too. It is important to be thoroughly consistent at all times, not to over-react when things do not go to plan and to explain to the child fully what is expected of him. It is best to be positive at all times and to praise good behaviour rather than to punish naughty behaviour. Occasional rewards can be helpful in encouraging compliance, but on the other hand you do not want to negotiate over every little thing. A tempting 'I'll give you a special treat if you do this' policy is not always such a good idea, simply because if the child refuses to cooperate he will not get what you have promised and this can lead to further tantrums and yet more bad behaviour. It is far better and much less risky to reward the child once he has achieved what you want.

WHAT CAN THE DOCTOR DO?

The doctor and health visitor have a great deal of experience in dealing with common behavioural problems in children. They may listen to the problems which the parents have experienced and supply specific recommendations designed to improve the situation. They can also exclude any underlying medical disorder which could be contributing such as glue ear with partial deafness or delayed coordination skills, with all the associated frustration and anger. The GP is also very well placed to assess any psychological disturbance in the child as a result of parental or domestic disharmony, school phobia or sibling rivalry. In severe cases of behavioural difficulties, psychological counselling in child and family guidance clinics for suitable cases can be arranged, sometimes with very good long-term results.

IF YOU REMEMBER NOTHING ELSE, REMEMBER THESE THREE THINGS

1   Behavioural problems in children are common and usually short lived.

2   A regular daily routine and consistent management imposed at a young age may prevent the development of many behavioural difficulties.

3   Psychological help in family guidance clinics is extremely useful in appropriate cases.

Birthmarks

Although birthmarks are common, the majority of them tend to disappear, without medical intervention, within the first few years of life. This usually comes as a huge relief to concerned parents whose child has a large, noticeable birthmark on his face, for example.

Strawberry Birthmarks

Otherwise known as a strawberry naevus, these birthmarks can appear anywhere on the body, often on the top of the head or face. They are bright red, lumpy and soft to the touch. They start to appear within a few days of the infant's birth and gradually enlarge over the next few months. They are particularly common in premature babies. They are caused by a bundle of abnormal

COMMON BIRTHMARKS

* Strawberry birthmarks

* Stork marks

* Port wine stain

* Moles and freckles

* Café au lait patches

* Mongolian blue spot

blood vessels which have enlarged in response to oestrogen, the female sex hormone, which is passed to the baby before delivery from the mother. Unfortunately, the blood vessels remain swollen and full of blood for some considerable time. But however large they are, the good news is that the vast majority clear up completely leaving no residual mark or scar. As time goes on, the birthmark becomes paler and flatter, and it is the small, dimpled, white spots on the surface of the birthmark which give it its strawberry appearance. It is extremely rare for a strawberry naevus to be still present by the age of six and it usually shows signs of getting smaller.

Stork marks

Stork marks are perhaps the commonest birthmarks seen, being particularly common on the back of the neck at the hairline and between the eyebrows. They are flat, pink areas which become redder when the baby wriggles or cries. Again, they are a collection of abnormal blood vessels which are present at birth but these fade more quickly than strawberry birthmarks, disappearing almost invariably within two years.

Port Wine Stain

In this condition the skin looks as though a deep red wine has been spilled upon its surface. The birthmark is purple in colour and is flush with the surface of the skin. Again, abnormal blood vessels are responsible but in this case the condition is permanent. Nowadays, treatment with lasers can be carried out with extremely good cosmetic results even as soon as in the first year of life.

Moles and Freckles

Freckles and moles start to appear at the age of about two, and go on appearing until adulthood by which time most people can boast a total of about two hundred or so on the surface of their skin. They are collections within the skin of the pigment melanin and are generally harmless. Moles, however, are capable of undergoing malignant change, particularly when exposed to strong ultraviolet light for prolonged periods. Some specialists believe that short periods of excessive exposure to sunlight, on holidays for instance, can be just as damaging. Any change in a mole or freckle should be instantly reported to the doctor.

Café au Lait Patches

These are light brown patches of discoloration on the skin which resemble huge, flat freckles. Many children have one or two, which is perfectly acceptable, but more than five can sometimes be associated with certain uncommon conditions of the nervous system such as neurofibromatosis. This is a condition where thickenings and lumps form on the surfaces of nerves and may or may not require medical intervention.

Mongolian Blue Spot

These grey-blue patches are generally seen on the buttocks of black or Asian babies. Although curious they are likely to disappear by the age of four or five and have no other medical significance. When they are first spotted they may be mistaken for bruises.

WHAT CAN YOU DO?

Although sometimes difficult, the main job of the parents is to remain patient until the more noticeable and brightly coloured birthmarks have cleared up on their own. Every parent expects a beautiful baby with totally unblemished skin, so they can suffer huge anxiety and disappointment when everyone's attention is drawn to a disfiguring bright red lump around the baby's mouth or eyes. But the baby is not even aware of it, so just loving him for what he is, in the full knowledge that the birthmark will clear up by itself and leave no scar or mark, is vitally important. In the meantime, for parents who are particularly concerned, the Red Cross offers a cosmetic skin camouflage service where the birthmark can be made to look as inconspicuous as possible. Skin camouflage cream can also disguise even the most obvious permanent birthmarks such as port wine stains.

Parents should watch any large moles or freckles which a child has and be ready to report any change to the doctor. If a mole is larger than the blunt end of a pencil, for example, if it changes in depth of colour, itches or bleeds, it could theoretically represent a sign of malignant change and needs to be examined and treated.

WHAT CAN THE DOCTOR DO?

In addition to reassuring concerned parents about the cosmetic outlook with regard to their child's birthmark, the doctor can advise about the Red Cross camouflage service and invite parents to consider laser treatment for older children with port wine stains. Laser treatment can target extremely accurately the dilated blood vessels under the surface of the skin, burning and scarring them to the extent that they shrink away to nothing whilst the overlying skin remains intact and unaffected. A number of treatments are required over a period of time, and the larger the birthmark, the more treatments are needed. The child should be reassured that such therapy is not painful, although a slight tingling sensation is often experienced.

IF YOU REMEMBER NOTHING ELSE, REMEMBER THESE THREE THINGS

1   Birthmarks are common and most disappear within the first few years of life.

2   The Red Cross offers an excellent skin camouflage service.

3   Laser treatment can now vastly improve the appearance of port wine stains.

Bow Legs

Many parents become quite concerned at the extent of their child's bow legs, but this shape is perfectly normal in toddlers aged between one and three. All babies are born this way and the bowing remains obvious as they take their first steps at the age of about one and start breaking into a trot at the age of about two. Some children with bow legs also have toes which point inwards, causing them to trip over their own feet as they run. This is usually the result of a certain degree of natural twisting of the bone in the lower leg, the tibia. In most cases it requires no treatment, as the legs correct themselves as the child grows older so that the toes point in a straight line. The only exception to this rule is the condition known as rickets, which is due to a lack of vitamin D and sunlight. Rickets can soften the bones to such an extent that bowing takes place, but thankfully it is now rare in this country. Unusual injuries or infections may also cause bowing but usually only in one leg and in most cases the underlying cause is obvious.

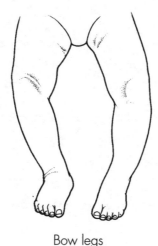

Bow legs

WHAT CAN YOU DO?

You only need to seek specialist help if:

* the bow legs persist after the age of three;

* there is severe toeing-in (see page 248);

* the bowing affects one leg only.

WHAT CAN THE DOCTOR DO?

A doctor only needs to be consulted if bow legs persist after the age of three. X-rays are usually sufficient to uncover any underlying abnormality and if one does exist surgery will usually be able to correct it.

IF YOU REMEMBER NOTHING ELSE, REMEMBER THESE THREE THINGS

1   Bow legs are normal in children aged one to three

2   The condition is self-correcting and usually requires no treatment

3   You only need to seek specialist help if the specific conditions mentioned previously exist.

Breath-holding Attacks

Breath-holding attacks are seen in about one to two per cent of toddlers and can be extremely alarming. They are most common between the ages of about eighteen months and two years, and tend to affect children with fairly wilful personalities; children, in other words, who like to get their own way. Through anger, frustration or pain the child first begins to cry or scream. He may then work himself up into such a state that when all the air has gone from his lungs he continues to hold his breath, going first red in the face and then blue. At this point normal breathing usually starts again quite naturally, though occasionally a brief episode of fainting or twitching resembling a convulsion can occur as the brain is briefly starved of enough oxygen. Thankfully, these episodes are quite harmless.

Breath-holding attacks are a form of infantile rage and, just like temper tantrums in an older child (see pagess 384–386), it is a mistake to pay too much attention to them. It is obviously important to make sure there is no serious underlying cause such as a true convulsion or fainting for other reasons, but once the correct diagnosis has been reached, ignoring the attacks and avoiding an escalation of the events that precede them as much as possible is the best solution. The more attention the child receives the more likely the attacks are to happen again.

WHAT CAN YOU DO?

The best approach to take is to be firm and consistent. There is no point in showing anger or frustration as the child will only interpret this as a form of parental attention. Be understanding and strong, but try not to let the child think you are impressed by his behaviour. Remember that by the age of four, breath-holding attacks almost always stop.

WHAT CAN THE DOCTOR DO?

The doctor needs to reassure worried parents about the nature of breath-holding attacks and to confirm that they are best ignored as much as possible. The most important job of the doctor, however, is to be absolutely confident that he or she has made the correct diagnosis. Where the child loses consciousness, as children very occasionally do, it is important to exclude any form of epilepsy or abnormal heart rhythm which, though rare, might be responsible. Once these conditions have been excluded, advising parents on how to manage the attacks is all that is necessary.

IF YOU REMEMBER NOTHING ELSE,
REMEMBER THESE THREE THINGS

1   Breath-holding attacks are commonest between eighteen months and two years of age.

2   Although disturbing for the parents, they are essentially harmless.

3   Firm and consistent handling by the parents is all that is required.

Bruising

Children are naturally clumsy and tend to fall over a lot, particularly when they first learn to walk or run. Consequently, small, almost imperceptible bruises are often seen on their bodies. Usually they are in areas which tend to be knocked regularly like the forehead, the elbows, knees and shins and usually there are no more than two at a time. Bruises are generally purply-blue in colour, darker in black-skinned people and more obvious in children with fair skin. They result from the escape of blood from blood vessels in or underneath the skin, and usually change to a yellow colour before finally fading altogether after ten to fourteen days.

Provided there is an obvious reason for the bruise, there is generally no need to worry although often the actual incident that resulted in the bruise may not have been witnessed by the parent. Bruising in unusual places such as under the arms, on the buttocks or on the insides of the thighs is unusual and should be investigated further especially since it also raises the possibility of physical abuse. More importantly, if there is no apparent reason whatsoever for bruising, and if bruising is regular or widespread, urgent investigation of the cause is required. In this instance a disorder of the blood vessels themselves, of the components of the blood or of the clotting factors within it, could be responsible. This type of bruising may very occasionally be the first sign of a serious blood condition such as leukaemia, so the doctor should be contacted without delay.

WHAT CAN YOU DO?

In most instances of normal bruising, simple reassurance and the immediate application of a cold compress to restrict further bleeding is all that is required. If the bruising appears to enlarge despite these measures, or if the bruising is widespread and has occurred for no obvious reason, a doctor should be consulted immediately.

IF YOU REMEMBER NOTHING ELSE, REMEMBER THESE THREE THINGS

1   Bruising is commonly seen after mild to moderate knocks.

2   Bruising in unusual or unlikely places on a child's body requires thorough examination.

3   Bruises which are widespread or unexplained need urgent blood tests to rule out serious blood disorders.

WHAT CAN THE DOCTOR DO?

The doctor is used to seeing children with normal, scattered bruises and will quickly recognise a situation where bruises are abnormally large, are in unusual locations or are multiple. In these instances a blood test to measure the cellular components of the blood and the quantity of blood clotting factors present is urgent and essential. Treatment will depend on the underlying cause.

Clumsiness

All small children are a little clumsy because their nervous system is struggling to keep pace with the development of their muscles and bones. But about ten per cent of children seem unusually clumsy. Boys are more often affected than girls for some reason, and the awkwardness is noticeable in a variety of ways. Parents may find that when their child begins to feed himself, he makes an especially unholy mess. When learning to dress himself, he may progress incredibly slowly, struggling particularly with buttons, zips or laces. He may fall more often than the average child so that he almost always has bruises on his arms and legs, and lumps and bumps on his head. He may be generally awkward with his hands and unable to perform tasks requiring fine dexterity such as building a tower of bricks (*at age three*) or pushing a peg into a peg board. The teacher at his school or nursery may notice that the child's writing is messy and untidy (*at age five to six*), that he is in the habit of breaking objects accidentally and that in physical activities he misjudges distances and has trouble catching (*at age five*) or throwing (*at age three*) a ball.

A large number of clumsy children find it difficult to distinguish their right from their left and more often than not they are often overactive, impulsive and have poor concentration spans. Many of these children start walking quite late (*eighteen months or more*) and when they do they take much longer than usual to become steady and confident.

Some children with poor coordination ability will have inherited this tendency from their parents. Often, if the parents of a clumsy child ask their own parents what they were like as children, they will be told that they were equally as clumsy or even more so. For some reason, the maturation of physical skills is delayed in these children, although in general they tend to catch up as they get older. In children without such a family history, there may be emotional reasons for the problem. If they are unhappy, distressed or worried about anything their concentration will be easily diverted, allowing frequent mishaps to occur.

Occasionally, a child may exhibit symptoms of clumsiness after an injury or an accident. If he is conscious of discomfort or pain in any area of the body, again this will act as a distraction and inhibit normal function. Children with head injuries are particularly prone to this, though any disorder within the skull such as a cerebral tumour, which may produce unsteadiness and clumsiness with more serious implications, is extremely rare.

Babies who are born small apparently tend to be more clumsy than normal birth weight babies, and there is growing evidence that minimal brain damage, perhaps due to influences within the womb or at birth, play an important role in this problem. There is no doubt, for example, that children with minimal cerebral palsy exhibit all of the symptoms associated with clumsiness described above, and many have learning or reading difficulties as well. In fact, in the USA all clumsy children are referred to as having 'minimal cerebral palsy'.

WHAT CAN YOU DO?

It is important to realise that a clumsy child will be more prone to behavioural problems as a direct result of his clumsiness. If the symptoms are frustrating for his parents and teachers, they are many times more frustrating for the child. Any child who is not good at doing something will tend to avoid that particular activity or throw a tantrum when he attempts it unsuccessfully – it is no fun always to be the last chosen for the team because of your ability to score own goals.

It is easy for parents, teachers, and doctors too for that matter, to regard clumsy children as 'normal but naughty', however there is now much evidence to suggest that such children are, in fact, not entirely normal due to subtle neurological deficits. These children need special consideration and encouragement. They need to practise tasks involving fine manual dexterity with somebody possessing ample understanding and patience. Clumsy children become much worse if they are scolded or reprimanded, and it is because they are ridiculed by other children and sometimes teachers, at school that they tend to play up in the classroom, become disruptive or play truant. Socially they may become unduly shy and some are prone to the development of stuttering or bedwetting. They may find ways of hiding their disability, one of which is by 'playing the fool' to attract positive rather than negative attention from other children.

It is difficult sometimes, especially for parents of a clumsy first-born, to know quite what is normal and what is not. For this reason, and because neurological disorder can certainly play a part in causing some of these children's problems, a consultation with the doctor is important.

WHAT CAN THE DOCTOR DO?

The doctor needs to listen carefully to what the parents have to say about their child's development and why they think clumsiness is a problem. At first glance the child may look perfectly well and healthy and sometimes he may even have a particularly high IQ. Some form of assessment needs to be carried out, and to begin with simple, fine tasks such as putting a peg into a peg board, building a tower of bricks or completing a simple jigsaw puzzle or drawing can be attempted in the doctor's surgery. Standing on one foot is another useful test – most children at the age of four can stand steadily on one foot, whereas a clumsy child may remain unsteady in this position up until the age of seven. More detailed assessment can be carried out at the child development centre – most district hospitals have one – where a paediatrician, occupational therapist and educational psychologist may make a joint assessment.

In the vast majority of cases, no serious underlying problem will be found, and many of these apparently normal children fit into the category of 'minimal brain damage clumsiness'. It is important for parents to understand that such children tend to catch up in terms of their motor development as the years go by, and if this condition is recognised it often makes life at school easier for the child. A good teacher can boost a clumsy child's self-esteem by reminding him, and the rest of the class, of the things he does well and easily.

With regards treatment, physiotherapy can certainly help in instances where unsteadiness is particularly poor, and there is much interest in the developing field of paediatric osteopathy, or cranial osteopathy as it is sometimes known, which is a branch of complementary medicine based on the hypothesis that nine out of every ten babies are born with some kind of birth trauma which can be treated by a physical, manipulative approach. Within conventional medical circles, however, it remains highly controversial, most doctors believing that it simply doesn't work.

IF YOU REMEMBER NOTHING ELSE, REMEMBER THESE THREE THINGS

1   About one child in ten is abnormally clumsy.

2   Understanding and patience are needed as these children become worse if scolded, ridiculed or reprimanded.

3   When medical assessment excludes physical disease, occupational therapy may help in assessing the extent of the problem and finding practical ways of alleviating it, such as practising fine manual tasks.

Constipation

People mean different things when they use the word 'constipation'. Some people say they are constipated when they cannot go when they want to. Some people believe it means the passing of small, solid, pebble-like motions. Others simply regard it as the infrequent passage of motions, sometimes as seldom as once a week. But the truth is it is as normal for somebody to pass a motion once a week as it is for another to do so twice a day. The only important consideration is whether there is also any pain or discomfort. So if a child's usual bowel habit of, say, going to the toilet every second day to pass a soft stool, suddenly changes to passing small, hard stools every fourth day, and this is accompanied by abdominal pain and discomfort in the bottom area, then it is safe to say that the child is constipated.

There are one or two other symptoms sometimes associated with constipation, namely the presence of blood and the leakage of a watery, brown fluid known as soiling. Motions as hard as rocks can lodge against the sensitive wall of the last part of the intestine and rectum, producing a small tear with bleeding when the motion is passed. The blood tends to be fresh, red blood and is seen on

CAUSES OF CONSTIPATION

* Diet

* Genetic factors

* Constitutional problems

* Faulty potty training

* Anal fissure

the outside of the motion. Much darker blood mixed together with the motion is indicative of bleeding from much higher up the intestine. The tear itself is known as an anal fissure and the pain which results from this can easily discourage a small child from going to the toilet, leading to further constipation. Consequently a troublesome vicious circle is set up. Soiling occurs when hard stools obstruct the intestine, producing a leak of watery fluid around it over which the child has no control.

Diet

In the vast majority of cases, the cause of constipation is dietary, and the age of the child is highly relevant.

An infant who is fully breast-fed will often only pass a motion every three to five days, although the stools passed will still be soft or semi-fluid. An infant fed with infant formula milk, on the other hand, may become constipated as a result of not being given adequate amounts of fluid or milk feeds generally. Infants fed too soon on undiluted cow's milk may also become constipated as a result of the unbalanced dietary components of the milk.

Older children rapidly develop an unhealthy taste for high carbohydrate, sugary foods and drinks which are low in fibre, a habit which many parents allow to happen as it is often the easiest option. Unfortunately, sufficient amounts of fibre are essential in a child's diet. Chronic constipation in a child fed a poor, unhealthy diet can lead not only to the symptoms described above, but also to a lazy, distended bowel which may never recover, resulting in many years of unnecessary laxative abuse.

Many of the naturally occurring sources of fibre, for example fresh fruit and vegetables, brown rice, wholegrain bread and cereals, are extremely healthy and should form an important part of a child's diet. If these foodstuffs are introduced to a toddler at an early age so that he becomes accustomed to their flavour and texture, an essential, healthy dietary habit is established for life. An adequate fluid intake is also important. One of the functions of the large bowel is, in fact, the reabsorption of water from the bowel. When a child becomes slightly dehydrated, for example after exercise, when wearing too many clothes during hot weather or in association with a fever or vomiting, the body will naturally hang on to any source of water possible, and that includes water contained within the intestine. So the adequate replacement of water lost from the body through perspiration or any of the above causes is essential.

Genetic Factors

There is almost certainly variation between people in how much water is reabsorbed from the stools by the gut and in the motility of the large intestine. The automatic, rhythmic squeezing action of the muscular wall of the intestine continually pushes the motions along until they are excreted – a process known as peristalsis. Its level of activity and efficiency in a child is likely to follow a similar pattern to that of his parents, so if mum or dad has always had a tendency to constipation, their child is likely to develop it too.

There is one well-known but rare condition called Hirschprung's disease, in which a short section of bowel is apparently devoid of the usual nerves which generate peristalsis. Chronic constipation and bloating result and surgery is required to remove the offending portion of intestine.

Constitutional Problems

If the intake of liquid or food is inadequate, or if excessive fluid is lost from the body, due, for example, to a hot climate, wearing too many clothes, a high temperature or vomiting and diarrhoea, a child may easily become constipated. Fluid replacement is, of course, the answer.

Faulty Potty Training

There is no doubt that over-enthusiastic, incorrect or ill-timed potty training can be a cause of constipation in children. It is essential to wait until the child is ready, since attempts to potty train too early will be regarded by the toddler as a highly unpleasant experience and something to be avoided at all costs. The potty should never be allowed to represent some form of punishment or trial, as punishment will merely serve to inhibit the reflex to pass motions. Also, the older the toddler becomes, the more he will realise how much attention and power he can wield over his parents by not cooperating. This is a battle well worth avoiding. If in doubt, ask your health visitor or doctor for advice.

Anal Fissure

This is a tear in the sensitive lining of the rectum, usually as a result of passing very hard, dry motions. It is very uncomfortable for a child and leads to tight spasm of the muscular ring around the anus which, together with the pain, will strongly discourage the child from passing any further motions. The fissure will heal providing the constipation is treated, although occasionally an anaesthetic and lubricating ointment or suppository may need to be used.

WHAT CAN YOU DO?

In babies and infants who are constipated, it is important to increase their fluid intake and a little freshly squeezed orange juice or brown sugar in water can be very effective. Once weaned, small children will respond well to some mashed-up stewed prunes or other high fibre fruit.

Constipation is common in children over eighteen months and is often associated with poor eating habits. It may be easily prevented or remedied by improving the child's eating pattern and including each day:

* Foods from each of the food groups: milk, cheese and yoghurt; cereals, bread and rice; meat and fish; fruit and vegetables; butter and polyunsaturated margarine or oils.

* High-fibre foods which provide bulk in the bowel and help stimulate a bowel action.

* Sufficient fluids to help soften the faeces.

* Regular exercise such as walking, running, outside games or sport to stimulate the muscles of the bowel.

* A regular time to go to the toilet to encourage emptying of the bowel, for example just after breakfast, after main meals, or after a warm bath in the evening.

The following are fibre-containing foods and need to be provided in your child's usual diet. If your child is not used to having these foods, you may need to introduce them gradually as snacks in place of sweets, sweet biscuits, cakes and soft drinks. Remember that high-fibre foods are good for all members of the family.

* Fresh vegetables with the skins left on where possible, for example jacket potatoes.

* Dried fruit such as sultanas, apricots or prunes.

* Fresh fruit with skins left on where possible.

* High-fibre cereals such as Shreddies, Weetabix, All-bran, porridge or muesli.

* Wholegrain bread and biscuits.

* Wholemeal flour in home cooking.

* Brown rice and wholemeal pasta.

* Whole nuts for children over four years, or crunchy peanut butter is a good alternative for all children.

Each day your child needs to drink several glasses of fluid, which should include; plain water, unsweetened fruit juice and milk. *Eating the right foods, drinking sufficient fluids, regular exercise and regular toileting will help remedy and prevent constipation.*

Although constipation is a frequent source of abdominal gripes and pains, you should not assume it is necessarily the cause. The colicky, aching pain of constipation tends to come and go. The child usually points to the bellybutton, but is not unduly distressed. A child with appendicitis, on the other hand, may start with a mild pain around the bellybutton area, but it soon becomes much more severe and moves towards the lower, right-hand side of the abdomen and produces a temperature and vomiting. If your child is constipated, therefore, be on the look out for these additional symptoms and consult the doctor if necessary.

If you feel over-zealous potty training may be the root of the problem, take advice from your health visitor as to how to restructure this. Similarly, a child of school age may hate using cold, unclean school toilets, but have too little time at home in the morning to empty his bowels. If the call of nature is ignored repeatedly, a distended, lazy bowel and chronic constipation can ensue. Getting up a little earlier in the mornings to avoid having to rush, having a high-fibre breakfast and regular exercise throughout the day will all help to overcome the problem.

On the whole, laxatives should be avoided except in established constipation, and in particular their regular use in children without the supervision of a doctor is inexcusable.

WHAT CAN THE DOCTOR DO?

When pain or discomfort is the problem, the doctor will want to exclude other causes such as appendicitis, wind or anal fissure. The doctor will want to know what sort of a diet the child has, and whether any blood has been passed in the motions. An examination, often using his or her little finger whilst wearing a surgical glove, will confirm constipation and suggest the remedy. Treatment usually consists of dietary adjustment, but in the case of temporary constipation which has been brought about by a sudden change in the child's general health, a gentle laxative in the form of a soap-like glycerine suppository or a specially formulated oral preparation usually does the trick.

IF YOU REMEMBER NOTHING ELSE,
REMEMBER THESE THREE THINGS

1 Constipation has more to do with pain and discomfort than how often a child passes a motion.

2 Over-enthusiastic or premature potty training can often trigger the problem.

3 Dietary adjustment is the most important part of the treatment.

Coughing

Coughing is a reflex action designed to clear the breathing passages of phlegm, smoke, dust, particles, gases, foreign objects and other inhaled irritants. A cough is described as 'productive' if mucus or phlegm is brought up, and 'unproductive' or dry if it is not.

Children who cough may do so repeatedly and persistently and yet seem totally oblivious to it. At other times a cough can be part of a more serious problem when it may be accompanied by a fever, loss of appetite and breathlessness.

CAUSES OF COUGHS

* Infection

* Asthma and allergy

* Inhaled foreign body

* Attention-seeking

COUGHING DUE TO INFECTION

By far the commonest reason for a child coughing is a simple cold, or a viral upper respiratory tract infection. A number of different germs may attack the respiratory system, and the symptoms will depend entirely on which part of the system is affected.

The common cold tends to produce symptoms restricted to the nose, throat, tonsils and adenoids. Other viruses attack further down as well, affecting in descending order the larynx (laryngitis and croup), the epiglottis (epiglottitis), the trachea (tracheitis), the bronchi (bronchitis), the bronchioles (bronchiolitis) or the lung tissue itself (pneumonia). All of these conditions produce a cough of varying intensity and severity. The further down the respiratory airways the infection takes place, the more serious the condition tends to become.

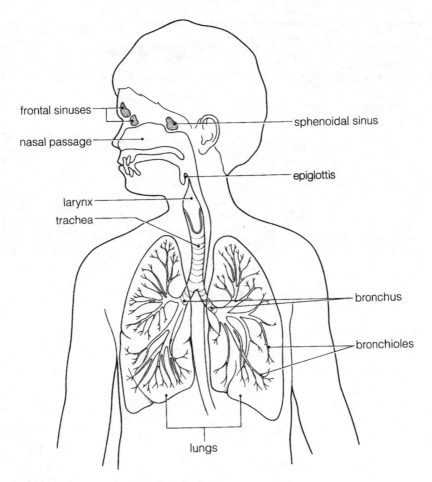

frontal sinuses

sphenoidal sinus

nasal passage

epiglottis

larynx

trachea

bronchus

bronchioles

lungs

Cross-section of the respiratory system

Colds

With a simple cold there is irritation at the back of the nose and throat with enlargement of the adenoids, tonsils and other glands. There is also irritation as a result of the trickle of mucus from the nasal cavity downwards towards the larynx. These two sources of irritation trigger the sensitive cough reflex which is designed to clear the windpipe of any obstruction or unwanted substance.

Coughing not only reduces the number of germs moving downwards towards the lungs but it also gets rid of the infected mucus which has already 'wrapped up' the invading micro-organisms in

CAUSES OF INFECTIVE COUGHS

* Colds

* Croup

* Epiglottitis

* Laryngitis

* Tracheitis

* Bronchitis

* Bronchiolitis

* Pneumonia

* Measles

* Whooping cough

order to prevent them spreading further. Many doctors believe that cough-suppressant medicines should not be prescribed for children because they do away with these protective functions of the cough reflex. However, if the incessant coughing brought about by the perpetual dripping of mucus at the back of the child's throat produces loss of sleep or breathing or speech difficulties, then symptomatic relief in the form of nasal decongestants and antihistamines are worth considering.

Croup

A child with a croupy cough sounds like a performing seal barking for fish. It is a sound which is very characteristic and unmistakable. So much so, that doctors are sometimes able to diagnose it over the phone. It is caused by a virus infection of the larynx or voice-box at the opening to the windpipe. In addition to the barking cough, there is a harsh, rasping sound when the child breathes in again afterwards, which suggests partial obstruction of the airway. Often there will also be the associated symptoms of a cold with a temperature and sore throat, but usually the infection does not last more than two or three days. Sometimes croup is difficult to distinguish from epiglottitis (see below), and both conditions may require urgent resuscitation in hospital.

Epiglottitis

The epiglottis is a flap of tissue which acts as a valve separating the windpipe from the gullet. This stops food going down the wrong way, as well as air going down into the stomach. When the epiglottis becomes inflamed, there will again be a croupy type of cough, but in addition the child may be generally unwell and requires urgent medical attention. With epiglottitis, which is caused by a bacteria called *Haemophilus influenzae*, there is a much more worrying 'gasping for breath', producing a strangulated noise, when breathing in. This is an alarming sound and warrants the urgent attention of a doctor.

Sometimes croup and epiglottitis are difficult to distinguish, so if in doubt ask your doctor's opinion straightaway. In any event, both conditions may require urgent resuscitation techniques in hospital. These include intubation, in which a flexible rubber tube is inserted into the windpipe to facilitate breathing until the child recovers. Signs that a child might need hospital admission include blueness of the lips and tongue, sucking in of the ribs and windpipe when breathing and general exhaustion.

Laryngitis, Tracheitis and Bronchitis

These affect the larger tubes of the air passages. They normally begin with the production of large amounts of phlegm following on from a simple cold. The child's temperature is often raised, he breathes more rapidly than normal (usually more than 40 breaths per minute) and does not want to eat. The cough may produce nausea or even vomiting, and sometimes a distinct wheeze can be heard. In severe cases there may be breathing difficulties or blueness around the lips and mouth. These latter symptoms suggest that the doctor is required urgently.

Bronchiolitis

The bronchioles are the smallest airways at the end of the bronchial tree, and this is where bronchiolitis strikes. It affects children under the age of one year, and occurs as epidemics during the winter along with the usual increase in colds and coughs. Symptoms start with those of the common cold, but the child's temperature will be raised and he will be struggling for breath, sometimes at a rate of more than 60 breaths per minute. Small children and infants with bronchiolitis must be observed carefully and are therefore usually admitted to hospital.

Pneumonia

Pneumonia is an infection of the lung tissue itself, and is more common in schoolchildren between the ages of four to twelve. The infection may begin with all the symptoms of a common cold, but usually it arises without any warning whatsoever. The child will have a high temperature, may feel nauseous or even be vomiting, and may complain of pain in the chest. The child will be generally ill, his breathing will be much faster and shallower than normal, and there may be added noises like wheezing, rattling or a little grunt at the end of each breath.

Bronchopneumonia is a similar type of infection which affects most of both lungs as opposed to one small portion of a lung. It is rare in childhood, and it used to occur after whooping cough or measles, both of which are now extremely uncommon due to the immunisation programme. The symptoms are rapid breathing, a dry cough and general floppiness and drowsiness.

Whooping Cough

Whooping cough merits special attention because it is such a dangerous childhood disease. It starts an ordinary cold and cough, but over a period of about a fortnight it often becomes much more persistent and severe, with spasms of coughing lasting for several minutes at a time. Between coughing bouts the child gasps in an attempt to breath air into his lungs again, but the swollen and clogged passageways interfere with the intake of breath producing the characteristic 'whoop' sound at the end of a prolonged spasm of coughing. The child may vomit and lie exhausted after coughing.

Whooping cough is a highly infectious disease, and is most dangerous when caught in the first year of life. Vaccination is mandatory for all children unless there is a specific reason for not having it, such as a previous severe reaction. Despite vaccination, however, some children still remain susceptible, though the disease is likely to be much milder than if vaccination had not been performed.

The cause of the infection is a bacterium known as *Bordetella pertussis* hence the medical name for this condition, pertussis. The spasms of coughing interspersed with whooping, and the vomiting that occurs following the unrelenting spells of coughing, are exhausting and alarming, not only for the child but for the parents as well. This phase of whooping cough may persist for as long as two to three months, by which time the entire family will have had enough.

Complications of whooping cough include haemorrhage as a result of blood vessels popping during coughing episodes, dehydration due to the child being unable to eat or drink, and ear infections associated with the original infection. In addition, infections of the lungs in the form of bronchopneumonia and bronchiolitis can occur, and convulsions are not unknown.

Any cough which is worse at night and which regularly makes the child sick should be considered as whooping cough until a doctor proves otherwise. Unfortunately, there is no specific treatment once the 'whoop' has developed, although the antibiotic erythromycin will reduce the likelihood of the infection spreading to others.

WHAT CAN YOU DO?

Coughs which are produced as a result of infection are often accompanied by a fever, so it is well worth taking the child's temperature regularly. The cough itself is often triggered by mucus dripping down from the nose and sinuses, or from the glands lining the respiratory passages themselves. This may be reduced by using children's formulations of nasal decongestants if the nose is congested or particularly runny, and expectorant cough linctus in an attempt to encourage loosening and expectoration of the mucus.

Cough suppressants should not be used if the cough is productive since mucus can then collect without being coughed up and spread further down into the lungs. Any kind of exertion should be avoided, and at night the child should be lying either propped up on several pillows or flat on his stomach or side, whichever is the most comfortable. The room in which the child is nursed should be warm and humid, and people should obviously avoid smoking in the vicinity. Sometimes, helping your child to bring up phlegm is useful, and this can be done by lying the child over your lap, head downwards, so you can gently pummel the back of his chest to loosen the mucus. Soothing drinks also help.

A worsening cough should be reported to the doctor, especially if the sound of the cough is suggestive of whooping cough. Croup may respond to steam inhalations, but for a young child this is best achieved by continuously boiling a kettle in the room to create a very humid, warm atmosphere for the child to breathe in. A small infant with bronchiolitis often needs to be admitted to hospital for observation and possible oxygen therapy, but it is usually possible to stay overnight with your baby in most paediatric wards. It is also worth keeping other children well away from the affected child in hospital in order to prevent further spread of the infection. Also, older siblings and adults may be asymptomatic carriers and pass the illness on to other children on the ward.

If the child has already been poorly for two to three months it is better to nurse him at home if possible. Because both the parents' and the child's nights will be disturbed, it is well worth a parent sharing a bedroom with the child, and offering small drinks and little snacks in-between the bouts of coughing or vomiting in order to keep the child's strength up and to prevent dehydration.

WHAT CAN THE DOCTOR DO?

Doctors are often asked to see a child with a cough if it has been persisting for several days, if fever is high and has not abated, or if the child shows general signs of ill-health. The doctor will examine the ears, nose and throat, and will listen to the chest to determine whether the infection has spread downwards into the respiratory passages and lungs. Symptomatic relief may be prescribed in the form of paediatric decongestant nose-drops, anti-histamines or cough expectorants. Antibiotics are usually prescribed if bacterial infection is suspected.

For whooping cough the doctor may take a per nasal swab (a swab on a wire is pushed down one nostril to the back of the throat) to confirm the diagnosis. Sedation has not been shown to be effective in the treatment of whooping cough, despite the obvious anxiety experienced by the child. Sedatives depress the ability to breathe, and this is certainly not required in this case.

A doctor faced with an infant with bronchiolitis may well admit the child to hospital as this is a potentially serious disease, and treatment includes oxygen therapy and antibiotics. In croup, the doctor may keep the child at home, but if he or she suspects epiglottitis, the child will be admitted to hospital for observation and urgent treatment. Antibiotics and intubation to maintain the airway may be necessary.

IF YOU REMEMBER NOTHING ELSE,
REMEMBER THESE THREE THINGS

1 Infections producing a cough may affect any part of the respiratory system.

2 Any cough which becomes associated with breathing difficulties, blueness around the lips and tongue, vomiting or persistent exhaustion will require emergency treatment.

3 Treatment usually consists of symptomatic relief in mild cases, or antibiotics, oxygen therapy and hospital admission for more severe cases.

NON-INFECTIOUS CAUSES OF COUGHING

Asthma and Allergy

Many people still believe that asthma is just another word for wheezing. However, although wheezing is an important additional symptom in asthma, especially in adults, the commonest way that asthma begins in childhood is in fact through persistent coughing at night. Wheezing does not even have to be present. Where there has also been no previous cold or runny nose, and where the symptoms have been going on for more than two to three weeks, an infectious reason for the cough becomes less likely, and the diagnosis is more likely to be asthma. If, in addition, the cough is brought about by exercise and is accompanied by wheezing or

211

breathlessness, particularly first thing in the morning, asthma is the probable diagnosis. Asthma is covered in detail in the section on Wheezing (see pages 444–455).

IF YOU REMEMBER NOTHING ELSE, REMEMBER THESE THREE THINGS

1   A persistent, dry cough at night may be the first and only sign of asthma in a young child.

2   Effective treatment is available to prevent as well as relieve asthma, and any child with persistent asthma symptoms needs to have his medication reviewed.

3   Asthma should be no bar to the enjoyment of sport and other normal children's activities.

Inhaled Foreign Bodies

When a child suddenly develops a severe cough, it is worth thinking about the possibility that he may have inhaled a small object, particularly if he has never had asthma or any other condition predisposing him to a cough. Children are forever putting things into their mouths – the eyes from dolls, buttons and so on – and it only takes a moment when they are falling, rolling or running about for such objects to be inhaled and become lodged in one of the smaller branches of the respiratory passageways.

Peanuts and small sweets are the commonest culprits, so remember the age of the child when offering these. Sometimes the cough may subside, only for a temperature to develop along with a slightly different type of cough, this time suggestive of infection. Depending on the site and size of the foreign body, it is also quite possible that the child will have a wheeze rather than a straightforward cough.

WHAT CAN YOU DO?

The best thing to do is to try and avoid your child inhaling a small object in the first place by removing all such objects from his reach. If, however, your child suddenly starts coughing, particularly if you notice that he was recently playing with suspiciously small, hard objects or eating peanuts or small sweets, tell your doctor that an inhaled foreign body could be a possible cause.

IF YOU REMEMBER NOTHING ELSE, REMEMBER THESE THREE THINGS

1   Coughing due to inhaled foreign bodies comes on suddenly.

2   Peanuts and small sweets are the commonest culprits and should not be given to young children.

3   X-rays are sometimes needed to diagnose the presence of an inhaled foreign body.

WHAT CAN THE DOCTOR DO?

A physical examination of the chest may give clues as to what has happened, but a chest X-ray is a more accurate indicator. What the X-ray may show is a collapse of the part of the lung blocked off by the obstruction in the airway, and surrounding signs of infection. If a foreign body is found, it will be removed under general anaesthetic using a special flexible telescope passed through the nose or mouth called a bronchoscope. The infection is treated in the normal way with antibiotics.

Attention-Seeking Cough

Children aged two and over know when they are onto a good thing. They quickly learn that they can grab all their parents' attention by feigning some kind of ailment, and a troublesome, persistent cough is a particularly easy one to imitate. Very often it will start as a genuine infective cough, but then persists long after the infection has been completely eradicated. The parents naturally remain worried, however, and the child, sensing this anxiety, milks it for all it is worth. The cough may become a nervous kind of tic, and start to occur almost automatically.

This manipulative behaviour is usually subconscious and will stop when the child gets the attention he seeks. The solution is to provide that attention in a more appropriate and satisfactory way, and usually that means the parents spending a little extra time with the child on an exclusive one-to-one basis.

WHAT CAN YOU DO?

You first need to be sure that other causes of a persistent cough are not responsible. Some degree of attention-seeking frequently coexists with asthma, and treatment for this is often needed to break the vicious circle. Mild whooping cough or an inhaled foreign body can also not be overlooked. Ask yourself if there are any signs of your child being ill such as a raised temperature, shortness of breath or wheezing. If not, is he running around and eating normally? Does he stop coughing when he is distracted by something more interesting? If the answer to both these questions is yes, then your child probably has an attention-seeking cough. In most cases, the attention-seeking cough will settle down as the child tires of the habit, but unfortunately the parents will often tire of it long before he does. If in doubt, ask your doctor to check him over.

WHAT CAN THE DOCTOR DO?

The doctor will want to exclude any physical cause for the cough. Keeping the child under review and seeing him again in about one month's time is a reasonable precaution, but on the whole reassurance is the key.

IF YOU REMEMBER NOTHING ELSE, REMEMBER THESE THREE THINGS

1   Most coughs are due to infection or to asthma.

2   Children will sometimes cough to gain extra attention from their parents.

3   Once diagnosed, an attention-seeking cough can usually be 'cured' by giving the child the attention he craves in a more positive way.

Diarrhoea

Diarrhoea is the frequent passage of very runny motions. It is important to be quite sure of what is meant by diarrhoea because many babies, especially breast-fed ones, pass several loose stools every day and some parents will mistake this for diarrhoea. Doctors restrict the term 'diarrhoea' to motions which are either liquid or semi-formed and which therefore take up the shape of any sample container they are collected in.

Usually, diarrhoea comes on suddenly and is short lived. If, however, in small infants it lasts for more than a few hours, especially where there is also vomiting and fever, there is a real risk of dehydration which, in this age group, may be very serious indeed. If diarrhoea persists and becomes a constant feature, if there is blood mixed with the motions or abdominal pain, the doctor should be consulted.

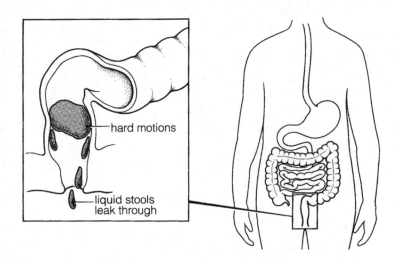

hard motions

liquid stools leak through

Diarrhoea/encopresis: showing how chronic constipation can lead to soiling

One of the most important questions to ask in cases of chronic diarrhoea is whether or not the child is putting on weight normally. Any persistent failure to gain weight or actual weight loss can be a sign of a significant underlying disorder and should be investigated. On the other hand, children will often lose or fail to put on weight during an acute illness, but they catch up again within a few days of their recovery.

CAUSES OF DIARRHOEA

* Gastroenteritis (tummy bug)

* Emotion and anxiety

* Encopresis (constipation overflow)

* Appendicitis

* Enterocolitis

* Intussusception

* Failure to absorb:
     Coeliac disease
     Cystic fibrosis
     Cow's milk protein intolerance
     Lactose intolerance

Gastroenteritis

The commonest of all causes of sudden-onset diarrhoea is infection of the intestine, otherwise known as gastroenteritis. Viral infections frequently produce diarrhoea, but often bacterial contamination of food or drink is responsible, in which case the gastroenteritis is known as food-poisoning.

The infection produces an inflammation of the lining of the bowel from which water is normally absorbed into the body, and as a result normal bowel function is interrupted. The intestinal contents are hurried through producing frequent, watery stools. When, in small babies, vomiting and fever also occur, this brings with it a serious risk of dehydration. So if the symptoms persist for more than several hours, a doctor should be consulted. Antibiotics are not recommended in most cases, as they will not eradicate the germs responsible for most cases of gastroenteritis, and they may in fact make the diarrhoea worse by killing off 'healthy' bacteria in the gut. Similarly drugs which are designed to 'dry up' diarrhoea merely prevent the natural process whereby infective organisms are excreted, thus allowing the micro-organisms to remain in the body for longer and protracting the course of the illness. Since the cause is almost invariably infective, it is very important to pay close attention to hygiene – the child should wash his hands frequently and, in babies and infants, whichever parent changes the nappy should do likewise. Failure to do so may result in the rest of the family coming down with the bug, although this may still happen despite your best efforts to avoid it.

Sometimes viral illnesses produce diarrhoea as well as infections of the ear (otitis media) and tonsillitis. There may be a tempera-ture, and the child often complains of pain in whichever part of the body is affected. Diarrhoea from this cause is usually short lived.

Emotion and Anxiety

Toddlers and schoolchildren may respond to fear and worry in the same way that adults do when they become nervous, for example about sitting an exam or running a race. Usually the cause of a child's anxiety is obvious and the resultant diarrhoea can therefore be explained easily.

Encopresis (constipation overflow)

Ironically, a child who has been constipated for a few days may soil his pants with motions resembling diarrhoea. The hard, pebble-like motions of constipation effectively block the child's intestine and as a result fluid leaks around the blockage and escapes to the outside. This is known as encopresis and occurs outside the child's control. So any expression of anger or impatience towards the child is inappropriate and counterproductive. Treatment consists of remedying the constipation rather than the soiling.

Appendicitis

The commonest symptoms of appendicitis are abdominal pain, loss of appetite and vomiting. Sometimes, however, especially if the inflammation within the appendix has spread to the lining of the abdomen which overlies it (peritonitis), or if the bowel itself has become inflamed, diarrhoea may occur. These particular symptoms are highly suggestive of appendicitis and the doctor should be called right away.

Enterocolitis (inflammatory bowel disease)

This condition is a form of inflammation of the intestine which is not due to infection. If the colon is predominantly affected, the condition is known as colitis, and if the small intestine is inflamed it is known as enteritis. When both parts of the intestine are involved the disorder is referred to as enterocolitis. It is thought to be due partly to a disorder of the immune system. For some reason, in children with enterocolitis, an autoimmune reaction in the gut occurs which suggests that some irritation or allergy from outside may be responsible. Since no specific causes have yet been identified, it may well be that the body produces antibodies in the gut to part of the intestine itself, almost as if the immune system recognised its own tissues as 'foreign' in some way. The diarrhoea in this case is often tinged with blood and there may also be weight loss and pain. Treatment is designed to reduce the inflammation and consists of dietary measures and special anti-inflammatory medicines. Sometimes, in severe cases, surgery is necessary.

Intussusception

In this uncommon condition the motions passed are quite characteristic, consisting of a combination of blood and mucus typically resembling redcurrant jelly. It generally follows symptoms of severe abdominal pain and vomiting and the failure to pass any stools at all.

The condition occurs when part of the child's intestine 'telescopes' into the next part. Why this happens is not fully understood although swelling of the tiny glands in the wall of the intestine may be partly responsible. Sometimes the condition corrects itself spontaneously but in more severe cases surgery is required to relieve the problem. It is seen most commonly at or around the age of weaning, although it can occur at any age.

Failure to Absorb

Coeliac disease

This condition may produce more frequent, pale, greasy motions which are not typical of normal diarrhoea. In coeliac disease there is a sensitivity to gluten in the diet, which is found in wheat and rye products. The symptoms begin when these are introduced to the diet as cereals at the age of about six months. Persistent diarrhoea and vomiting with failure to gain weight occurring at about six months are typical symptoms.

Cystic fibrosis

In cystic fibrosis, other siblings may be affected by the condition, and the failure to absorb food properly results in loss of weight, greasy motions and diarrhoea. This is because the pancreatic tubes get clogged up with secretions that are thicker than usual. The same thing happens in the lungs, producing a persistent cough with tenacious phlegm.

Cow's milk protein intolerance

Most infant formula milks come originally from cow's milk where the animal fat has been removed and replaced by vegetable fat. In casein-dominant baby milks (like Cow & Gate Premium, Wyeth's SMA Gold and Milupa's Aptamil) the protein in the cow's milk is also modified, whereas in whey-dominant milks (like Milupa's Milupril, Wyeth's SMA White and Cow & Gate Plus) it remains relatively unmodified.

A very few babies may develop an intolerance to the protein content of cow's milk (modified or not), in which case soya-based milks can be used instead. The symptom of diarrhoea caused by cow's milk protein intolerance begins soon after cow's milk is introduced to the baby's diet, clears up when it is discontinued and recurs if it is tried for a second time. This remains the best way of confirming this difficult and controversial diagnosis.

Lactose intolerance

Any temporary inflammation of the wall of the intestine from gastroenteritis upsets the normal process of digestion for a short period. As a result, certain enzymes (the molecules made by the body to help digest food) are not produced in sufficient quantities to break down particular substances in the diet, so diarrhoea occurs as a consequence. One of these substances is the sugar lactose found in milk, so it is well worth avoiding milk and other dairy products for a few days if diarrhoea persists after what appears to be an ordinary tummy bug.

WHAT CAN YOU DO?

Small babies are most at risk from diarrhoea as they can become dehydrated very quickly. This is especially so if vomiting and a fever coexist. Any baby who has had persistent diarrhoea for more than a few hours should be referred to a doctor. In older children, manageable diarrhoea where there is no distress or discomfort will usually settle down within a few days. But where there is blood or mucus in the motions, persistent weight loss or the motions are particularly fatty or greasy, there is a good case for urgent referral to the GP.

It is always worth taking the child's temperature to see if there is fever, and food and milky drinks should be avoided as these are likely to make the diarrhoea worse for a while. Instead, fluid intake should be maintained using special rehydrating fluids, though these should only be used for 24 hours as they contain little in the way of calories. The ideal fluid, known as Dioralyte, is a combination of salt and sugar and can be bought ready made in the right quantities at the chemist. The powder merely needs to be dissolved in the right amount of water. In bottle-fed babies, milk feeds should be temporarily discontinued and clear fluids given instead. Breast-fed babies may continue to breast-feed, though in fact gastroenteritis is very rare in breast-fed babies because of the protective effects of breast milk. As a child improves, gradually and gently reintroduce the components of their normal diet, in older children starting with bland foods such as porridge, rice and soups.

Clearly, most cases of diarrhoea are due to infections so it is imperative that stringent hygiene rules are followed. Always wash your hands after changing a nappy, and older children with diarrhoea should wash their hands thoroughly after using the toilet. Make sure that all food you prepare and handle remains uncontaminated, and remember that sterilising babies' feeding equipment is vitally important at all times.

WHAT CAN THE DOCTOR DO?

The first thing the doctor needs to do is assess the child for any serious underlying conditions, including dehydration. If he or she can ascertain the exact cause of the diarrhoea, so much the better, but this will require a thorough examination that includes looking at the ears, throat, chest and abdomen. The doctor may decide to send off a sample of the motions for investigation, especially if the diarrhoea has persisted for a few days and the type of organism responsible remains uncertain. He or she can advise on the amount of fluid the child should have over a 24-hour period according to his weight, and will keep an eye on the situation over the next few days. Very often the child will continue to suffer from sporadic diarrhoea for up to two weeks, so parents will need constant reassurance and the doctor will need to be satisfied that the normal pattern of the illness is being followed.

IF YOU REMEMBER NOTHING ELSE, REMEMBER THESE THREE THINGS

1   The commonest cause of diarrhoea in children is gastroenteritis.

2   Babies with severe diarrhoea, especially with fever and vomiting, should be referred to the doctor straightaway.

3   Troublesome diarrhoea persisting for more than a week in any child requires further investigation.

Earache

Earache is one of the most common reasons of all for parents bringing their children to the doctor's surgery or asking for a house call in the middle of the night. An older child may tell you directly that his ear hurts and it may be obvious that he has become slightly deaf in that ear. Sometimes there may be a fluid discharge from the outer ear canal, which is a sign that the eardrum itself has been perforated.

A younger child may show signs of an earache in more subtle ways. He will usually be obviously unwell and miserable, and may be whimpering, crying and pulling or rubbing the affected ear. The ear may look red and be painful if touched in any way. Often the child will also have the symptoms of a cold, with a runny nose, swollen glands at the front of the neck under the jaw and a red throat where the tonsils are inflamed. The temperature is often raised at about 38°C or above.

CAUSES OF EARACHE

* Infection of the middle ear (otitis media)

* Inflammation of the ear canal (otitis externa)

* Foreign body

* Boils

* Injury

* Teething

* Tonsillitis

* Mumps

Infection of the Middle Ear (Otitis Media)

This is by far the commonest cause of earache in children, and is due to a viral or bacterial infection of the middle ear cavity which has spread usually from the throat or nasal passages. Adults suffer in much the same way, but in children the communicating tube from the back of the throat, the Eustachian tube, is much shorter and straighter and consequently the infection spreads more easily. It is for this reason that otitis media is most common in children under the age of about six.

When a doctor examines the eardrum of a child with otitis media using a special torch and speculum (called an auriscope), the drum will appear a dull, red colour and it may be bulging outwards as a result of fluid collected behind it.

Complications of otitis media include a perforated eardrum, or permanent damage to the middle ear cavity or the little bones that

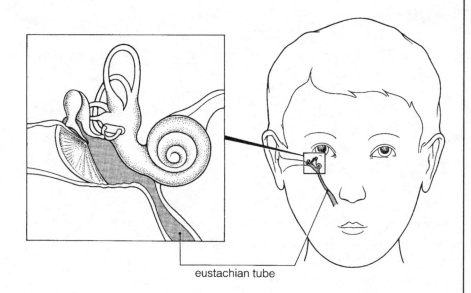

eustachian tube

Cross-section of the middle ear cavity and Eustachian tube, which can fill with fluid through infection or allergy

lie within it and which conduct sound. For this reason every child with earache should be examined by a doctor so that the appropriate treatment can be commenced.

Inflammation of the Ear Canal (Oitis Externa)

This is an infection or inflammation of the outer canal of the ear. The skin within the canal is reddened, flaky and sore and may well be weepy and infected. Viruses, bacteria and fungi may all be present and the condition is a lot more common in children with generalised skin problems, particularly eczema. Itching is a common additional symptom.

Foreign Body

Children are fond of poking small, round objects into their own or their siblings' ears, particularly things like beads, marbles and sweets. These can become stuck, leading to partial deafness, irritation and infection.

Boils

Just as spots and boils can develop on the skin, they can also develop within the ear canal itself. However, because the skin of the ear is stretched so tightly over the surrounding bone, any inflammation or swelling produces intense pain. The ear is therefore particularly tender to touch when this occurs.

Injury

Falling onto the side of the head or a blow to the side of the face can damage the ear both outside and within. Usually the ear itself is reddened and swollen, giving the parents a clue as to the reason for the earache. If, on the other hand, the inside of the canal has been scratched or damaged in some way with a sharp object, the cause of the earache may not be so obvious.

Teething

Often a child who is teething will experience earache rather than dental pain (see pages 382–384). This is because the pain is transmitted along nerve pathways which supply both the teeth and the ears with feeling and sensation. As a result, the brain may confuse the two. So when your child pulls at his ear and the doctor finds nothing wrong when he or she examines it, a look inside his mouth and appropriate treatment for teething pain will often do the trick. Another clue to the correct diagnosis is that teething is often associated with a mild fever and loose stools as well.

Tonsillitis

In the same way that teething can result in earache, so can tonsillitis. Tonsillitis is also likely to allow infection to spread along the Eustachian tube to the middle ear cavity, so tonsillitis and otitis media often occur hand in hand. Luckily, antibiotics and painkillers can be used to treat both conditions simultaneously.

Mumps

Mumps, now rare due to the immunisation programme, causes inflammation and painful enlargement of the salivary gland which lies just in front of and slightly below the ear. Swelling is therefore often associated with earache, and the ear lobe may be seen to be pushed up.

WHAT CAN YOU DO?

Take your child's temperature. If your child has a temperature, an infection is the most likely cause. Look at the outside of the ear. If the ear itself is reddened or any discharge is emerging from the ear canal, this also suggests a middle ear infection. However, in most cases of otitis media there will be no outward signs of infection and without looking directly at the eardrum it is almost impossible to be sure.

Is your child hearing all right? If your child appears to be slightly deaf in the affected ear it suggests a number of possibilities. There could be a foreign body in the ear canal, there might be a build-up of wax or, again, infection may be to blame.

Has your child got a cold? Earache often goes hand in hand with a runny nose, sore throat or tonsillitis. So if your child's throat is red and he is sneezing and spluttering, then again infection is most likely.

All this information is useful when you come to speak to your doctor, but in the meantime refrain from poking anything into the child's ear, including the all-purpose cotton bud, do not allow the ear to come into contact with any water from a bath or shower, and avoid using any ear-drops unless advised to do so by the doctor. The best course of action is to apply a warm hot-water bottle against the ear to ease the discomfort, and give paracetamol syrup or tablets if the temperature is raised or if pain is present.

WHAT CAN THE DOCTOR DO?

Every child with earache should be examined by a doctor, and usually the child is able to travel to the doctor's surgery for this examination to take place. The doctor uses a special torch and speculum, called an auriscope, to examine the ear canal and eardrum, and by taking a direct look he or she can diagnose otitis externa, otitis media, the build-up of fluid behind the eardrum (serious otitis media) or the presence of a foreign body. If all appears normal, the examination will then concentrate on other areas, including the teeth, tonsils and salivary glands.

Most earaches are caused by otitis media and consequently antibiotics are usually prescribed in order to eradicate any bacterial infection that is either present or may occur later. In the past, when antibiotics were not available, the spread of such infection producing very serious conditions such as mastoiditis, abscesses and encephalitis was quite common. Thankfully, this is now rare. In addition to antibiotics, pain relief in the form of paracetamol is usually advised, although applying a hot-water bottle to the side of the face is valuable too.

IF YOU REMEMBER NOTHING ELSE, REMEMBER THESE THREE THINGS

1   The commonest cause of earache is a middle ear cavity infection.

2   A doctor should always examine a child with earache to discover the cause. Untreated otitis media can lead to permanent hearing loss.

3   Treatment usually consists of a combination of paracetamol and antibiotics.

Eyesight Problems

A child who has visual difficulties will in most cases have a problem located within the eyes themselves rather than any form of general disease. The checks which all pre-school children should receive will almost certainly pick these up.

Short-sightedness, where a child can see close-up objects easily but struggles to focus on distant objects, tends to develop in late childhood. There is often a family history of short-sightedness, and so regular eyesight tests are vital for children whose parents or siblings suffer from the condition. Long-sightedness is usually present at birth, and both short- and long-sightedness are almost always correctable with the use of glasses.

Visual problems caused by a squint must be treated as soon as possible since, if neglected, the lazy eye may eventually become permanently blind. Whatever treatment is used to correct the squint, it should be carried out before the age of six or seven.

WHAT CAN YOU DO?

Most babies develop binocular vision, which means that both eyes focus together on the same object, by the age of about three months. Parents can test this by holding a brightly lit, coloured object in front of the baby's eyes at a distance of about 9–18 inches (20–40 cm) and, when it is moved slowly up or down or side to side, the baby's gaze should attempt to follow it. After the age of three months any squint should be brought to the attention of the doctor. The same applies if a child has been bumping into objects such as doorframes or furniture. This suggests a problem in the peripheral vision and again requires investigation.

It is common for a child to play up and misbehave when being tested by the optician, and this may mean that he is conscious of being unable to do a test because of some underlying problem. If this is the case, it is well worth making another appointment. Remember, however, that even a condition unrelated to the eye such as partial deafness caused by a recent ear infection can interfere with a reliable eye test.

By and large, most visual problems can be corrected with the use of patches worn over the good eye, orthoptic exercises for the bad eye or glasses. The most important thing a parent can do for the child who needs to wear a patch or has been prescribed glasses is to reassure him that his eyesight is well worth the effort of wearing them, and to prepare him for any teasing at school. Glasses should have plastic lenses, which are lighter and less likely to break than glass ones, and the child should always have a spare pair and be encouraged to keep the lenses clean. For times when he is very active, an elastic strap around the head fixed to the frames will make playtime a lot less frustrating.

WHAT CAN THE DOCTOR DO?

The doctor can test each eye in turn and both eyes together for any visual disturbance. He or she may confirm the presence of a squint and examine the eyes for any form of soreness, irritation,

IF YOU REMEMBER NOTHING ELSE, REMEMBER THESE THREE THINGS

1   Visual problems in children are almost always due to problems within the eye itself rather than to internal disease.

2   Regular pre-school eyesight checks are vital for all children.

3   Parental support and encouragement for a child wearing newly prescribed glasses is especially important in the early days.

allergy or infection. Simple eye tests involve asking a child under the age of three to match pictures on a card with identical pictures on cards held by the doctor. Older children can usually manage the illuminated charts that are used for adults, read from a distance of six metres. The doctor will also examine the individual structures of the eye – the clear cornea at the front, the pupil, the lens, the light-sensitive retina at the back, and the blood vessels which supply it. The optic nerve head can also be seen through the doctor's ophthalmoscope, and should the doctor find anything untoward he or she will refer the child to the ophthalmologist.

Failure to Thrive

There are enormous variations in the normal growth patterns of children. Some children are big, some are small, some are obese some are thin. None of these are average, but all of them are normal. Many parents become anxious when their child is not like most other children, but even if they are below or above average

CAUSES OF FAILURE TO THRIVE

* Genetic

* Low birth weight

* Early illness

* Underfeeding

* Malabsorption

* Other physical disorders

height and weight, they may still be perfectly healthy provided they are full of energy and are happy and well. In fact it is healthier to be slightly below average weight than above it. On the other hand, the further away a child becomes from the average, the increased likelihood there is of an underlying disorder.

Genetic

Small parents tend to produce small children who later go on to become smaller than average adults. This is especially true if both parents are small. The child will be of normal height and weight but may still be some way below average. He is likely to have a smaller appetite and eat smaller quantities compared with other children. There should, however, be steady growth in both height and weight over a period of time and, provided this growth velocity is maintained, there is usually no problem whatsoever. Attempts to overfeed the child in order to encourage him to catch up with children of the same age merely results in him becoming chubby and overweight, which is unhealthy. Far better to accept that his size is inherited, and to let him eat as much (or as little) as he needs. Like his parents he is simply a small person, and what is good enough for them should be good enough for him.

Low Birth Weight Babies

Babies who are born small for their gestational age are more likely than other babies to remain small in the future, especially if any growth retardation occurred early on in the pregnancy. There are, of course, some notable exceptions, and it is impossible to predict which children will grow faster and to a greater degree than others. But if a child has not caught up with the average by the age of two, it is probable that he will remain comparatively small.

Early Illness

Any kind of illness which stunts the growth of a small baby may mean that they will never fully catch up in size. Again, this is not always the rule but there seems to be a critical period during which growth must accelerate or it will never quite manage to make up for the poor start.

Underfeeding

A baby who, for any of the following reasons, is not fed enough calories is certainly going to fail to grow to his maximum potential. Firstly, one of the few disadvantages of breast-feeding is that breast-fed babies are more likely to be underfed than bottle-fed babies since it is easier to see if a bottle-fed baby is not taking enough (enough being approximately 150 millilitres per kilogram per day). Nowadays, scales are accurate enough to measure a breast-fed baby's weight before and after a feed to estimate how much he has taken, but this can cause added anxiety and is not generally recommended. Secondly, it is easy to imagine that premature babies need less milk than full-term babies, but in fact they need more since the growth that should have occurred inside the womb is massively more than can be attained out of the womb. Thirdly, not all babies cry when they are hungry so parents cannot always assume that a baby is satisfied and well fed purely because it is quiet. This is the one disadvantage of demand feeding.

In older children, underfeeding can be self-imposed. If, for example, a child is separated from his parents because of illness or admission to hospital, he may become emotionally withdrawn and refuse to eat. Finally, in some cases of child abuse, underfeeding may be deliberate or be due simply to neglect and here the failure to gain weight will be compounded by associated emotional factors.

Malabsorption

Children can fail to absorb many of the constituents of a normal diet due to various conditions. In cystic fibrosis and coeliac disease the child passes pale, bulky, foul-smelling stools which tend to float on the surface of the water (see page 440). Fat and other components of the diet including proteins, calories, vitamins and minerals are not absorbed properly and growth becomes restricted.

Carbohydrate, which is the most immediate energy source for children, fails to be absorbed in children with certain enzyme defects. These enzymes are chemicals in the body which break down the carbohydrate, allowing it to be absorbed across the gut wall into the bloodstream. These defects may be inherited (primary) or can follow on from a sudden tummy bug infection (secondary). They can also develop in association with cystic fibrosis, coeliac disease or cow's milk protein intolerance (see pages 220–221). Lactose intolerance is the commonest condition caused by enzyme deficiency and occurs due to absence of the enzyme lactase which breaks down a sugar called lactose present in the diet. In the inherited form it may be noticed as soon as the newborn baby is put to his mother's breast but more often the condition develops temporarily after a bout of gastroenteritis.

Other Physical Disorders

There are a number of relatively uncommon physical disorders which, when everything else has been excluded through medical investigations, may turn out to be the underlying reason why a child is not growing. Some of these are due to chronic infection, kidney infection being one of the most significant. Sometimes, disorders of a single organ in the body such as the heart, liver or kidney may be responsible. In other children, anatomical problems or a chromosomal abnormality present from birth could be the reason. Whether or not the child will catch up in size with his contemporaries will depend entirely on the underlying cause.

WHAT CAN YOU DO?

Any parent worried that their child is not growing should first ask themselves whether the child is active and happy. If he seems perfectly fit and well, it is unlikely that there is a serious underlying physical problem and it may be that he is destined to below average height and weight for genetic reasons. If both parents are on the small side, the child may be expected to be small too, and small children tend to have smaller appetites. If you are breast-feeding and you are concerned that your baby may not be taking enough or is not satisfied, the health visitor or GP can advise about supplementation with bottle feeds if necessary, although this can have the effect of reducing the breast-milk supply further (see page 14). Expert advice is all the more important if your baby was born prematurely or was born small for his dates. For an older child, ask yourself whether he could be anxious about any problems at school or at home, and especially whether he might be picking up on any domestic disharmony.

If you suspect that there may be a physical problem, then seek urgent consultation with the doctor. Frequent episodes of diarrhoea and vomiting, perpetual crying, thin arms, legs and buttocks in the presence of a swollen tummy are all suspicious signs.

WHAT CAN THE DOCTOR DO?

Doctors are often faced with the problem of a child who, as far as the parents are concerned, does not seem to be growing adequately. Thankfully, in the majority of cases, full evaluation reveals no underlying disorder and the child turns out to be quite normal. But a full physical examination should, nonetheless, be carried out, and blood and urine samples should be analysed. Urine tests can detect previously undiscovered infection and the presence of abnormal protein or sugar. Blood tests can uncover evidence of malabsorption, chronic inflammation, infection, chromosomal abnormalities, diseases in individual organs of the body and rare metabolic conditions which interfere with the way the body uses food. Disorders such as coeliac disease require special tests such as an intestinal biopsy, but these would be carried out under specialist supervision in hospital. If the GP is not able to find a simple explanation for a child who fails to grow, he or she will refer him to a local consultant paediatrician.

IF YOU REMEMBER NOTHING ELSE,
REMEMBER THESE THREE THINGS

1   Small children who have plenty of energy
    and are happy are usually quite normal.

2   In the majority of cases, the reason for a
    child being small is genetic.

3   In a small number of cases, underfeeding,
    malabsorption or other physical conditions
    may be responsible.

Fainting

Fainting occurs when the blood pressure suddenly drops
temporarily, depriving the brain of sufficient oxygen. This is more
common in girls and older children and adolescents, and is relatively rare in children under the age of ten. Although it generally
occurs out of the blue, there are a number of trigger factors which
make the possibility of fainting more likely. Standing up quickly
from a lying or sitting position will suddenly reduce the blood pressure, and strong emotional reactions or shock have the same effect.
Children seem particularly vulnerable to fainting when they are
tired or run down, and sometimes a persistent cough can pre-
cipitate a fainting bout. The other major factor is heat. Any
infection producing a fever or even the warmth of a hot summer's
day will bring about a drop in blood pressure. When the body is
hot, blood is diverted to the skin in an attempt to lose heat and

there is less blood remaining in the central circulation which feeds the brain. Keeping the patient cool after a faint is therefore important.

Any child heading for a faint may experience useful warning signs. Initially he will feel hot and sweaty. The head will start to swim, he may see 'dancing spots' in front of his eyes and hear a buzzing in the ears. If he is sitting at the time and puts his head between his knees, he may well be able to avoid fainting. He may also achieve this if he is standing, by lying down quickly with his head back and his knees raised. Sometimes, however, the child is just too late and will black out, fall to the floor and briefly lose consciousness. This loss of consciousness seldom lasts more than one to two minutes and it is not unusual for the child to twitch slightly during this time. During a faint the child will look pale, lie still and have a fast weak pulse.

It is important to make the distinction between a simple faint and an epileptic fit. Both cause the child to fall to the ground and lose consciousness, but they are quite different conditions and require quite separate treatment. In an epileptic seizure a rigid contraction of the limbs occurs for a short while, followed by a period of frantic thrashing around and then a prolonged period of unconsciousness. The child recovering from a seizure will then only be semi-conscious and confused for quite a long time, whereas the child recovering from a simple faint will be back to normal within seconds of coming round. During a seizure it is quite common for the child to involuntarily wet himself, froth at the mouth or bite the tongue whereas this never happens during a faint. Finally, a fainting child will be able to remember exactly what happened immediately before the faint whereas a child having a seizure will not. Any parent witnessing a child apparently fainting should observe carefully what happens (if that is possible despite their obvious concern) so that they can describe the episode clearly to the doctor and enable him or her to reach a correct diagnosis.

WHAT CAN YOU DO?

There is no doubt that some children are more prone to fainting than others. Those who are more susceptible to fainting should avoid the many trigger factors which can cause it. Keeping cool at all times and remembering to rise slowly from a sitting or lying position are the two most important things. On a warm day it is a good idea to drink plenty of fluids to keep the blood pressure up and to avoid wearing tight, restrictive clothing.

Once a child has fainted it is probably more important for a parent to remember not what to do, but what *not* to do. The child should not be sat up or supported in an upright position. Rather, he should be allowed to lie completely flat with his head back and the legs slightly raised on two or three cushions. This brings the blood pressure back up and allows increased blood flow to the brain. The child should not be unconscious for more than one to two minutes, and after the first few seconds the child should be placed in the recovery position as described on page 102.

WHAT CAN THE DOCTOR DO?

Doctors rarely see a child who has fainted because recovery is so fast. The time they are likely to witness such an episode, however, is when visiting a sick child with a fever who jumps out of bed quickly and suddenly becomes dizzy and faints. Doctors are more likely to become involved when a child appears to be particularly vulnerable to fainting, having perhaps more than three episodes in a year. GPs should always ask the parents to describe carefully what actually happened during a fainting attack, since it is important to exclude the possibility of an epileptic fit.

GPs should be able to reassure parents when their child faints, but they should also keep the possibility of epilepsy at the back of their minds and carry out further investigations if appropriate. These would be justified if the child is under ten, if the loss of consciousness lasts more than a couple of minutes, if the child cannot remember exactly what happened before the episode and particularly if the child wet himself or bit his tongue whilst unconscious.

IF YOU REMEMBER NOTHING ELSE, REMEMBER THESE THREE THINGS

1 Being aware of the warning signs may enable a child to avoid fainting.

2 During a faint the child should be laid flat on the ground with his legs slightly raised.

3 It is important to distinguish a faint from an epileptic fit.

Fever and High Temperature

The usual cause of a high temperature or a fever in a child is some kind of infection. The commonest examples are the viruses that cause colds, sore throats and ear infections. Very often there will be symptoms of pain and discomfort as well. The normal core temperature is between 36 and 37 degrees Celsius (°C), and anything above 37.7°C (or 100°F) is classed as a fever. Children have a less well developed temperature-regulating mechanism than adults, and this is why their temperatures can rise and fall so quickly and so sharply. A high temperature in a baby under six months is particularly serious as dehydration can occur so fast, but any child with a temperature of above 40°C should be seen by a doctor as soon as possible.

A high temperature is due to the effect of substances, called pyrogens, released by the bacteria or viruses causing the infection. It is part of the body's defence mechanism working to combat the infection, so in some ways it can be regarded as a good thing. Unfortunately, the effect of a high temperature on a child is to make him miserable, and when it becomes excessively high, certain potentially serious consequences need to be avoided.

High temperatures lead to headache, lack of energy, nausea and vomiting, hot, sweaty, clammy skin, dry mouth and lips, and shivering. In addition to these unpleasant symptoms, some children under the age of seven are prone to convulsions or fits as a direct result of the effect of the fever on the brain. These are known as febrile convulsions and although relatively common and benign (about one in every twenty children are affected), they are extremely alarming for the parents. However, very few children who experience febrile convulsions go on to develop epilepsy in adult life, the vast majority growing out of them as they get older. It is particularly important for any child who has had a febrile convulsion in the past to have treatment for a fever as soon as it begins.

CAUSES OF FEVER AND HIGH TEMPERATURE

* Colds and coughs

* Chest infection

* Influenza

* Glandular fever

* Rashes

* Kidney infection

* Tummy bug

* Meningitis

Colds and Coughs

The commonest cause of a temperature is a common cold. There will often be a runny and blocked nose, sore throat and earache. Coughing may be present too. In a small child who may not be able to tell you exactly where the pain is, he may simply rub or pull at his ear or refuse to eat his food since swallowing is uncomfortable. His throat will be red to look at, as may his ear, and sometimes it is possible to feel large glands just under the jawbone at the front of the neck.

Chest Infection

Bacterial chest infections requiring antibodies are extremely uncommon in children. A child suffering from a chest infection looks unwell, has a high fever and his breathing may be fast and shallow. A chest infection can follow on from a cold, or can occasionally begin without warning.

Viral asthma is very common in children under two, affecting as many as one in four. Coughing, wheezing and more rapid breathing are the usual symptoms if the swelling and increased secretions are principally in the windpipe, there may be a croupy type of cough, but if the lower airways are affected, wheezing is the predominant feature (see page 444).

Influenza

Contrary to popular belief, influenza is not just a severe cold. In true 'flu the temperature is much higher, often up to 40°C or above. The child is completely listless and without energy, refuses to eat or drink much and complains of aching all over, particularly in the muscles and joints.

Glandular Fever

Although glandular fever occurs more often in teenagers, it is also fairly common in younger children. It usually starts with a sore throat, just like tonsillitis, but in glandular fever the soreness and fever persist for much longer than a few days and do not respond to antibiotics. In fact, some antibiotics (ampicillin) must be avoided as they can often produce a characteristic rash when given during glandular fever. Enlarged glands will be present, not only in the neck but also in the armpits and groin, and occasionally there will be a rash and tummy discomfort. The child may take several weeks to recover to full health.

Rashes (see pages 115–167)

Both measles, which is now uncommon due to the immunisation programme, and chickenpox will produce a fever, usually a higher one in the case of measles. The chickenpox rash consists of a number of small blisters containing clear fluid which appear first on the trunk. As the blisters enlarge, they burst leaving the top to crust over, and the surrounding skin becomes reddened and slightly sore.

The child with measles has all the symptoms of a very nasty cold with red eyes, a very runny nose and a sore throat. He is always miserable and has a bright red, blotchy rash, particularly on the face and upper body. Other infectious rashes can also coexist with a fever and these are described on pages 115 to 130.

Kidney Infection

In some children, especially girls, the infection causing a fever may be situated in the bladder or kidneys. Symptoms to look out for are a child who is wanting to go to the toilet much more often than usual or who complains of burning or scalding when he does, particularly if they have abdominal pain as well. The urine may have an odour that is stronger than normal, and occasionally it may be pink or blood stained.

Tummy Bug

Occasionally a child with diarrhoea and vomiting will have a temperature as a result of gastroenteritis. If abdominal pain is present, or if an infant is pulling his knees up towards his chest in obvious discomfort, a doctor should always be called, as abdominal pain combined with a temperature could be a sign of appendicitis.

Meningitis

This is a very serious inflammation of the meninges, the membranes which cover the brain and spinal cord. It may be caused by a virus or bacteria, the bacterial type being the most dangerous. In older children, the fever is accompanied by headache, neck stiffness, nausea or vomiting, a dislike of bright lights and increasing drowsiness and confusion. Sometimes there is a purply rash under the surface of the skin. This occurs when the infection gets into the bloodstream and produces blood-poisoning or septicaemia. This is a medical emergency and requires immediate transfer to hospital. In babies, the signs to look for, along with a high temperature, are a weak, high-pitched cry, refusing feeds, staring, sunken eyes, floppiness and vomiting. A rash similar to the one sometimes seen in older children may also be present.

If you have even the slightest suspicion that your child may have meningitis, do not hesitate. Call the doctor immediately, explaining the symptoms, and convey your worry that it might be meningitis. Do not worry about being mistaken because a good doctor will be keen to visit a child with these symptoms, knowing full well that meningitis can progress swiftly and become life-threatening if not treated without delay. Early treatment is the key.

What If My Child Has A Raised Temperature For No Apparent Reason?

Doctors call this a PUO, a pyrexia (fever) of unknown origin. Often the underlying cause of the fever becomes obvious within a few hours, but now and again no apparent cause reveals itself even after several days. Sources of hidden infection include the kidneys or liver in the case of pyelonephritis or hepatitis, but there are hundreds of possibilities ranging from deep-seated abscesses and blood disorders right through to brucellosis from drinking unpasteurised milk, tuberculosis and even exotic conditions such as malaria.

Children with long-standing PUO are generally admitted to hospital for full investigation so that the underlying cause can be diagnosed and treated. Investigations commonly include blood cultures, urine tests, swabs from various sites, stool specimens and blood counts.

WHAT CAN YOU DO?

A child's temperature may fluctuate rapidly and dramatically. A single reading may be normal when you first take it and rise dramatically within fifteen minutes, and vice versa. So it is well worth checking the temperature regularly. Once you have established that the temperature is consistently raised, it is sensible to take steps to reduce it, not only to reduce the unpleasant symptoms that accompany high temperature, but also to reduce the risk of febrile convulsion. Contrary to the old-fashioned – and incorrect – treatment consisting of wrapping the child up in several layers of clothing to 'sweat out the fever', it is imperative that the child's body is cooled. The following steps are important in all cases of fever, but are especially so in a child who has a history of febrile convulsions. Such children are always likely to have fits accompanying fever, so as soon as their temperature has spiked, all of these steps should be undertaken.

1 Avoid overheating. Strip the child off, leaving him in just a single cotton vest and covered by a single cotton bedsheet. The body loses heat by radiation and evaporation from the skin, so keeping the skin in contact with the air is important.

2 Encourage fluids. The child should be encouraged to drink fluids. With a high temperature, a child is unlikely to want to eat or drink very much, but regular sips of cool or even iced drinks are refreshing. More importantly, they reduce the risk of dehydration which occurs much more quickly in children than adults, especially in the presence of fever. Water is as good as anything, but if your child prefers squash or soft drinks, they are fine too.

3 Keep the room cool. The body is better able to lose excess heat if the surrounding temperature is kept low, so turn down the central heating and open the windows.

4 Tepid sponging. If the child's temperature remains high despite the above measures, soak a flannel or sponge in tepid water and wipe the child down from head to foot in soothing, gentle movements. The water should not be too hot or too cold; water that is too hot prevents adequate heat loss, and cold water is not only unpleasant but tends to constrict the blood vessels under the skin, preventing them from losing heat. Tepid sponging encourages the evaporation of water from the skin, which gradually and effectively cools it down. The child's temperature should be rechecked after ten minutes or so, after which the tepid sponging can be repeated if no improvement has taken place.

5 Medication. Paracetamol in either syrup or tablet form is readily available as an over-the-counter remedy, and is effective and safe for children when used in the correct dosage. It should be used in conjunction with steps 1 to 4 in cases where the temperature remains raised. The dosage depends on the child's age, and the manufacturer's recommendations should be followed. If in doubt, or if you are worried about a baby under three months with a fever, your doctor should be consulted. It is reasonable to continue paracetamol treatment for up to 24 hours, with the dosage being repeated every four hours, but after this time the doctor's opinion should be sought. Aspirin should not be used in children under twelve unless prescribed by a doctor because of the very small risk of Reye's syndrome which has been linked with this medication.

WHAT CAN THE DOCTOR DO?

It is difficult to generalise about when to call the doctor for a child who has a fever, as a lot will depend on the presence or absence of other symptoms. A fever can be a useful sign of the progression of an infection, but the height of the fever does not necessarily reflect its seriousness. In general, a doctor should be called out to a baby under six months old with a temperature of over 37.7°C, as babies are most at risk. Similarly, any child who has had febrile convulsions or a family history of these should be treated by a doctor as soon as possible. A fever persisting for more than 24–48 hours where there is no obvious cause should also be investigated by a doctor.

Finally, if additional symptoms point to the possibility of a more serious underlying illness such as meningitis, then immediate and emergency referral to a doctor or casualty unit is essential. The nastier bacterial forms of meningitis can, in some instances, prove life-threatening within a few hours if left untreated, so it is always better to err on the side of caution and seek a medical opinion.

A doctor can assess the child and, by way of a thorough medical examination, will generally be able to pinpoint the source of the infection and the cause of the fever. He or she can then advise on treatment which, in the case of bacterial infections, may or may not include prescribing antibiotics. The doctor will also instigate any necessary tests and investigations should the underlying disorder remain unidentified.

IF YOU REMEMBER NOTHING ELSE, REMEMBER THESE THREE THINGS

1   Check the child's temperature regularly to monitor progress.

2   Keep the child in cool surroundings and use paracetamol to reduce the fever and hence the risk of dehydration and febrile convulsion.

3   If the fever is linked with the symptoms of meningitis, then call the doctor without delay. Also call the doctor if your child is under 6 months and has a temperature of over 40°C.

Foot Problems

Parents often become concerned about a variety of problems concerning the shape and position of their children's feet, but the good news is that most of these minor deformities, which are in fact very common in small babies and infants, cure themselves without any treatment whatsoever.

COMMON FOOT PROBLEMS

* Talipes or club-foot

* Toeing-in

* Toeing-out (pigeon-toes)

* Toe walking

* Crooked toe

* Flat feet

* Athlete's foot

* Verrucae

Talipes or Club-Foot

This is a relatively common condition where there may have been pressure exerted on the position of the feet whilst the child was developing in the womb. The foot is either twisted downwards and inwards (like a horse's hoof), in which case it is called talipes equino-varus, or twisted upwards and outwards in which case it is called talipes calcaneo-valgus. Most cases will correct themselves in the course of time, usually fairly soon after the child begins to walk. In more severe cases, however, or in cases where walking is impossible because of the deformity, treatment with exercise or splinting may be required and occasionally surgery is necessary. By and large, with the equino-varus form of club-foot, if a parent can take the child's foot and bring the toes up far enough to touch the front of the leg there will be no need for future treatment. A doctor's opinion should always be sought, however, if parents are worried.

Toeing-in

In this condition the feet point inwards towards each other. This is usually caused because the whole limb is rotated inwards from the hip joint downwards, and if parents look they will see that the child's knees are almost facing each other. Although it looks awkward, this condition is in most cases self-curing by the age of eight.

Toeing-out

In this condition the feet point outwards away from each other. It is caused by an outward rotation of the limb from the hip downwards and is usually self-correcting by the age of two.

Toe Walking

Some children when they start to walk like to walk on their toes, and there is no physical problem whatsoever. If asked to they can put their heels firmly on the floor and walk quite normally. Other children who have previously walked normally may toe walk if they have a painful heel. This may be due to bruising following jumping onto hard ground or a pebble, or there may be a blister or verruca in the heel area which is tender.

In rare instances there is congenital shortening of the Achilles tendon sufficient to prevent the child from getting the heel right down to the floor. In severe cases of this condition surgery may be required to elongate the tendon, although most cases are mild and will self-correct as the tendon gradually lengthens when the child begins to walk. A very few toe-walking children have a degree of cerebral palsy with some spasticity in one or both lower legs with contraction and shortening of the calf muscles and the Achilles tendon. Physiotherapy and surgery in these instances are worth considering.

Crooked Toe

This is a common complaint in which one toe bends to one side and lies either above or beneath the neighbouring toe. This does not interfere functionally with the child's walking in any way, but if it is neglected corns or calluses may develop. If it is going to be corrected, and it should be, it should really be done at as early an age as possible. In the old days the crooked toe would be strapped to its straight neighbour to encourage it to develop in a straight line, but this was ineffective. These days a chiropodist will be able to provide a simple device known as a toe prop which is simply a soft pad of cushioning which lies beneath the toes lifting the crooked one up into straight alignment with the others. It is simply held onto one of the straight toes by means of an elastic ring. It is very comfortable to wear and is worn inside the socks and shoes for as long as is necessary to correct the condition.

Flat Feet

All babies have flat feet at birth, and the characteristic inside arch of the foot seen in adults does not develop fully until the age of about six. Flat feet can be identified easily by looking at the wet foot imprint on a tiled or stone floor – flat feet will produce an imprint in which the whole of the sole of the foot is seen to be in full contact with the ground. It used to be thought that untreated flat feet were a major source of problems in later life, but this is not the case. In fact other than insoles to support the non-existent arch, no other treatment is required.

Athlete's Foot

Athlete's foot is a fungal infection occurring between the toes (see page 153). It produces a soggy, white, itchy skin rash which if neglected will spread to the webs of other toes. It is made worse by wearing plastic shoes or trainers which do not allow air to get to the feet and which therefore encourage the build-up of moisture in which the fungus thrives.

Verrucae

Verrucae are simply warts which occur on the soles of the feet (see pages 164–165). They are quite contagious amongst children and once they arise they form hard, gritty nodules in the skin which are pushed into the deeper layers of the flesh through the pressure of walking.

WHAT CAN YOU DO?

If your child has a club-foot, it is well worth using the simple test described above to see whether your child has the type which is self-correcting. If the toes can be brought up to touch the front of the leg then generally speaking no treatment will be necessary. If not, or in cases where the feet are twisted upwards and outwards, then a doctor's opinion is certainly worthwhile.

Crooked toes respond very well to the provision of a toe prop which can be obtained from a chiropodist, but the provision of comfortable and well-fitting shoes is vital too. Athlete's foot responds to the regular application of antifungal creams, powders or ointments and there is no doubt that leather shoes or even open-toed sandals are healthier than trainers. Verrucae are sometimes difficult to eradicate completely without medical help, and most cases should be seen by the doctor or chiropodist.

WHAT CAN THE DOCTOR DO?

Although the doctor knows that most cases of mild club-foot will get better on their own, he or she still needs to keep an eye on the problem so that the few that do not self-correct are referred for an orthopaedic opinion. This is specially so in cases where the child is tripping over constantly and where walking is either a problem in itself or fails to fully correct the club-foot. Children who toe-in after the age of eight and children who toe-out after the age of two may again require assessment by a specialist. Flat feet are not serious in themselves, if anything merely requiring the provision of a special insole which will support the non-existent arch of the foot so that aching and discomfort does not arise in later life.

Verrucae may be treated in a variety of ways, but the old-fashioned method of applying acid and then rubbing off the dead skin with emery paper or a pumice stone is both messy and ineffective. A far quicker method of treatment involves the use of freezing and is known as cryotherapy. It uses liquid nitrogen and can be used in most children over the age of five or six.

IF YOU REMEMBER NOTHING ELSE, REMEMBER THESE THREE THINGS

1 Most foot deformities are self-curing during childhood.

2 Occasionally a severe case of club-foot may require exercises, splinting or surgery.

3 If parents are uncertain about a foot problem, a chiropodist or GP should be consulted.

Foreskin Problems

The foreskin is the loose fold of skin covering the bulb-like tip of the penis or glans. When a boy is born the foreskin is attached to the glans and gradually separates over the course of the next three or four years. Parents often make the mistake of trying to retract the foreskin, but there are no hygienic reasons for doing so and infection or damage can occur. If a tight foreskin persists after the age of five there is still no urgent need to consult a doctor unless the child is unable to pass urine normally or suffers from frequent infections. Signs of obstruction to the flow of urine include a very fine stream, and ballooning of the foreskin.

The main medical reasons for surgical removal of the foreskin, or circumcision, are phimosis or balanitis described below. Circumcision is also carried out on religious and cultural grounds, but in these cases not under the NHS.

COMMON FORESKIN PROBLEMS

* Non-retractile foreskin

* Balanitis

* Phimosis

* Paraphimosis

Non-Retractile Foreskin

A non-retractile foreskin is normal up to the age of five or six. No attempt should be made to force the foreskin back because there is no need to clean under the foreskin at this age and in fact it can cause infection or mechanical damage.

Balanitis

This is an infection of the foreskin and the glans penis beneath it. The tip of the penis is red and sore and often there is a whitish yellow discharge. Predisposing factors include nappy rash and sometimes a mild allergy to soaps, bubble baths or biological washing powders in which terry nappies or underpants have been washed. Untreated balanitis can lead to phimosis (see below).

Phimosis

In this condition, the hole at the tip of the penis is pinhole in size and the whole of the foreskin balloons outwards when the child attempts to urinate. When he does, the stream may spray, as if from a watering can, in all directions. As the child grows older, pain on erection can occur since the foreskin cannot retract over the enlarging penis.

Paraphimosis

In this condition the foreskin has been retracted backwards over the ridge of the glans penis and has become stuck in this position, leading to painful swelling of the tip of the penis. It is a good reason for not forcibly retracting the foreskin in the first place, and sometimes the foreskin needs to be pulled forwards again gently by the doctor using local anaesthetic cream.

WHAT CAN YOU DO?

Do not be tempted to retract a young boy's foreskin since it is not designed to retract until the ages of between three and six. There is no need to clean underneath for hygienic reasons, and the best way to keep the area clean is to bathe the child regularly in ordinary warm, soapy water. Babies who develop a red tip to the foreskin and who cry when they urinate should have their nappies changed frequently to reduce the risk of nappy rash, and should be kept as dry as possible. Barrier cream should be applied if necessary to avoid the skin coming into contact with the nappy contents. Older children should be allowed to run around with no pants on at all. If soap, detergent or biological washing powders appear to be partly responsible, these should be avoided. If the redness doesn't respond to simple measures such as a barrier cream or there appears to be any discharge at the tip of the penis, antifungal, antibacterial and mild steroid cream may be applied after the foreskin has been gently and fractionally pulled back. A warm bath in hot, salty water is probably the most soothing treatment.

Where the stream of urine is held back by an over-tight foreskin or where frequent infections occur, the doctor should be consulted.

WHAT CAN THE DOCTOR DO?

Doctors can often relieve pain and remove any obstruction to the flow of urine by reducing any swelling and redness which is the

IF YOU REMEMBER NOTHING ELSE, REMEMBER THESE THREE THINGS

1   Most worries are caused by an over-tight foreskin, but this rarely requires surgery.

2   Retraction of the foreskin in children up until the age of five or six is unnecessary.

3   Severe phimosis and recurrent infections may require circumcision.

result of nappy rash. In many cases an antifungal cream is all that is required. Where bacterial contamination has occurred, antibiotics in cream form will often cure the problem, but, rarely, where recurrent infections are a problem, circumcision may be required. This operation is also carried out in cases of severe phimosis. Circumcision is a straightforward operation requiring general anaesthetic and a 24-hour stay in hospital. In paraphimosis, the foreskin may be gently manipulated back with the use of local anaesthetic cream or KY jelly.

Groin Lumps

Medically speaking, the groin refers to the junction of the top of the thigh and the base of the abdomen. The crease in the skin here is called the inguinal ligament and important anatomical structures run along, above, below and underneath it. Many people also use the term 'groin' when referring to a male, to include the scrotum, the loose bag of skin which contains the testicles. For this reason, lumps in both the groin and the scrotum are included in this section.

CAUSES OF GROIN LUMPS

* Enlarged lymph glands

* Inguinal hernia

* Undescended testicle

* Scrotal swellings

Enlarged Lymph Glands

Usually, when lots of little lumps are felt in the groin, they are enlarged lymph glands. The lymphatic system is designed to 'mop up' infection, and when this occurs special white blood cells are concentrated in the lymph glands which swell and become slightly tender. These lumps can be felt in the groin after colds and coughs, but will also appear if any local inflammation is present. A cut, graze or eczema anywhere on the leg which becomes infected can cause this reaction, but so can any kind of medical injection in the bottom or thigh. Such enlargement of the lymph glands is normal but should gradually settle down over the course of two or three weeks in most cases.

Inguinal Hernia

This type of hernia produces a lump just above the crease of skin at the top of the thigh where it joins the lower abdomen, and the lump may continue right along the crease and down into the scrotum. It is caused by a weakness in the muscular wall of the abdomen through which a loop of bowel extrudes, producing the swelling. The lump may be very small, in which case the tough lining of the abdomen which is pushed through the muscle merely contains fluid, or it may be quite large in which case the lump will contain a loop of bowel.

Inguinal herniae are sometimes present in babies from birth, usually on one but occasionally on both sides. Increased abdominal pressure through crying will make the swelling more prominent, and because of the risk of strangulation when the blood supply to a loop of bowel becomes cut off, surgery is required.

Undescended Testicle

Sometimes there is a lump in the groin because one of the testicles has not descended fully from the abdomen down into the scrotum at birth and has become lodged in the inguinal canal, a narrow structure just behind the inguinal ligament at the top of the leg. Sometimes the testicle can be gently manipulated down into the scrotum from the inside part of the inguinal canal using the fingers. This is easiest after a hot bath. Where this is not possible, surgery is required by the age of four or five to prevent long-term complications including possible infertility or malignant change. Parents should never jump to conclusions about an undescended testicle, however, since a normally descended testicle can often be pulled back up to the top of the scrotum in certain conditions such as moderately cold surroundings or anxiety and can be easily coaxed down again by careful manipulation.

Scrotal Swellings

When parents notice that their son's scrotum is swollen, they generally tend to think of the testicles first. A testicle may be injured, for example through rough play or falling astride a fence, and sometimes the testicle can twist upon itself cutting off the blood supply. This is known as testicular torsion. Both of these are accompanied by moderate to severe pain.

A painless swelling, on the other hand, may be due to a hydrocele, a collection of fluid around the testicle. Many boys are born with a hydrocele, often suggesting to the proud parents that their child is particularly 'well endowed'. This is absolutely normal and settles within the first few weeks after birth. When it occurs later in childhood, it is a sign either of recent injury or of an inguinal hernia (see above).

WHAT CAN YOU DO?

In most cases, swollen lymph glands in the groin are due to infection somewhere in the body. If this is the case, it is worth checking for enlargement of other glands such as those in the neck and armpits. Often the infection may be obvious, such as infected eczema, athlete's foot, an infected graze of the knee or a boil on the thigh. Sometimes a vaccination has been given into the thigh or buttock where a local reaction with redness and pain has occurred. Again, this is very likely to produce enlargement of the lymph glands in the groin. Such swellings are fairly small, mobile and rubbery and clear up within two to three weeks at the most. When they do not, where the child is also unwell, his glands are swollen in many different parts of the body or a single larger swelling is present, the doctor should be consulted. As far as groin lumps caused by inguinal hernias, undescended testicles and scrotal swellings, are concerned, a precise diagnosis is required before the child's parent can do anything significantly helpful. So the first task is to take the child with the lump to the doctor.

WHAT CAN THE DOCTOR DO?

Often the doctor is able to diagnose the condition through examination. Where enlarged lymph glands are present in the groin, the doctor needs to keep them under observation to make sure that they clear up within two to three weeks, or if other glands around the body are swollen he or she may need to investigate to find the source of the infection. Once the cause of the problem has been identified, the doctor can organise appropriate treatment. Very occasionally, a single lymph gland can be the first sign of a malignant condition of the lymph glands such as Hodgkin's disease.

Hydroceles in babies require no treatment as they settle spontaneously, but when they occur in an older child they suggest the presence of an inguinal hernia which will require surgery. Undescended testicles also need surgical treatment before the age of five to prevent long-term complications.

A hernia which becomes 'strangulated' is a surgical emergency requiring urgent admission to hospital, and all parents of children with herniae should be warned about the rare possibility of this happening. A hernia which is hard and tender and which cannot be pushed back inside the abdomen is potentially strangulated and should be seen immediately by the doctor.

IF YOU REMEMBER NOTHING ELSE, REMEMBER THESE THREE THINGS

1   Most lumps in the groin are due to swollen lymph glands.

2   A single lump in the groin or a group of very swollen lumps should be referred to the doctor.

3   A strangulated hernia is a surgical emergency.

Hair Loss

Parents are usually more concerned about their own hair loss than that of their children. However, hair loss does occur in childhood, although thankfully it almost always grows back. The most frequent type of hair loss is that which occurs in patches, and a great deal depends on the age of the child.

Babies
Babies can be born with a full head of hair or be virtually bald. In either case, the hair is generally very fine and the attachment of the fair follicles to the scalp is fairly weak. Much of the initial hair can be lost just after birth, and it is not unusual for children to remain bald for the first few months of their lives. After the age of one the hair starts to grow thicker and darker, much to the relief of anxious parents. A common cause of patchy hair loss at the back of the baby's head is contact with the pillow or mattress as

he sleeps. This frequent and mechanical pressure is sufficient to rub away the fine hair leaving a bare patch, and this seems to happen however soft the padding is behind the head and has no lasting consequences for the child. This form of hair loss in babies has become more common now that we lay babies to sleep on their backs rather than their sides or tummies.

Toddlers and older children
Some children when they are anxious or when they are busy concentrating, will subconsciously twiddle their hair around their fingers and pull it. This is no more than a nervous tic which the medical profession endow with the grand title of trichotillomania and which may result in bald patches if continued. Another cause of patchy baldness is alopecia areata which is a lot more dramatic in that there can be several completely bald areas scattered over the scalp. This condition often begins following a simple illness or some kind of emotional upset, and although it looks alarming it settles down by itself within a few months and the hair all grows back. Ringworm is a fungal infection producing small areas of hair loss which are scaly, reddened and slightly itchy.

In a few cases there can be an inherited abnormality of the hair itself, and drugs used in chemotherapy for serious blood disorders and malignant conditions are well known to produce temporary hair loss right across the scalp in most instances. Any severe illness, it has to be said, particularly when there is a fever, will result in the shedding of large numbers of healthy hair follicles simultaneously leading to temporary thinning.

WHAT CAN YOU DO?

There is not a great deal that parents can do to correct the above conditions other than to identify the cause and reassure the child. Children at school can be easily teased by their peers so being alert to that possibility and helping the child to cope with any psychological problem is important.

Children should generally be discouraged from pulling on their hair, and a child suffering from temporary hair loss can be supplied with a fashionable hat of some kind to cover any obvious bald patches. A soft night bonnet may help the baby who has rubbed hair from the back of his head leaving a bald patch. If ringworm is suspected the doctor should be consulted.

WHAT CAN THE DOCTOR DO?

The doctor's job is usually to reassure and offer advice to the worried parents. However, ringworm of the scalp requires treatment involving simple antifungal cream, which will cure the condition when applied regularly.

IF YOU REMEMBER NOTHING ELSE, REMEMBER THESE THREE THINGS

1 Loss of hair in children is usually temporary.

2 Hair loss in children is usually patchy.

3 Ringworm of the scalp requires treatment with antifungal cream.

Headache

Headaches in children are really quite common. In junior schools they affect one child in every five, and this increases to 85 per cent of children attending secondary school. By and large the symptoms are trivial and short lived.

CAUSES OF HEADACHE

* Psychological factors and tension

* Infection

* Environment

* Hunger and tiredness

* Head injury

* Migraine

* Toothache, earache, sinusitis and eye problems

* Brain tumour

* Medication

Psychological Factors and Tension

In many cases of headache, no physical problem exists. Psychological reasons include worries about school, fear of being bullied and separation anxiety from having to be parted from parents. Such 'headaches of convenience' are usually easily identified because they only occur when the source of the anxiety is imminent, such as in the mornings on school days, and disappear afterwards. If parents become overly concerned about the child, he may then use headaches as a way of seeking more attention from mum and dad.

Sometimes, significant and persistent anxieties can produce

muscular tension in the head, neck and shoulders, leading to the physical condition known as tension headache.

Infection

The commonest physical reason for a headache is infection, particularly if it causes a fever. Adults know only too well how a temperature and dehydration can produce a thumping headache, and the same is true for children. Colds, coughs, 'flu and measles are all likely to lead to headaches.

One particular infection worth mentioning above all others is meningitis. Here the headache is accompanied by nausea and vomiting, increasing drowsiness and confusion, neck stiffness, and discomfort when looking at bright light. This collection of symptoms in association with severe headache is highly suggestive of meningitis, some forms of which are life threatening and demand the most urgent medical attention.

Environment

Children do not like being kept too long in a hot, stuffy room and prefer to be outdoors in the fresh air. Many headaches are merely due to lack of activity and unhealthy confinement in a stuffy atmosphere.

Hunger and Tiredness

Many children develop headaches when they are tired and hungry. Some may even develop low sugar levels in the blood just before mealtimes which may predispose them to headaches. Healthy snacks between meals and plenty of sleep is the answer.

Head Injury

A bang on the head, particularly from a height, will obviously cause a headache. Your child may feel sick or actually vomit from the shock of it. In most cases, vomiting occurs just once and the child then gradually perks up again. If vomiting continues, or if the child lapses into increasing drowsiness, immediate medical attention is required. If a headache comes on some days after a significant head injury, this is also important as on rare occasions it may be a sign of raised pressure within the head as a result of the blow. Again, this requires urgent medical attention.

Migraine

Many children develop a headache along with abdominal pain if they suffer from migraine. Migraine in children is different from that in adults, and may not be confined to one side of the head. Nausea and vomiting can occur, and the symptoms may be triggered by tiredness, exercise, stress or worry, or by factors in the diet such as chocolate, cheese or fizzy drinks. There is usually a family history of the condition, with one or other parent suffering from classic migraine.

Toothache, Earache, Sinusitis and Eye Problems

Any of these conditions, which usually cause localised pain in one area of the head or face, may be interpreted by a young child as a headache. A recent cold or cough or tenderness over the teeth and gums are all helpful clues in this case.

Brain Tumour

This is perhaps something which all parents worry about when a child complains of recurring headaches, but it is reassuring to know that brain tumours are in fact extremely rare. Most children are perfectly well in-between headaches, and this is always a very encouraging sign, but on the other hand, if your child should be uncharacteristically lethargic, has lost his appetite and is unduly clumsy (perhaps walking into doorways or falling over for no apparent reason), the doctor should be consulted urgently. A headache which is accompanied by vomiting and occurs first thing in the morning is a particularly worrying sign.

Medication

Some medications can cause headache. There are not many which children take that do this, but amongst them the anticonvulsants used for epilepsy, anti-inflammatories and some antibiotics can prove problematical.

WHAT CAN YOU DO?

If your child complains of headache, ask him where the pain is. Younger children will often say that it is all over the head, although older children may describe pain at the back of the head or just behind the eyes if they have developed a tension headache. Obviously, if the child has had a bang on the head, there will be localised pain at that site. A parent can feel for any tender spots if they suspect a minor head injury has occurred, and it is always worth checking a child's temperature since infection is often the cause of a headache.

If the headaches are related to school attendance, then it is well worth asking the child sympathetically if he has any concerns or worries. Sometimes teachers can be helpful in this situation. If either parent suffers with migraine, then headaches associated with nausea and vomiting in your child could well be due to the same condition, and any trigger factors will be worth avoiding. Certain aspects of the diet could be triggering the migraine, so a chat with the doctor or dietician would be useful.

There is no reason why paracetamol should not be used in most instances of headache, but first try giving your child a drink and a snack if the headaches seem to occur before meals when he is hungry. There are certain conditions, however, which can produce characteristic headaches, that require urgent attention from the doctor, and all parents should be aware of these. Meningitis is perhaps the most important one, so if fever, neck stiffness, confusion, drowsiness and dislike of bright light accompanies the headache, contact your doctor without delay. If your child has a headache and you have already tried using paracetamol to relieve it to no avail, again your doctor should check things out. Also, any child who is continuously vomiting, complaining of blurred or double vision, or has a headache that wakes him at night, again needs a full physical examination to discover the exact cause. Recurring headaches in children under the age of five and headaches which become progressively worse at any age should never be left unexplained.

WHAT CAN THE DOCTOR DO?

Doctors need to work through all the possible causes of sudden or recurrent headache in order to come up with an explanation. A full physical examination should be carried out, including a look at the back of the eyes using a special torch called an ophthalmoscope which can identify the signs of any raised pressure from within the head. The blood pressure should be checked, and if necessary referral to hospital for further investigations can be arranged. Treatment will depend on the underlying cause.

IF YOU REMEMBER NOTHING ELSE, REMEMBER THESE THREE THINGS

1   Headaches in children are common but seldom serious.

2   Headaches associated with vomiting, neck stiffness and drowsiness require immediate medical attention.

3   Recurrent or worsening headaches always require full physical examination and tests.

Hearing Problems

Hearing problems will affect as many as fifteen per cent of children at some stage. Some will have hearing difficulties from birth, but others will have entirely normal hearing until they run into trouble later on. Hearing loss at any time is extremely serious in children, since it may significantly affect their speech development and, to a greater or lesser extent, disrupt their education at school. In an older child who is already at school, the onset of deafness may affect not only the quality of school work, but also the child's general behaviour. Any child who does not hear well becomes frustrated, angry and bad-tempered and obviously misses a great deal of what is being said around him. Such a child will tend to turn the radio or TV up very loudly and miss simple commands that his parents give him. On the other hand, if you are suspicious about your child's hearing, you must first make absolutely sure that the child is listening attentively since young children become easily engrossed and preoccupied in toys and games, and although they may hear the sound of your voice, they do not necessarily register what you are saying. This is known as selective deafness. In younger children and babies, any hearing problems are harder to spot and deafness in a child can easily be missed unless regular checks are carried out and the parents remain vigilant.

Developmental checks in babies

A newborn baby should hear normally and may jump or appear startled in the vicinity of a loud noise. As a reflex action the baby may raise his arms, as he does to any sudden stimuli. By the time the baby is just a month old, he is quite capable of quietening and listening to familiar sounds. He may blink his eyes, stop sucking his dummy (if he has one) and may even find listening to the sound more interesting than crying. At three months, a baby who can hear will generally babble away quite happily, listening to the sound of his own voice and smiling at the reassuring sound of his mother's voice. At this stage he can also turn towards the source of a sound. At nine months, a baby will listen attentively to familiar sounds, will make a variety of different noises himself, and will move his head to locate even fairly quiet sounds. By eighteen months he should be able to say about half a dozen words clearly.

This pattern of hearing development is normal and is one which the health visitor will check for regularly, performing hearing tests at eight months, eighteen months and if there is any doubt about the child's speech or hearing, at three years. A child's speech is highly indicative of how well a child hears, and at eighteen months a toddler should be able to say single words clearly, by two and a half will start to run words together, and by the age of three will be able to speak in short sentences. *Any child who has delayed or defective speech must have his hearing checked by an expert as deafness could well be the reason speech has not fully developed.*

CAUSES OF DEAFNESS

* Glue ear (serous otitis media)

* Wax

* Foreign body

* Nerve damage

* Medications

Glue Ear

Glue ear is the commonest cause of loss of hearing in children under twelve, affecting as many as one in every five at one time or another. Even in minor degrees it can affect the child's speech, language and learning ability. In this condition the middle ear cavity becomes filled with a glue-like fluid which significantly reduces the transmission of sound from the eardrum, across the middle ear space to the inner ear. There are often no other symptoms at all, such as earache or discharge, although this may have occurred at various stages in the past, especially if the eardrum became perforated. Some older children may, however, complain of popping noises or ringing in their ears.

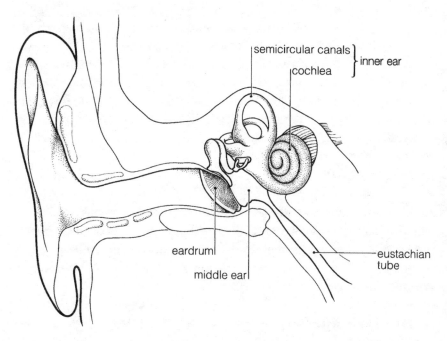

Cross-section of the ear and the hearing apparatus within

Glue ear occurs when the Eustachian tube becomes blocked as a result of infection or allergy, and the air pressure in the middle ear behind the eardrum can no longer equalise with the air pressure of the outside atmosphere. As air is gradually absorbed into the bloodstream from the middle ear cavity, the pressure decreases and draws fluid into the cavity. This situation may occur as a result of regular middle ear infections, frequent colds and coughs, enlarged adenoid glands, allergies such as hay fever and having parents who smoke. Premature babies are particularly susceptible and often there is a tendency for glue ear to run in families. It is also more common in children who have cleft palate, Down's syndrome or other congenital problems such as autism or cerebral palsy.

Wax

Some children produce more wax in their ear canals than others. If it builds up to the extent that it completely blocks the ear canal, then sudden hearing loss will result. Softening the wax with olive oil or sodium bicarbonate drops followed by gentle ear syringing by the doctor will generally solve this problem, although it is worth knowing that when wax is seen discharging from a child's ear the cause may often be a middle ear infection. The inflammation and heat caused by this condition tends to liquefy the wax, enabling it to run out of the ear. This may be accompanied by an infective discharge of pus, but only if there has been perforation of the eardrum.

Foreign Body

Small children have a penchant for inserting small objects into their ears such as beads and sweets. Sudden hearing loss in a child, particularly in one ear, will often turn out to be due to this unfortunate habit, so careful examination by the doctor should be arranged as soon as possible.

Nerve Damage

Any condition leading to damage of the nerves responsible for hearing, or that part of the brain which interprets sounds, may result in deafness. Most problems of this type are congenital, so the child is born with them, and a critical time in the development of hearing is the first six weeks after conception.

Something like twenty-five per cent of all children with cerebral palsy have some degree of deafness, and thirty per cent of children born to mothers who had rubella infection in the first three months of their pregnancy will be similarly affected (see page 116–117). Other infections, such as meningitis, can cause nerve damage at any age. Severe jaundice in a newborn child may also be responsible for deafness, and this is why urgent treatment is necessary for this condition. In older children, head injuries are not uncommon causes of hearing loss due to nerve damage.

Children with autism or ADD (attention deficit disorder) may appear to have hearing difficulties, but this is much more likely to be due to decreased social responsiveness in these children than to true deafness.

Medications

Certain medications administered to a child, or even to the child's pregnant mother prior to delivery, may be responsible for deafness as a side-effect. Examples include chloroquine used for the treatment of malaria, streptomycin used in the treatment of tuberculosis, gentamicin used in the treatment of septicaemia, (blood-poisoning) and vincristine used in the treatment of leukaemia.

WHAT CAN YOU DO?

The most important thing that a parent can do is to detect the hearing problem as early as possible. The longer any deafness continues, the greater the effect on the development of speech, language and learning. Although hearing loss will not always be obvious, a baby that does not seem to babble happily by itself at three months or an older child who turns the TV up loudly and misses half of what you say could well have problems. Similarly, a child whose behaviour deteriorates, who becomes irritable and bad tempered and whose school work takes a turn for the worse may well be suffering from hearing loss. If your child complains of frequent earaches, picks up coughs and colds easily, snores at night (suggestive of enlarged adenoids) then they will be more susceptible to hearing loss.

The health visitor will test small children routinely at about eight months and three years of age, but a parent should have their child examined by the doctor at any time if they suspect any degree of hearing loss. If some loss of hearing is found, then parents should also have a word with the teachers at school to explain the problem so that allowances can be made and the child seated nearer the front of the class.

WHAT CAN THE DOCTOR DO?

The doctor should liaise routinely with the health visitor when there is any suspicion of deafness in a child. The GP may carry out simple hearing tests and may look into the child's ear canal to detect problems both in the outer ear canal itself and in the middle ear cavity. He or she is also able to identify problems such as enlarged tonsils or adenoid glands at the back of the nose which, in turn, can block the Eustachian tubes, leading to otitis media. If there is any doubt about the size of the adenoids, a special soft tissue X-ray of the back of the nose and throat can be organised which will confirm any significant enlargement. Even small babies can now have their hearing tested in a specially designed instrument known as an acoustic cradle, and referral to an ear, nose and throat specialist can be organised by the GP if this is considered appropriate. An oto-acoustic emission test is an even more sophisticated test which, in the future, will probably be the first one carried out.

Glue ear is probably the commonest cause of deafness in children, and there is some debate as to how this should be treated. In the earlier stages, where infection seems to have been the trigger, antibiotics are often used to eradicate any persisting germs. Where allergy might also be involved, antihistamine tablets or syrup are often prescribed for several months at a time, and these have the additional benefit of reducing the outpouring of the fluid from the middle ear cavity which is responsible for much of the hearing loss. Where enlarged adenoids are a problem, these may be removed surgically in an operation known as an adenoidectomy, and at the same time grommets (tiny, hollow, dumb-bell shaped tubes) can be inserted into the eardrum to enable the fluid in the middle ear cavity to drain away and for it to aerate and become dry again.

Wax or foreign bodies in the outer ear canal may be removed, either with a special ear syringe or with tiny forceps, but you should never attempt this yourself. Medicines which are known to produce hearing loss as a side-effect should be avoided if at all possible.

Even in cases of permanent nerve damage, hearing aids (usually used in both ears) can be helpful from the age of six months upwards. Those children who do not benefit even from hearing aids can now be offered a cochlear implant for the worst ear, a device which bypasses the middle ear and sends amplified sounds direct to the organ of hearing itself, located deep within the skull. Special needs schools, and other facilities are now available for children with hearing difficulties to maximise their learning and general development.

IF YOU REMEMBER NOTHING ELSE, REMEMBER THESE THREE THINGS

1   Fifteen per cent or more of children will suffer from a degree of deafness at some stage, usually due to middle ear infections.

2   An older child who becomes bad tempered and whose school work deteriorates may well have a hearing problem.

3   Every child with delayed or defective speech should have his hearing tested by an expert.

Hyperactivity

Hyperactivity is a fashionable term often banded around these days, though true hyperactivity is rare. Most children can be over-active at times, their natural energy and exuberance spilling over into over-stimulated and excited behaviour. Any active and restless child can be difficult to cope with, particularly in a large family living in cramped or unsuitable accommodation. Usually, however, these episodes of frenetic agitation are short lived and temporary.

True hyperactivity is another thing entirely. Such children are also overactive, excitable and constantly restless but their concentration is poor, their attention span short and they are slow learners as a result. They seem never to be able to finish one task before going on to the next, their mood changes suddenly, they exhibit frequent temper tantrums and may be aggressive and bully other children. As they grow older, they touch and break things frequently and are generally destructive. They find it hard to cope with criticism, they are distracted easily, impulsive, and frequently seem clumsy and poorly coordinated. Hyperactive children may also be unaffectionate towards other children and may sleep particularly badly.

Such unmanageable symptoms are seen in as few as one to two per cent of all children and for some reason boys seem to be affected about five times as often as girls. Interestingly, there may also be a family history of such behaviour. The problem is present when the child is still a baby and he may sleep little and cry a lot. Otherwise known as hyperkinetic syndrome, attention deficit disorder (ADD) or minimal brain dysfunction, these symptoms are best corrected at an early stage since there is growing evidence that neglected hyperactive children may otherwise go on to practise criminal activities as adults.

Nobody really knows what causes the symptoms of hyperactivity but there is undoubtedly both a genetic and environmental component. Some authorities favour minimal brain dysfunction as a cause, although there is no physical evidence that this exists. Allergies and sensitivities to pollen, dust and chemicals have also been incriminated. Twenty per cent of hyperactive children experience a true food allergy, and in the last few years there has been intense interest in the idea that food 'intolerance' as opposed to 'allergy' accounts for many of the other cases.

Dr Feingold in San Francisco first hypothesised that food additives and preservatives might be to blame for hyperactivity, and he also suggested that something like eighty per cent of such children might improve with dietary adjustment. Some scientists have wondered whether a deficiency of the enzymes in the intestine that detoxify food additives could lead to behavioural changes in a child, in the same way that certain foods may trigger migraine or gout in adults. Those who support the idea of a dietary cause of hyperactivity point to the rise in incidence of the condition in the last twenty years which has coincided with the increased consumption of convenience foods which are rich in artificial additives and preservatives. Most doctors, however, believe that even if foodstuffs are a cause of hyperactivity, it is only in a small number of cases (five per cent).

The truth is that all children, hyperactive or not, can exhibit many of the symptoms of hyperactivity to some degree at some stage of their childhood. Many will demonstrate emotional misconduct of some kind, though more as a result of family tensions, lack of discipline or an unsettled home life or school environment than from any reaction to what they are eating or drinking. It is important for parents not to feel guilty about this. We all do our best, but no-one is perfect and our children are bound to suffer a little from the ups and downs of normal life. Whatever the causes, parents need some guidance as to what they can do about it.

WHAT CAN YOU DO?

All children respond well to a regular routine and this is particularly true of hyperactive children. It is because they are extremely restless and have a short concentration span that they respond to having their daily life organised largely for them. This can be difficult and time-consuming, but it works.

Part of the regular routine should be the provision of 'quality time' which the parents can enjoy with their child. The child will benefit from a methodical and patient approach to learning, for example following a story through, finishing a jigsaw puzzle or completing a drawing. There is no substitute for parental guidance in this, and occasionally the parent may in fact be the only person who has the commitment and patience to do it. Many hyperactive children are clumsy and badly coordinated anyway, so practising fine tasks requiring manual dexterity is especially important.

Hyperactive children characteristically flit from one activity to the next, leaving a trail of wreckage behind them. Try to fix their attention on one thing for longer periods so that they become constructive rather than destructive. Attempt to discover which things they are most interested in and concentrate on these.

You cannot restrain a hyperactive child all the time. In fact, there are considerable advantages in putting by a set period every day, as part of the regular routine, for totally wild, undisciplined and frenetic activity. This acts as a safety valve – a means of blowing off sufficient steam so that a more sedate and organised existence can subsequently be achieved. It also gives the parents or teachers a break and interrupts the constant cycle of restraint followed by rebellion which hyperactive children otherwise experience.

WHAT CAN THE DOCTOR DO?

The GP may not witness to any great extent the nature of the hyperactive child's behaviour, but he or she can certainly imagine what is going on from the accounts of the child's parents and teachers. Hyperactive children in my surgery usually make themselves known by constantly fiddling with all the medical equipment, emptying the toybox all over the floor, opening all the filing cabinets and constantly pestering their parents. Much can be gained by observing how the parents themselves react – some may be totally unaware that there is a problem, whilst others appear to have given up the unequal struggle long ago.

Psychologists may be sceptical about the existence of true hyperactivity and the value of dietary change, but since some allergists, or clinical ecologists as they increasingly like to be called, are claiming to improve up to eighty per cent of such children, referral to these hospital clinics is worth considering. There is little else to offer medically – except perhaps the use of ritalin for a trial period in certain cases. Ritalin is a central nervous system stimulant which many parents of children with attention deficit disorder report great success with. If allergists decide that there may be a dietary problem, the complex process of elimination diets can begin, requiring at least three weeks of painstaking work on behalf of the parents whereby an attempt is made to discover which dietary factors may be responsible for the child's problem.

IF YOU REMEMBER NOTHING ELSE, REMEMBER THESE THREE THINGS

1   Hyperactive behaviour is much more likely to be due to heredity and problems within the family than to diet.

2   Hyperactive children should be allowed a set time each day for wild and uncontrolled activity within a framework of organised and disciplined routine.

3   Clinical psychologists and clinical allergists can offer help to most hyperactive children and occasionally drug therapy may be indicated in certain cases.

Itching

Itching is a common symptom in children, and it may be widespread or confined to one specific area of the body. Itchy spots are usually due to allergies, insect bites or infections such as chickenpox (see pages 115 to 130). Less often, there is itching all over the body with no rash or spots whatsoever to show for it. In such cases, both psychological and physical factors may be responsible.

GENERALISED ITCHING

CAUSES OF GENERALISED ITCHING

---

* Allergy

* Eczema

* Infection

* Scabies

* Fungal infection

* Chilblains

Allergy

By far the most common cause of generalised itching is some form of allergy. This may produce individual spots, say after an insect bite, or more generalised spots or rashes after eating a specific type of food, taking certain types of medication or being in contact with an allergenic chemical. All told, there are a vast number of trigger factors which may produce allergy, the commonest being dietary factors, medicines, wool and nylon materials in clothing, biological washing powders, detergents in the form of soaps and shampoos, fur from domestic animals, plants and the house dust mite (see page 449)

Urticaria (hives) is a very characteristic form of allergic rash where there are swollen, pink weals as well as red blotches which come and go very quickly. It is common in the under fives.

WHAT CAN YOU DO?

The first thing to do with an itchy allergic rash is to try to identify the cause. This can be difficult as there are so many trigger factors, and also because when the skin becomes sensitised to one source of irritation it can become sensitive to others as well. Once a trigger factor is identified, it should obviously be avoided, and this may mean not using synthetic fibres such as nylon, woollen garments, biological washing powders, soaps, bubble baths, shampoos and sometimes avoiding contact with pets as well.

The environment can be made less allergenic with help and advice from your health visitor and doctor, and there is no reason why you cannot treat the itching symptomatically before your doctor is consulted. The skin should generally be kept cool, as the warmer it is the greater the itching is likely to become. Calamine lotion is very soothing, and the addition of a little sodium bicarbonate to the bath water may be worthwhile. Antihistamines can be bought over the counter in syrup and tablet form to stop skin irritation, and these will also help if your child is not sleeping because of the itching. Some of the older forms of antihistamine are particularly useful in this situation as they quickly induce drowsiness.

WHAT CAN THE DOCTOR DO?

Often the doctor may be able to identify the cause of the allergy so that the allergenic substance can be avoided. This can be done in a number of ways.

Skin prick tests involve placing spots of selected allergen solutions on the soft skin with the tip of a tiny needle. This allows a small amount of each allergen into the outer layer of skin, and the reaction is looked at after 15 to 30 minutes. Common allergen challenge solutions include cat and dog fur, grass pollen and house dust mite, although specialist centres may also test for allergens such as other animals' fur, feathers, tree pollens and a range of fungi.

Skin contact tests involve placing allergens directly onto the skin, or on skin that has been thinned by single sellotape application and then removed, without the need for any needle-pricking. These are used especially for contact allergies and suspected food allergies, and for other types of reaction where pre-prepared allergen solutions are not easily available.

Other tests include food challenge tests and provocation tests, but these are potentially dangerous and should always be conducted under strict supervision in specialist centres where treatment for anaphylaxis is immediately available.

Generally speaking, any doctor should try to diagnose the cause of the allergy from the child's symptoms and circumstances. Despite the fact that allergy testing is available, there is no strong evidence that it can successfully predict clinical allergy, and even less that it can influence useful and effective therapy. It should also never be forgotten that some tests are potentially hazardous. Because of this, and the fact that time and resources are limited, most doctors rely mainly on symptomatic relief of the itching using oral, non-sedating antihistamines and steroid creams.

IF YOU REMEMBER NOTHING ELSE, REMEMBER THESE THREE THINGS

1   Allergy is the commonest cause of generalised itching.

2   Once the trigger factor is identified, the allergen may be avoided.

3   Treatment involves antihistamines, calamine lotion and steroid creams.

Eczema

Eczema is a chronic inflammatory condition of the skin producing intense itching (see pages 142 to 150). The distribution of the rash is usually typical, with the surfaces where the joints flex being most severely affected. Dry, scaly, thickened and sometimes weepy patches occur at the front of the elbows, the back of the knees, the front of the wrists and over the face and neck. Sometimes the itching is so severe that intense scratching leads to bleeding and secondary infection of the areas with bacteria.

WHAT CAN YOU DO?

In most cases there is a strong family history of eczema, but there are a number of exacerbating factors which can make the symptoms worse. If these can be avoided, the discomfort suffered by the child can be reduced. Dietary restrictions, and avoiding biological washing powders and medicated soaps and shampoos are helpful. Cotton clothes should be worn against the skin as opposed to wool or synthetic materials, and the child's home should be made as allergy-free as possible.

WHAT CAN THE DOCTOR DO?

Once every effort has been made to prevent the occurrence of the eczema as far as possible, the main treatment of established eczema involves the use of antihistamine syrups and tablets, antibiotics to eradicate bacteria and the use of aqueous cream and emollients to moisturise the skin. In addition, hydrocortisone cream can be applied to reduce inflammation within the skin itself.

IF YOU REMEMBER NOTHING ELSE, REMEMBER THESE THREE THINGS

1 Itching caused by eczema occurs in characteristic areas of the body.

2 Trigger factors make the itching worse.

3 Treatment requires the use of antihistamines, emollients, hydrocortisone cream and antibiotics.

Infection

Certain infections may produce itching, especially chickenpox, cold sores and shingles (see pages 155 to 160). All of these begin with tingling and itching, swiftly followed over the next few days by a crop of sore, water-filled blisters which burst and then crust over. In shingles and cold sores, the irritation is limited to a localised area of skin, but in chickenpox the blisters may occur all over the body.

WHAT CAN YOU DO?

The itching produced by viral infections may be treated symptomatically with the use of warm salt-water bathing and the application of calamine lotion. In cold sores and other herpes-type infections where the problem is recurrent, the application of antiviral cream as soon as the symptoms start is helpful.

WHAT CAN THE DOCTOR DO?

In chickenpox, if the blisters begin to ooze and weep there is the strong possibility of secondary infection with bacteria, in which case antibiotics can be prescribed. In shingles and cold sores, the doctor can prescribe antiviral creams which will reduce the severity and duration of attacks considerably.

IF YOU REMEMBER NOTHING ELSE, REMEMBER THESE THREE THINGS

1   Certain infections may produce blisters which itch.

2   Antihistamines relieve much of the itching.

3   Antiviral and antibacterial preparations help to limit infection.

Scabies

Scabies produces an intensely itchy rash, particularly in the skin creases at the front of the wrists, in the webs of the fingers and in the groin area. The itching is caused by an allergy to the scabies mite which burrows under the skin to lay its eggs. In addition to the tiny, pearly-grey lumps below the skin, there may be small, red tracks where the burrows lie. The itching is characteristically much worse at night when the child is warm in bed. World-wide, scabies infestations are widespread in most communities.

WHAT CAN YOU DO?

If you suspect your child's itching is due to scabies then he should be examined by the health visitor or doctor, who may be able to see the burrows with a magnifying glass. Specific treatment with an insecticide lotion will be necessary and the child's clothing and bedclothes will need to be washed at high temperature and then hot-ironed to prevent recurrences of the infection. Other children living in the house should also be examined carefully, as close physical contact can pass the infestation on.

WHAT CAN THE DOCTOR DO?

Once the doctor has confirmed the diagnosis, he or she can supply

---

IF YOU REMEMBER NOTHING ELSE, REMEMBER THESE THREE THINGS

1   The typical scabies itch is much worse at night.

2   Scabies is often first seen on the front of the wrists, in the webs of the fingers and in the groin area.

3   Insecticide skin lotion will eradicate the problem, but steroid creams and antihistamines will reduce the immediate symptom of intense itching.

---

the special insecticide lotion for use at home. After a warm bath, the lotion is applied from the neck downwards and left on for a period of 24 hours before it is rinsed off. Parents should be warned that although the first application usually kills off all the mites, a second application just to make sure is recommended after seven days, and the itching may continue, despite successful treatment, for up to a fortnight.

Fungal Infection

Fungal infection may produce a mild itching of the skin, whether it is thrush producing a form of nappy rash, ringworm producing athlete's foot, a groin rash or scalp problems. There is generally a characteristic rash and the condition is easily treated.

WHAT CAN YOU DO?

Most fungal infections thrive in a warm, moist environment. If the skin can be kept dry at all times, fungal infection may be prevented. Applying talc to the skin and wearing clothes and shoes which allow the skin to breathe are a good idea. Simple antifungal foot powders may be sufficient to eradicate early infections.

WHAT CAN THE DOCTOR DO?

If there is any doubt about the diagnosis, skin scrapings of the rash can be taken and the presence of the fungus confirmed by examining them under the microscope. Antifungal treatment in the form of cream is effective.

IF YOU REMEMBER NOTHING ELSE, REMEMBER THESE THREE THINGS

1   Fungal infections may produce a mild itch.

2   Diagnosis can be confirmed by the doctor taking skin scrapings and examining them under the microscope.

3   Antifungal cream is generally effective within a week, but if symptoms persist a localised allergy becomes more likely.

Chilblains

Chilblains are caused basically by a hypersensitivity to cold conditions. First of all the child's fingers become blanched and numb, but then as they warm up again, for example when the child comes indoors, they become red and itchy. Chilblains generally affect the hands and feet, but the ankles and the back of the legs can suffer too.

WHAT CAN YOU DO?

A child who is prone to chilblains should obviously keep his extremities warm by wearing thermal gloves and socks and using thermal insoles in his shoes whenever he plays outside. Sometimes talc can be soothing once the chilblains have started, but the child should be prevented from scratching as breaks in the skin will merely make the condition worse.

WHAT CAN THE DOCTOR DO?

Other than giving the above advice, the doctor can prescribe special vasodilator cream for severe cases which prevents the spasm in the small blood vessels of the skin that triggers the problem in the first place. These creams contain menthol and camphor amongst other things and are sometimes known as rubifacients.

IF YOU REMEMBER NOTHING ELSE, REMEMBER THESE THREE THINGS

1   Chilblains are caused by a sensitivity to cold weather conditions.

2   They are seen predominantly on the fingers and toes.

3   If thermal gloves and socks do not prevent the condition, vasodilator creams may help.

Anal Itching

The commonest cause of itching around the anus is threadworm infection. The threadworm is a tiny, slender, white worm about a centimetre long and which resembles a short piece of dental floss or white thread. The worms live just inside the anus and emerge mostly at night to lay eggs on the skin outside. Itching is therefore usually more severe at night and the child may be seen scratching through his pyjama bottoms. Scratching leads to the threadworm eggs being stuck under the fingernails which, if not washed and scrubbed, may contaminate food which is then eaten either by the child himself or by other people with whom he is in close contact. When this happens the eggs will hatch out in the human intestine within a fortnight, and thus the lifecycle of the threadworm is completed.

Sometimes the tiny worms can be seen when the child goes to the toilet, as little threads wriggling on the surface of the stool. Usually, however, the worms are not seen, and the only symptom is the child frequently scratching his bottom.

WHAT CAN YOU DO?

If you suspect that your child has threadworms, you can either obtain anti-worm treatment over the counter at the chemist or obtain a prescription from your doctor. The important thing to do is to make sure that all members of the family are treated at the same time and then again ten days later, as the condition may have inadvertently already been spread. Also, make sure that the child's fingernails are cut really short. Everyone should be scrupulously hygienic, washing and scrubbing their nails regularly. Girls as well as boys should be encouraged to wear pyjama bottoms if infection is suspected as this helps to prevent transmission.

WHAT CAN THE DOCTOR DO?

If there is any doubt about the diagnosis, the parents can apply a little Sellotape to the child's anal margin first thing in the morning, transfer it to a slide provided by the doctor, and then have it examined under the microscope. The existence of threadworm eggs can then be confirmed. Treatment consists of an anti-worm or anti-helmintic preparation which should be taken by every member of the family in case the infection has already spread.

Sometimes the doctor can determine that threadworms are not the cause of the itching, and that a localised form of dermatitis or fungal infection is responsible. If this is the case, anything which irritates the skin such as perfumed soaps and bubble baths should be avoided. Emollients and hydrocortisone cream are useful in localised forms of dermatitis, and antifungal creams are effective in treating conditions such as thrush or ringworm.

IF YOU REMEMBER NOTHING ELSE, REMEMBER THESE THREE THINGS

1   Persistent anal itching is almost always caused by threadworm.

2   All members of the family need to be treated if threadworm is the cause.

3   Localised dermatitis or fungal infections should be excluded before starting treatment for threadworm.

Itching of the Scalp

There are a number of conditions that can lead to an itchy scalp, the commonest in children being infestation with head lice. But seborrhoeic eczema, fungal infections and psoriasis may cause it too.

CAUSES OF AN ITCHY SCALP

* Head lice

* Seborrhoeic eczema

* Fungal infection

* Psoriasis

Head Lice

These live on and suck blood from the scalp. They leave very small red spots on the skin which are intensely itchy and lead to scratching. Sometimes the skin can become inflamed and infected with bacteria, in which case oozing and weeping may be seen as well. The female lice lay batches of eggs or 'nits' which attach themselves firmly to the individual hairs close to the scalp. They hatch in about seven days and live on the child's scalp for several weeks at a time. Contrary to popular belief, all social classes of children are affected by head lice and clean, regularly shampooed hair is more vulnerable to the lice than unwashed, greasy hair.

Epidemics of head lice infestation commonly occur in schools, so if your child is affected you should certainly let the teachers know so that they can warn other parents and encourage consultation with health visitors and doctors.

WHAT CAN YOU DO?

If your child is perpetually scratching his head, examine his hair and scalp carefully for evidence of nits and spots. The nits are easily confused with dandruff or dust, so if in doubt consult your health visitor or doctor.

Once head lice have been diagnosed, treatment should begin

immediately, and all hairbrushes and combs which the child uses should be boiled to eradicate any attached eggs.

Resistance to some types of insecticide can occur, so if the treatment you are using appears to be ineffective consult your health visitor or doctor for further advice.

WHAT CAN THE DOCTOR DO?

The visual appearance of the nits and of the scalp is so character-istic that a doctor can usually make the diagnosis by clinical examination alone. Lotions containing malathion or carbaryl kill the lice and the nits very quickly. It is applied to the hair and scalp and should be washed off after about twelve hours. The hair should then be combed thoroughly with a special fine-toothed comb to remove all dead nits and lice.

IF YOU REMEMBER NOTHING ELSE, REMEMBER THESE THREE THINGS

1   Head lice are the commonest cause of an itchy scalp in children.

2   Head lice can occur in children with clean or dirty hair.

3   Insecticide lotions and shampoos are effective in treating head lice.

Seborrhoeic Eczema

Seborrhoeic eczema is not nearly as itchy as ordinary eczema and occurs usually in the first three months of life, clearing within a few weeks of its onset. It occurs anywhere where there are numerous sebaceous or oil-producing glands in the skin, and it may well be the presence of maternal hormones in the baby's body which stimulates the activity of these glands. The scalp is commonly affected, other areas being the groin (where it may look like extensive nappy rash), the armpits, the neck, the cheeks and behind the ears. On the scalp, there is typically yellowish, greasy scaling, a condition more commonly known as cradle cap.

WHAT CAN YOU DO?

It is tempting to want to pick off the greasy-looking crusts, but it is better to use a special cradle cap shampoo which you can buy from the chemist to remove the dead skin scales more easily. Olive oil is a simple home remedy, though it has no active ingredient and merely softens the skin making the scales easier to remove. Some creams containing salicylic acid and sulphur cream can prove more effective than shampoos, (I recommend Pragmatar) and another very effective cream contains a mixture of mild hydro-cortisone and ten per cent urea (Calmurid HC).

WHAT CAN THE DOCTOR DO?

The doctor should reassure parents that although the appearance of seborrhoeic eczema is unattractive, it will start to clear up within two to three months and be gone by six months. He or she can recommend skin softeners for mild cases and prescribe more potent creams if necessary.

IF YOU REMEMBER NOTHING ELSE, REMEMBER THESE THREE THINGS

1   Seborrhoeic eczema produces a mildly irritant honey-coloured crust of dry, dead skin on the scalp.

2   It may also affect the cheeks, the neck, the armpits, behind the ears and the groin.

3   Urea and hydrocortisone creams are amongst the most effective remedies.

Fungal Infection

Fungal infections of the scalp usually produce circular, well-localised patches of reddened skin with overlying loss or thinning of hair. Close examination may show shortened hairs which have broken at a centimetre or so above the scalp. There may also be other areas of fungal infection on the body, particularly in the groin and between the toes.

WHAT CAN YOU DO?

Have a look for other possible areas of fungal infection on your child's skin and take him to the doctor if in doubt.

WHAT CAN THE DOCTOR DO?

If the diagnosis is uncertain, skin scrapings can be taken for micro-scopic examination. If fungal elements are seen, antifungal creams applied regularly for at least two weeks after the rash seems to have completely faded will cure the problem. The rash is only mildly itchy, so usually no antihistamine medication is required.

IF YOU REMEMBER NOTHING ELSE, REMEMBER THESE THREE THINGS

Fungal infections of the scalp:

1   produce patchy hair loss;

2   are only mildly itchy;

3   can be treated effectively with antifungal cream.

Psoriasis

As well as affecting the back of the elbows and front of the knees, psoriasis most commonly affects the scalp. There is usually a positive family history and the condition is often triggered initially by a sore throat or other mild infection. It generally tends to clear up within three months of its onset, although it is likely to recur at some stage within the next five years.

Nobody is clear as to what causes psoriasis, but the underlying problem is an over-rapid production of skin cells which heap up in thick layers. The appearance is of an oval patch of reddy-pink skin with silvery flaking scales over the surface.

WHAT CAN YOU DO?

Psoriasis is unusual in children below the age of five so a doctor should certainly see the scalp rash in order to exclude other conditions. Normal exposure to natural sunlight is helpful, and the regular and fastidious application of the prescribed creams will hasten improvement.

WHAT CAN THE DOCTOR DO?

In children, the mildest ointments which control the skin condition should be used, but in severe cases hydrocortisone cream and coal-tar preparations may be necessary. Dithranol is particularly useful in the more resistant forms of psoriasis, and short-contact regimes, where the cream is applied for thirty minutes every evening and then any excess cream wiped off, improve efficiency and reduce any possibility of burning or staining of the skin. Coal-tar solutions can also be prescribed for use in the bath.

IF YOU REMEMBER NOTHING ELSE, REMEMBER THESE THREE THINGS

1   Psoriasis of the scalp is mildly itchy.

2   It produces reddy-pink patches with overlying silvery scales.

3   Hydrocortisone and coal-tar preparations are effective treatments.

Jaundice

Jaundice is the medical name given to yellowing of the skin and the whites of the eyes due to the build-up of bilirubin, a yellow pigment produced by the breakdown of red blood cells in the body. Usually bilirubin is dealt with by the liver and excreted, however, when the liver is unable to handle all the bilirubin, it will build up in the bloodstream and become deposited in the eyes and skin. This may happen because of excess breakdown of red blood cells, failure of the liver cells to excrete the bilirubin into the bile ducts, or because there is an obstruction to the outflow of waste products from the liver itself. The most likely causes depend on the age of the child.

JAUNDICE IN NEWBORN BABIES

CAUSES OF JAUNDICE IN NEWBORN BABIES

* Physiological factors

* Rhesus disease

* Liver abnormalities and infections

Physiological Factors

In the first few days after birth, the majority of babies will develop a slight degree of jaundice because of the relative immaturity of the liver. This is known as physiological jaundice. Babies' livers do not possess enough enzymes to break down the normal amounts of bilirubin in their bodies, resulting in jaundice. For this reason, premature babies are especially vulnerable to this condition. The jaundice is usually noticed within a day or two of birth and normally lasts for four to five days, but slightly longer if anything in breast-fed babies. Any newborn baby who becomes jaundiced has a tiny blood sample taken through a simple heel prick test for bilirubin analysis. If the level rises too high, treatment can be instigated to reduce the level of circulating bilirubin which, if left untreated, could produce potential brain damage and convulsions. Treatment consists of encouraging the baby to drink plenty of fluids and lying the naked baby under a special blue light – a treatment known as phototherapy.

Rhesus Disease

In this condition the baby's red blood cells are prematurely destroyed by the mother's antibodies. This occurs where there is a hereditary mismatch between the mother's blood and that of her baby, and in the past 'rhesus incompatibility' was a common cause of stillbirth and neonatal disease. Today, thankfully, the condition is rare since rhesus-negative women are given an injection of anti-D immunoglobulin soon after the birth of a rhesus-positive baby. They should also have this injection following miscarriage and any surgical procedure during pregnancy such as amniocentesis. This is to prevent rhesus incompatability problems in future pregnancies – the first baby will not be affected. During childbirth there is risk of the baby's blood entering the maternal blood circulation. If the baby is rhesus-positive and the mother is rhesus-negative, the maternal blood then develops antibodies to destroy the 'alien' positive blood cells, and these antibodies remain permanently in her circulation. Consequently, should she then fall pregnant with another rhesus-positive baby, the antibodies in her circulation would cross the placenta and destroy her baby's positive blood. When rhesus disease occurs, the baby's liver is unable to handle the large quantities of bilirubin produced from destroyed blood cells and jaundice as well as anaemia occurs.

Liver Abnormalities and Infections

Congenital abnormalities of the liver and its bile ducts through which waste materials are excreted sometimes occur. The urine is dark and the stools quite often light in colour, and this kind of jaundice classically produces itchy skin from a build-up of bile salts. Any jaundice that persists after ten days should be rigorously investigated.

JAUNDICE IN OLDER CHILDREN

CAUSES OF JAUNDICE IN OLDER CHILDREN

* Infectious hepatitis

* Glandular fever

* Inherited blood disorders

* Solvent abuse

Infectious Hepatitis

This infection of the liver is due to a virus which is generally contracted from contaminated food or water supplies. It is common in those parts of the world where sanitation and hygiene are inadequate, although it is certainly seen in Britain too. The illness can occur without symptoms, particularly in young children, but may begin with loss of appetite, nausea and vomiting, a general feeling of malaise and mild abdominal pain. About a week after these symptoms, the jaundice begins. Since there is also a failure to excrete bilirubin, the stools become pale and the urine dark. When the doctor examines the child he or she will generally feel for the liver in the upper right-hand corner of the abdomen, and the edge of it may occasionally feel tender. The child will continue to feel weak and tired for some time, ranging from as little as a fortnight to up to six months. Most children are better off resting up completely in bed until they are really well, and most are off school for a period of about a month.

Glandular Fever

Glandular fever, or infectious mononucleosis, is a viral infection that is not uncommon in older children, and which begins with a typical sore throat with enlarged glands at the front of the neck. It may persist much longer than normal tonsillitis, however, and the child often feels noticeably exhausted. Being a generalised virus, it affects not just the glands in the neck but also the spleen and liver, resulting in a few instances in mild jaundice. A simple blood test confirms the diagnosis.

Inherited Blood Disorders

Sickle-cell anaemia and thalassaemia are both examples of inherited blood disorders which occur as a result of a defective gene. Sickle-cell anaemia is seen mainly in Afro-Caribbean people and occasionally in people of Mediterranean origin. The red cells themselves are abnormal and they distort into a sickle shape when the amount of oxygen in the blood is reduced. As a result of the breakdown of these cells, jaundice may occur along with tiredness, headaches, breathlessness on exertion and pallor.

In thalassaemia which is common in the Mediterranean region, the middle-east and south-east Asia, the genetic fault lies in the production of haemoglobin which is the oxygen-carrying pigment in red blood cells. Affected red blood cells are destroyed easily, leading to anaemia and jaundice. These symptoms usually occur in the first three to six months following birth.

Solvent Abuse

Regrettably, drug-taking in schools is very widespread and children as young as eight or nine are sometimes being led astray. At this age, the substances which are easiest to obtain and still relatively cheap are solvents, and regular abuse of these may occasionally produce jaundice. Other signs include ulcers around the mouth, personality changes including euphoria and moodiness, agitation and a flushed facial appearance. But the immediate signs of solvent abuse, namely the intoxication, are often totally absent as the effects wear off within a few minutes or so. The greatest risk to the child from inhaling solvent fumes, however, is sudden death from cardiac arrest, or from spasm of the vocal cords which effectively produces suffocation.

WHAT CAN YOU DO?

A parent with a newborn baby who develops neonatal jaundice merely needs to keep an eye on the depth of the yellow colour of the skin and to give the baby plenty of fluids. This can be difficult at times, because a jaundiced baby is often drowsy, and a drowsy baby is generally reluctant to feed. The midwife will carry out tests to keep an eye on the bilirubin level using a special visual monitor, and this will be done whether the baby is still in hospital or is at home. In rare instances, when the bilirubin level rises too much, the baby will be readmitted to hospital for phototherapy, a treatment in which a special blue light is shone on the skin. Milder cases merely need to be kept under observation as the level will fall naturally within a few days. In the meantime, placing your baby by a sunny window, where ultraviolet light can fall on the baby's skin, is a good idea. If at any time the jaundice continues for more than ten days, or if the baby is otherwise unwell, the doctor should always be consulted.

Older children who have previously been fit and healthy and who suddenly lose their appetite and become nauseous and jaundiced may well be showing the first signs of infectious hepatitis. Sometimes the family may have recently been abroad on holiday to a place where hygiene is wanting, but it is quite possible to contract infectious hepatitis from eating out in this country too. A child with this condition should be put to bed for complete rest, kept comfortable, and given plenty of fluids. It is imperative to pay careful attention to hygiene at home, since this is a condition that can be passed on to other members of the family if food and drink is contaminated. Children become bored quickly lying in bed, but by and large it is a bad idea to allow the child up too early as this can cause the condition to take longer to settle and fatigue can be considerable. In glandular fever, adequate rest is also necessary as too early a rehabilitation appears to produce a more protracted illness.

The inherited blood disorders – sickle-cell anaemia and thalassaemia – are potentially serious problems requiring specialist medical help in hospital. Solvent abuse is still relatively rare in children under twelve, but is certainly something that all parents should be aware of as it can occur in all parts of Britain and amongst all social classes. The parents are in the best possible position to prevent the problem in the first place and to do something about it once it occurs. Talking to your child about drug abuse at an early age is recommended, and should you suspect that your

---

IF YOU REMEMBER NOTHING ELSE, REMEMBER THESE THREE THINGS

1   Fifty per cent of all newborn babies develop a mild degree of jaundice in the first few days of life.

2   A newborn baby whose jaundice lasts for more than ten days or who is otherwise unwell should be referred to the doctor.

3   Any older child with jaundice must have the exact cause pinpointed by the doctor as a matter of urgency.

child is involved in it in any way, your doctor and many other professional and charitable organisations are available to help.

WHAT CAN THE DOCTOR DO?

The first thing the doctor needs to ascertain is the exact cause of the jaundice. If it is physiological jaundice or infectious hepatitis, the doctor can do little more than the parents, although he or she can certainly offer support and encouragement. Rhesus disease and liver abnormalities obviously require specialist intervention in hospital, as do the inherited blood disorders sickle-cell anaemia and thalassaemia.

Knock-knees

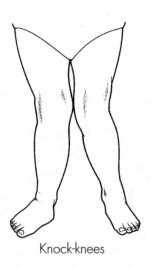

Knock-knees

Three-quarters of all children between the ages of three and five have knock-knees. That is to say, if they stand straight with their knees together their lower legs splay outwards so that their ankles do not touch. The gap between the ankles if measured will in almost all cases be less than ten centimetres. As the child grows older, and usually by the age of ten, the legs again change shape and become straight and parallel. If knock-knees remain to any significant degree after the age of ten, surgery can be performed. This involves breaking and realigning one of the longer bones in each leg, so it is reserved for severe cases only. In moderate cases wedges in the shoes can be used to achieve straightening. Doctors should always be aware of the possibility, albeit rare, of rickets, where the bones become softened as a result of vitamin deficiency. This is still seen in some Asian immigrant children as a result of inadequate diet and sunlight.

IF YOU REMEMBER NOTHING ELSE, REMEMBER THESE THREE THINGS

A specialist should always see a child with knock-knees if:

1 the knock-knees persist beyond the age of ten;

2 the measurement between the ankles, when the child stands straight with his knees together, is more than ten centimetres;

3 the inward bowing is in one leg only.

Limping and Leg Pains

Parents may be puzzled when they notice that their child is limping. The usual cause is some kind of injury, often resulting from a knock of some kind, but the child may not even remember how or when it occurred. Equally, there may be a joint sprain or muscle tear which the child does not immediately link to any particular activity or movement. These 'mechanical' causes of a limp are by far the most likely, but there are many others which may also be responsible.

Pain can cause a child to limp, and this may be the result of something as simple as excessively tight shoes squeezing the toe joints and pushing the toes themselves together. The skin may become chaffed and sore, and nipping and blisters may result. In older children, an in-growing toenail is another strong possibility. It is therefore well worth any parent looking for redness of the skin on the feet and double-checking to make sure that the child's shoes fit correctly. Looking at the child's legs for signs of cuts, splinters, swelling, bruising and redness, particularly over the joints, ankles

CAUSES OF LIMPING

* Injury

* Perthe's disease

* Slipped epiphysis

* Psychological problems

* Viral infections (especially 'flu)

* Joint conditions (arthritis)

* Bone disorders

* Congenital dislocation of the hip

and heels, may reveal the cause of the limp. It is also worth moving each joint in turn, particularly the hips and knees, to see if this triggers the pain. Occasionally lumps in the groin resulting from herniae or swollen glands (see pages 169 to 171) can produce discomfort, especially when the leg comes forward and the knee is raised high off the ground.

Usually, even where the cause of the problem is unknown, a child who limps will be symptom free after an overnight rest. If the problem persists the following day, then clearly the problem is not just one of a pebble in the shoe or a splinter in the heel and the doctor needs to be consulted.

Injury

The commonest cause of limping or leg pain is some kind of injury to any part of the lower limb. The trauma may be trivial or serious and although the event causing the problem is usually obvious it is not invariably so, especially in toddlers who sustain trauma during excited play and only notice discomfort the next day when swelling and bruising has occurred. For this reason it is advisable for any parent to have a good look for any sign of damage if their child is limping.

Perthe's Disease

Perthe's disease is a condition of the hip affecting children between the ages of two and ten. It happens when the blood supply to the top of the thighbone becomes insufficient, causing the ball part of the hip joint to become malformed. It varies in severity, and in advanced cases produces a permanent limp and unless it is treated leads to the development later on of osteoarthritis. A child complaining of a persistent limp should have not only the hips X-rayed, but also the knees, because sometimes this is where the pain is actually felt. X-rays are then carried out on a regular basis to monitor the progress of the treatment.

Slipped Epiphysis

Unlike adults' bones, which have stopped growing and are fully formed, children's bones are still enlarging and changing shape slightly. Growth occurs in a layer of cartilage attached near the end of the bone called the epiphysis. At the top of the thighbone, the epiphysis takes a great deal of weight and pressure, and the shearing forces produced are capable of causing the epiphysis to 'slip' so that it no longer sits neatly on top of the underlying bone. This is more common in boys than girls, is more likely in over-weight and tall individuals, and generally affects children aged between ten and fifteen. Again, pain and limping are the obvious signs and when the condition is confirmed by X-ray, surgery is required to correct it.

Psychological Problems

I have seen a number of children in my surgery whose anxious parents have brought them in because of a limp. Sometimes the limp may be quite dramatic, even melodramatic in fact, suggesting that there might be an element of 'acting' going on. If, after looking for swelling and redness and putting every joint in both legs through a full range of movement, nothing is found, it is well worth enquiring about any problems the child might have and how well he is getting on at school. It could well be that the limp is a devious way of avoiding having to go to school or playing games, although if the problem persists further investigations, including X-rays, should be carried out to exclude any underlying physical disorder.

Sometimes a child may develop a limp because of an acute sprain, but continues limping when this has got better because he enjoys the attention it attracts from his parents.

Viral Infection ('flu)

Viral infections commonly produce temperatures with aching muscles, weakness and pain in the limbs due to direct invasion of the body tissues by the virus. Sometimes there is an element of 'reactive' arthritis where the virus causes the body to produce inflammation in the joints themselves. This may happen in the hips, knees and ankles as well as anywhere else in the body, and sometimes occurs several weeks after the infection. In the acute illness there will usually be associated symptoms of runny nose, sore throat and cough, so the usual treatment consists of symptomatic relief in the form of paracetamol and bed rest. Any joint and muscle pain caused by viral infection will generally settle within three to seven days.

Joint Conditions (arthritis)

A number of different forms of arthritis may occur in children, although thankfully long-term, damaging arthritis is rare. Children often fall off their bicycles and play in dirty areas of the garden so infection from the skin may spread to joints producing septic arthritis, or osteomyelitis if the bone itself is affected. In both cases the area is extremely tender. Rheumatic fever is now very rare, although there is some evidence that it is on the increase again (see page 128). Pain, swelling and redness of the affected joints would be the signs to look for.

Bone Disorders

Occasionally disorders of the bones themselves can be responsible for a limp. Bacterial infection of bone, or osteomyelitis, is one example, although modern antibiotics are effective in both preventing and treating it. Another common condition is called Osgood–Schlatter's disease, which produces pain just below the knee around the knobble on the front of the lower leg. This is where the tendon of the thigh muscle joins the bone, and where the tendon becomes inflamed as a rapidly growing child becomes more physically active. In the past, people may have referred to this as an example of 'growing pains' and certainly the condition improves within a few months, although physiotherapy can speed up the healing process.

Certain blood disorders, including leukaemia, can produce pain in the bones, but this condition is relatively rare. At any rate the child would usually show other symptoms of this disorder such as anaemia and being generally unwell. Occasionally, benign cysts in bones, called osteomas, are present and these tend to produce pain at night and on exertion.

Congenital Dislocation of the Hip

This produces a long-standing and usually painless limp which has been present ever since the child first learned to walk, anywhere between the ages of eight and fifteen months. In general, a limp of this kind is due to something the child was born with, and although this might be muscular dystrophy, cerebral palsy or polio, congenital dislocation of the hip (CDH) is much more likely.

In CDH, the dislocated hip is present at birth, a condition affecting about 400 in every 100,000 babies. Girls are more commonly affected than boys, and it often runs in families. All newborn babies are examined at intervals in order to detect any signs of CDH, but if the diagnosis is missed a limp is likely to develop as the child begins to learn to walk. If the problem is corrected in infancy, using leg splints for about three months, there will usually be no long-term difficulties at all. When treatment is delayed, however, even traction or surgery entailing a long spell in hospital cannot guarantee normal walking in the future. So early detection and treatment is vital.

WHAT CAN YOU DO?

The first thing to do if your child has a limp is to look for any obvious injury. Is there any evidence of bruising, of tender muscles or joints? Is there a pebble in the shoe or sock, a cut anywhere, a splinter or even a blister from shoes that are too tight? Is there any redness, swelling or bruising? Does the child have a viral infection? If no mechanical problem can be found, look for any lumps in the groin and see whether it hurts to move the joints in any direction. If you think you have identified the source of the pain, allow 24 hours before doing anything, giving the child paracetamol if this helps. If, however, the pain and limp persists for longer than this, call the doctor so that further examination and investigation can be carried out.

WHAT CAN THE DOCTOR DO?

The doctor can examine each leg in turn, comparing one to the other, to attempt to identify any obvious abnormality. If he or she suspects an underlying physical problem or recent injury, the child can be referred directly to a casualty department or to an orthopaedic surgeon or rheumatologist for further evaluation.

IF YOU REMEMBER NOTHING ELSE, REMEMBER THESE THREE THINGS

1 Limping in a child is usually the result of an injury.

2 A child who limps for no apparent reason needs his hips and other joints examined carefully.

3 If the limp persists for more than 24 hours consult your doctor.

Loss of Appetite

'My child won't eat' is a common complaint made by parents. Complete loss of appetite for any length of time is unusual, the more common problem being dawdling over food or poor appetite in a constitutionally small child, since small children need less food to grow than big ones. The two central questions which need to be asked are: Has the child actually lost weight, and is the appetite considerably less than it has been recently?

Children often lose their desire for food quite suddenly when they suffer a simple illness such as an infection. This is especially true if the child has a temperature. Common infections such as sore throats, ear infections and gastroenteritis where there is diarrhoea and vomiting, are often responsible for loss of appetite. Sometimes an emotional upset can have the same effect. Appendicitis can have a sudden onset too, and in this instance the loss of appetite is accompanied by abdominal pain, vomiting, a slight temperature and, sometimes, constipation or slight diarrhoea. By and large, if the child wants to skip one or at most two meals within a 24-hour period, that is acceptable. But if the problem persists for longer than this, and particularly if the child is not drinking either, a significant physical cause should be sought.

Long-standing cases of loss of appetite will normally be associated with significant weight loss. Where no weight loss has occurred, it often turns out that the parents are merely being excessively anxious about how much and what type of food their child is eating. But this is a problem in itself and still needs to be addressed. It should never be forgotten, however, that in some cases there is a physical cause for loss of appetite, kidney infections and chronic asthma being two examples.

One of the important things for parents to understand is what constitutes a normal, healthy appetite in a child. It is also vital to realise that the growth rate of a baby slows down in the second six months of life. Mums and dads are often delighted at how much weight their baby puts on initially, and can become quite concerned when their weight gain slows down. At the age when children start to exert their own will and take control of their food intake, they become much more mobile and naturally leaner. You only have to look at their developmental growth charts to see this (see page 86). Some children inherit a constitutionally small build from their parents and their nutritional requirements will necessarily be smaller too. Others are naturally small or slow eaters compared with other children, but again this is not abnormal. There is a tendency in children between nine months and three years to have a rather negative approach to eating anyway. They like to play with their food and make a mess. They like to swill it around in their mouths and then spit it out. Most of all, they enjoy the extra attention they receive when their parents become concerned, irritable or extra affectionate in response to their apparent lack of appetite. The simple fact is that most children prefer to graze at regular intervals all day long rather than to sit down for three regulated, proper meals at set times.

WHAT CAN YOU DO?

If the child loses his appetite suddenly, or if a recent infection has brought it on, then clearly the doctor should be consulted and appropriate measures taken. If there has been any obvious weight loss, the same applies. On the other hand, if meal times have simply become a battle of wills between the child and his parent, some kind of strategy needs to be carefully worked out.

Force-feeding your child can be counterproductive. Any unpleasantness, threats or punishment simply become associated with food, and this will merely serve to make the problem worse. Bribing a child to eat should be avoided too. It does not take too long for the child to get used to such rewards, and he will soon start to eat nothing without some kind of negotiation with the parent. However tiresome it may be, it is worth remembering that children without underlying disease never starve themselves to death. It is incredibly frustrating at times to see food thrown around the room and smeared on the face, hair and clothing, but it is best to show no frustration or anger as this is likely to be interpreted by the child as extra attention which, of course, he desperately enjoys. It is better to calmly mop up any mess and end the meal after a set period of time.

Often parents find that a child with an eating problem will eat very much better in the presence of either other children who do eat well (particularly if they steal his food!), or a visiting adult they know, such as a grandparent. It is worth cutting down on snacks between meals as well, and sometimes it helps to eat as a family as the child is not then eating in isolation. It certainly helps if you give a child the food he prefers, though some children have a remarkably small repertoire of foods they enjoy, and these may not be sufficient to provide adequate all-round nutrition. If your child is finicky, other foods with different tastes and textures should sometimes be put on the plate or mixed with the foods with which he is already accustomed. The earlier this is achieved the better.

WHAT CAN THE DOCTOR DO?

The doctor should always see a child who has lost weight or whose loss of appetite may be caused by an underlying physical condition. In most cases the condition is short lived and trivial, but there are a number of serious disorders which will stop the child eating. A full examination should be carried out and any suspicion of weight loss or failure to gain weight should be kept under observation by using centile charts over a period of time. The doctor will often liaise with the health visitor who can visit the child at home regularly to see what goes on and how the child behaves at mealtimes. Any underlying condition will require the appropriate treatment.

IF YOU REMEMBER NOTHING ELSE, REMEMBER THESE THREE THINGS

1. Loss of appetite often just means that the child eats less than the parents want or expect him to.

2. Sudden loss of appetite is usually due to a simple infection.

3. Loss of appetite with weight loss requires investigation by the doctor.

Mouth Soreness

Although soreness in the mouth is quite common in children, it rarely causes severe problems unless the child is unable to feed or drink.

CAUSES OF MOUTH SORENESS

* Thrush infection

* Herpes infection (herpetic stomatitis)

* Hand, foot and mouth disease

* Aphthous ulcers

* Tooth bite

Thrush Infection

This fungal infection is particularly common in babies. Sometimes the mother's nipple may be quite sore and the child may have nappy rash as well as a result of widespread infection. The baby may appear quite fit and well most of the time but when he starts to feed, either from the nipple or the bottle, he sucks briefly and then starts to cry. The inside of the mouth is red and white spots may be noticed sticking to the lining. These can be distinguished easily from milk curds, which are often seen in the mouth after feeding and are much more easily removed.

Herpes Infection (herpetic stomatitis)

The herpes virus is the same one that causes cold sores and when a child comes across it for the first time it may produce large crops of ulcers inside the lips, on the tongue, over the gums and on the lining of the cheeks. The child, usually aged between four and twelve, will be quite unwell and tired and may complain of swelling and pain in his glands at the sides of his neck. If the ulcers are multiple and deep, drinking may become difficult, so the child may become dehydrated as well as suffering pain. In this case admission to hospital is sometimes required where general nursing care can be given and treatment with the antiviral agent Acyclovir given.

Hand, Foot and Mouth Disease

This infection is caused by a coxsackie virus and produces small epidemics. A trivial illness in children, it has nothing whatsoever to do with foot and mouth disease in cattle, merely producing a few flat, greyish blisters under the skin, particularly over the pads of the fingers and toes and sometimes inside the mouth. Occasionally, in older children and adults, the ulcers within the mouth can become a little sore.

Aphthous Ulcers

These tender, white ulcers are seen in older children, particularly when they are tired or run down. They may well be triggered by viruses, although crooked teeth and wearing braces may play a part. They tend to be short lived, clearing up on their own within four or five days, although the glands in the neck can be enlarged for a little while longer. Anxiety and stress can make them worse.

Tooth Bite

Children who accidentally bite the insides of their cheeks or their tongue may develop a small, whitish ulcer as a result. This is not uncommon, particularly in children who have crooked teeth, and recurrent problems should be referred to a dentist.

WHAT CAN YOU DO?

Babies who have thrush should have all their teats and bottles thoroughly sterilised. Dummies should have the same treatment, but are best not used at all until the thrush has cleared up. If the mother's nipples are sore, an antifungal cream should be applied to them to rule out the possibility of re-infection from this source. Antifungal gel is also available for the sore areas in the baby's mouth, but if a baby has nappy rash as well it suggests that there is thrush within the bowel which, if left untreated, can again re-infect the mouth. A better form of treatment is antifungal drops given to the baby by dropper in a dose of one millilitre, four times a day for five days. This eradicates thrush both within the mouth and within the bowel.

Older children with herpetic stomatitis may be relieved with the use of paracetamol and must be encouraged to drink as much as possible, even if it hurts to swallow. The teeth should be brushed gently and regularly, despite any minor discomfort, in order to avoid any secondary infection with bacteria. Hand, foot and mouth disease requires no treatment since the condition is trivial and short lived, but children who have tender aphthous ulcers in the mouth can have anaesthetic gel or tincture applied, or the doctor can prescribe tiny steroid tablets which are held against the ulcers with the tongue and will allow the ulcers to heal more quickly. Any tooth bites to the tongue or cheeks generally settle on their own, although salt-water gargles are helpful.

WHAT CAN THE DOCTOR DO?

Children with severe herpetic stomatitis who become dehydrated through not being able to swallow occasionally need to be treated with intravenous fluids in hospital, although this is rare. Most antifungal preparations are available on prescription and babies with thrush will generally require this form of treatment. Tiny steroid tablets are helpful for children suffering from recurrent aphthous ulcers, and where the child has enlarged lymph glands in the neck coupled with pain, the doctor will probably want to check that this settles down within a week or two.

Occasionally, recurrent soreness in the mouth, with or without ulceration, can be the first sign of a more serious underlying blood disorder, and blood tests and other investigations may become necessary.

IF YOU REMEMBER NOTHING ELSE, REMEMBER THESE THREE THINGS

1   The commonest cause of mouth soreness in babies is thrush infection.

2   In older children mouth soreness is usually due to aphthous ulcers.

3   Where dehydration or recurrent ulceration occurs, the doctor should be consulted.

Noisy Breathing

Breathing problems of one type or another are often reported in children, but the commonest reason of all for concern is that the breathing is noisy. Noisy breathing comes in many forms. It always suggests a degree of obstruction in the respiratory passages, and often the type of noise produced gives the doctor a good indication of the underlying problem. Snoring, for example, is a good example of the noise produced by obstruction at the back of the nose or within the nose itself (see pages 351–354). Rattley breathing, on breathing either in or out, is a sign of mucus collecting in the back of the throat and in the larger respiratory airways of babies and infants who do not have a good cough reflex and have not yet learnt to cough up the phlegm which is interfering with the flow of air. The more important factor in this case, however, is whether the infant is ill or not. Some can be quite lively, full of energy with a normal appetite and are rattling merely because of discharge from the nose trickling down the back of the throat. Others, on the other hand, may have a high temperature, be generally listless and may well be harbouring a more serious respiratory condition such as a patch of pneumonia or a form of bronchitis.

Stridor is the name given to a noise made in the throat on breathing in only. It is present in children who have inhaled a foreign object, in croup, and in epiglottitis, a bacterial infection affecting the flap of cartilage known as the epiglottis situated at the top of the windpipe. The epiglottis normally prevents swallowed food from going down the windpipe, directing it instead down the gullet. When it becomes inflamed through infection with a bacteria, the child will be generally unwell with a sore throat and have a croupy type of cough which sounds a bit like a performing seal barking for fish. Often swallowing is difficult and, as the epiglottis swells further, breathing too can become a problem. Any further swelling can obstruct breathing completely, therefore if you hear stridor the condition must always be regarded as a potential emergency.

Wheezing, on the other hand, is only heard when the child breathes out. It is a high-pitched, musical sound similar to the noise produced through the reed of a wind instrument. The commonest cause of a wheeze is asthma, although infection and an inhaled foreign object can sometimes be responsible (see pages 444–457). In infants aged between one and six months, one of the commonest reasons for wheezing in the winter is an infection called bronchiolitis. This is caused by the respiratory syncitial virus which is also seen frequently in older children and adults producing croup and colds respectively. In infants, however, it can become quite a serious problem since inflammation of the respiratory airways combined with phlegm production may easily lead to obstruction. Because of the potential dangers to breathing, such children are generally admitted to hospital for emergency care, and any sign of wheezing in this age group should always be taken seriously.

Recurrent episodes of wheezing in children are almost always due to asthma (see pages 444–455). Often there is a strong family history and the child may have hay fever and eczema as well. Something like one child in every five now suffers from a degree of asthma, and perhaps because of environmental pollution the condition is becoming increasingly common. Wheezing is an obvious indication of asthma, but in younger children the first sign is commonly a persistent, dry cough at night or a cough which is brought on by exercise in cold air. Parents often report that their child's colds always seem to go down onto his chest and that the wheezing is worse at night and first thing in the morning. There are many trigger factors for asthma, and as well as cold and exercise, infections, allergies and emotional factors have to be borne in mind.

WHAT CAN YOU DO?

If your child is having a problem with his breathing, ask yourself if he is at all unwell. Some alarming noises can be produced in a child's throat which may merely be due to a build-up of mucus and which may well be cleared by coughing. However, if a high temperature is present an infection is probably responsible, and some childhood infections can be potentially serious. Look to see if the child is struggling to breathe, perhaps resting his arms and shoulders on a piece of furniture in front of him. Often the muscles in the neck and the muscles between the ribs will stand out as the child uses extra muscles to facilitate breathing. Any blueness around the lips is a very serious sign and warrants urgent attention. Sometimes it is the rate at which a child pants which is of most concern. By and large, if the child is breathless, if noisy breathing is persistent and certainly if the child is also unwell, distressed or lethargic, you should call the doctor immediately.

WHAT CAN THE DOCTOR DO?

When the doctor examines a child with breathing problems, he or she can get some idea as to how serious the problem is just by looking at him. There is a world of difference between a child who is coughing whilst rushing about playing, and a child who is wheezing and lying quietly on the sofa wrapped in a blanket. The rate of breathing says a lot about how much oxygen the child is getting into his bloodstream, and the use of additional chest and neck muscles to aid breathing or any blueness around the lips are also important signs. The loudness of the noisy breathing may be misleading since the greater the obstruction, the quieter the noise will become. Examination of the child's chest with a stethoscope can reveal where any abnormal sound is coming from. If it is merely coming from the back of the throat the chest will sound clear, but if it is coming from the lungs themselves, tell-tale sounds will be heard in the chest.

The doctor's job is to diagnose accurately the cause of the breathing problem and to take the appropriate steps. Nasal congestion caused by mucus production or allergy may be treated simply with nasal decongestants or anti-allergy sprays. Epiglottitis is a serious bacterial infection which warrants admission to hospital where antibiotics and, if necessary, assisted ventilation and oxygen therapy can be given. Bronchiolitis in very small children again warrants hospital admission as breathing difficulties can increase and require assisted ventilation. Physiotherapy for the chest, antibiotics to prevent any secondary infection and oxygen therapy if needed can all be given.

The treatment of asthma involves not only the doctor and nurses, but also the parents and, most important of all, the child himself. In this condition it is important that the child learns to monitor his asthma day by day by means of a peak flow meter (see page 453) and then manages the treatment himself using all the various inhalers at his disposal (see pages 451–452). It is useful if he keeps a diary of his condition and tries out several of the different treatments available under the supervision of the doctor until he discovers the ones that suit him best.

IF YOU REMEMBER NOTHING ELSE,
REMEMBER THESE THREE THINGS

1   Noisy breathing is common and has a
     number of different causes.

2   Noise made when breathing in (stridor)
     requires urgent assessment and treatment.

3   Noise produced when breathing out
     (wheezing) is usually caused by asthma,
     particularly if recurrent.

Nose Bleeds

Nose bleeds are rare in infants but relatively common during child-hood. Thankfully they are usually trivial, affect only one nostril, and by and large are stopped easily. The real problem, however, is that they can often prove recurrent, which can be tiresome as well as messy. The commonest cause is nose-picking, which results in crusts being scratched off the sensitive lining membrane of the nose causing the fragile blood vessels to bleed. Occasionally, a bang on the nose, a mild infection or sneezing can be responsible. A less common reason is the presence of a foreign object up the nose. Children frequently push small objects like beads, buttons and sweets up their nostrils. Usually the type of bleeding from this cause is more watery, and the child's breath is usually bad too. Other causes include allergies which produce frequent sneezing fits, whooping cough and, much less commonly, certain blood disorders where the blood is not able to clot properly.

Children who have regular bleeding from one nostril tend to have a patch of very fragile blood vessels in one region called Little's area, which is found just inside the nose over the central partition. If more than three or four episodes of significant nose bleeding have occurred in a short space of time, treatment of these blood vessels with electrocautery (burning) under local anaesthetic to stop them bleeding is recommended.

WHAT CAN YOU DO?

Although some nose bleeds look alarming, it is important to keep your cool and not panic. Sit your child up and get him to lean forward slightly with the mouth open so that blood does not get in the way of normal breathing. Pinch the nose just below the bony part and continue pinching for about fifteen minutes. Collect any bleeding in a bowl to avoid further mess. After a maximum of twenty minutes, release the nostrils and discourage your child from touching the nose again. If the bleeding has not stopped by this time, take your child to the nearest accident and emergency department.

WHAT CAN THE DOCTOR DO?

The doctor may treat a nose bleed by repeating the first-aid measures which you may already have taken. If, after a further twenty minutes, the bleeding still has not stopped he or she will pack the nostril with gauze which maintains a constant pressure over the fragile blood vessels and will encourage the blood to clot. In severe cases where bleeding continues, a rubber balloon may be inflated within the nose but this is seldom required in children. At a future date, when all traces of blood and clot have disappeared, the child can be brought back to the GP or to the ear, nose and throat clinic at the hospital to have the area of fragile blood vessels in his nose treated. This may be done under local anaesthetic and involves either shrivelling the blood vessels up using a chemical such as silver nitrate, or cauterising them electrically with a special probe. The doctor will decide which method is most suitable for your particular child.

IF YOU REMEMBER NOTHING ELSE, REMEMBER THESE THREE THINGS

1   Nose bleeds are common in childhood.

---

2   The commonest cause is a bundle of fragile blood vessels on one side of the central partition of the nose.

---

3   Regular nose bleeds require treatment with chemical or electrical cautery.

Obesity

For some reason, many people still believe that a chubby baby is a healthy baby. That may well be the case, but it is not always true, and to some extent children who are slightly less than average weight for their age and height may be healthier than those who are overweight. Grandparents in particular like to see the cherubic features and rolls of fat typical of an overweight baby, and this is probably a hangover from the days, at around the turn of the century, when infant mortality was much higher as a result of poor nutrition. Children who are merely 'well covered', on the other hand, are not obese children, since obesity is strictly defined as weighing 20 per cent more than average for a child's height and age. In true obesity, rolls of fat are obvious on the upper arms and thighs and, in the vast majority of cases, this is simply due to over-feeding. It is tempting to settle a crying baby by putting it to the breast or giving him a bottle, but sometimes a drink of water, comforting, cuddling or changing the nappy is all that is required.

It is a fact that most overweight children are brought up by over-weight adults, and the problem is that they will become overweight adults themselves unless the spiral of unhealthy eating patterns is interrupted.

Fat children are often tall as well compared with other children of their own age, at least until puberty, but may well end up shorter as adults). There is growing evidence that overweight children also tend to develop more respiratory infections and problems from asthma. In addition, obese children are likely to have problems in the future, such as heart disease, high blood pressure and joint problems. It is therefore well worth doing something about a child's obesity as soon as possible. Fat children are often remorse-lessly teased at school; especially in the changing rooms, and may become self-conscious and withdrawn as a result. This can often alienate them from physical exercise and play which they may find difficult anyway, and merely serve to make their obesity worse. Too little exercise is a major contributory factor and a habit which, once learnt, is extremely difficult to break.

WHAT CAN YOU DO?

All parents should keep an eye on their children's weight espe-cially if they begin to look a little chubby. In the vast majority of cases, overfeeding is the underlying cause and dietary advice from your doctor, health visitor or a dietician is useful. Eating the wrong kinds of food can also lead to obesity. It is all too easy for chil-dren to develop a sweet-eating habit, and every parent knows that, given the choice, they will opt for confectionery, biscuits, fizzy drinks, squashes, chocolate, crisps, desserts, jellies, jam and honey rather than healthier more nutritious options. These foods are fine in moderation, but the major part of the diet should consist of much healthier foods such as fibre-rich wholemeal bread, whole-grain cereals, brown rice, pasta, fruit and vegetables. Added sugar should be avoided wherever possible, snacks between meals should be kept to a minimum and fried foods should be avoided in preference for steamed and boiled ones. Exercise is vital too and benefits health in a number of ways. For example it helps to prevent heart disease and encourages skeletal and muscle development. If a habit of regular, vigorous physical activity can be encouraged at an early age, it is much more likely to be continued into adulthood.

WHAT CAN THE DOCTOR DO?

The GP is in a very good position to look at an overweight child in the context of his environment. If the parents are overweight themselves this may be highly relevant, and the child's level of activity needs to be taken into account as well. The advantages of controlling the child's weight gain need to be made clear to everyone concerned. If any glandular problem is suspected the doctor can begin investigations, and if these prove negative, as they almost certainly will, precise advice regarding the child's diet should be given. The health visitor together with a practice or hospital dietician can provide a varied and wholesome diet for the child, but whether the parents adopt it or not is entirely up to them. All the doctor can do is advise the parents to encourage their child to stick to a healthy diet and to take plenty of physical exercise from an early age. By doing so as a family, they will reap huge benefits in years to come.

IF YOU REMEMBER NOTHING ELSE, REMEMBER THESE THREE THINGS

1   Most overweight children are simply overfed.

2   Too many sugary foods and too little exercise are also to blame.

3   Overweight children may suffer short- and long-term health problems.

Painful Neck

A child may have a painful or stiff neck for a variety of reasons, but by far the most important is that caused by meningitis. If parents can recognise the early symptoms of meningitis the child is offered the best possible chance of surviving. Early diagnosis and treatment is crucial, and neck stiffness is an important characteristic, particularly in children two years of age or more. However, it is reassuring to know that a painful or stiff neck is more often due to much less serious and sometimes trivial conditions.

CAUSES OF PAINFUL OR STIFF NECK

* Torticollis at birth

* Acute torticollis (wry neck)

* Infection other than meningitis

* Meningitis

* Medication

Torticollis at Birth

Otherwise known as congenital torticollis or a sternomastoid tumour, this is thought to be due to a minor birth injury resulting in a baby being born with a slightly swollen neck muscle on one side. The baby is unable to allow a parent or doctor to turn the head fully to one side, and a firm lump can be felt in the affected muscle. Usually, this problem settles down with some gently physiotherapy, but if it is neglected and is still present in an older child, treatment with injections and sometimes surgery may be required.

Acute Torticollis (wry neck)

This is seen in older children and is simply due to spasm in the muscle in one side of the neck. Often the child will wake up with pain on one side of the neck, probably triggered when a nerve is trapped between the bones in the neck through sleeping in an awkward position or possibly from sleeping in a draught. Treatment consists merely of rest and applying heat in the form of a warm bath or a hot-water bottle. The condition usually settles by itself within a week. Children with juvenile arthritis may also suffer with this form of torticollis as a result of inflammation within the joints in the neck.

Infections Other Than Meningitis

Many viral infections, particularly those affecting the respiratory system, can produce irritation of the covering surfaces of the brain and spinal cord (the meninges), although no infection of the nerve cells themselves takes place. Examples include ear infections, tonsillitis and pneumonia although a deep-seated kidney infection can occasionally have the same effect. Swollen lymph glands in the front of the neck can also cause discomfort, as can tension headaches in older children and head injuries. Virus infections of the nervous system itself, including polio, meningitis and encephalitis, are certainly the most serious causes of meningeal irritation and stiff neck, and are considered separately.

Meningitis

Meningitis is an inflammation of the membranes which cover the brain and spinal cord (the meninges) resulting from an infection with a micro-organism, usually a virus or bacteria. The symptoms of viral and bacterial meningitis are almost indistinguishable, but viral meningitis is relatively mild with few complications whereas bacterial meningitis is life threatening and may cause deafness, brain damage or death without urgent treatment. The symptoms in an older child include fever, intense headache, nausea and vomiting, intolerance of bright light and a stiff neck. In rare cases, where the organism gets into the bloodstream as well, there may be a purply-red, widely scattered skin rash as well. These symptoms may develop within a matter of hours, with increasing drowsiness and loss of consciousness occurring within a day.

In babies, nausea and vomiting take place and the baby becomes unresponsive and floppy. He may stare ahead with sunken eyes, refuse feeds and utter a shrill, high-pitched cry. The pressure within the head may be increased and the soft spot at the front and top of the baby's head, the fontanelle, may bulge.

It is often impossible to tell through examination alone whether meningitis really is the correct diagnosis or which type of micro-organism is responsible. Any child suspected of having meningitis needs urgent hospital admission for accurate diagnosis and urgent treatment.

Any parent genuinely worried about neck stiffness as a symptom may find these further details helpful. Lateral movement of the head from side to side will not necessarily cause the child any bother, but when the child's head is brought forward with the chin approaching the chest, resistance in the back of the neck and discomfort in the child is noticeable. It is well worth keeping an eye on the child's face too, since he may well wince when you gently test this out. Also, a child with genuine neck stiffness will very often be unable to kiss his knees because of discomfort.

Medication

Although rare, a few children who take anti-sickness and anti-travel sickness medication may develop a stiff neck as a side-effect. The problem disappears, I am glad to say, when the medication is discontinued.

WHAT CAN YOU DO?

At the very first possible suggestion of meningitis, a parent must obtain the most urgent emergency help for the child, especially if the child is also unwell. A child who is feeding normally, bouncing around complaining simply of tenderness on one side of the neck is unlikely to have this grave condition, but things can certainly change rapidly. In cases where the signs are obvious, the attention of a GP is reasonable, but only if this can be provided immediately. If this is not possible, the best course of action is to call an ambulance or take your child to the nearest emergency centre yourself.

WHAT CAN THE DOCTOR DO?

It is often difficult for even the doctor to diagnose meningitis in the early stages when its symptoms resemble those of a simple

IF YOU REMEMBER NOTHING ELSE, REMEMBER THESE THREE THINGS

1   Neck stiffness in a child who is unwell should be regarded as meningitis until proved otherwise.

2   There are many other causes of stiff neck other than meningitis.

3   Finding out the precise type of meningitis responsible is impossible without a lumbar puncture test in hospital. This is not always done, however, as the test can cause problems of its own and antibiotics are equally effective without it.

'flu-like infection or sore throat. He or she may well wish to observe the child over a period of time to see if the symptoms change or become worse, but as soon as the doctor is in any doubt, he or she should arrange urgent hospital admission, having first given an immediate dose of penicillin in injectable form to improve the child's chances of survival. Even if the diagnosis is later disproved, the penicillin will have done no harm and may well prove life-saving. Final diagnosis can only be made through a lumbar puncture, whereby a sample of cerebro-spinal fluid, the fluid which bathes the nervous system, can be obtained and examined for infection. Viral meningitis only requires supportive treatment and the occasional use of antiviral medications, but bacterial meningitis, on the other hand, is treated with large doses of antibiotics given directly into a vein.

Paleness

The colour of a child's face can change dramatically and suddenly. The face reddens and darkens when the infant cries, only to lighten again naturally during sleep. Part of the reason for this is the transparent thinness of the skin which is unable to disguise the colour change brought about by circulatory flushing when the child wriggles, cries or screams. This is true of all babies, but especially true of those who have a naturally pale complexion. Sometimes parents become alarmed at the deathly pallor of a baby who is naturally blond or red-haired, but this lack of pigment in the skin has nothing whatsoever to do with general health.

Having said that, unusual pallor in a child can certainly be a sign that he has acquired a medical condition requiring attention. Sudden paleness can be precipitated by a simple infection like a cold or 'flu, but a tummy upset or pain are also often responsible. A more permanent paleness is occasionally due to anaemia, where there is a reduction in the capacity of the blood to carry oxygen around the body. Children who are anaemic are always pale and generally physically tired with it.

CAUSES OF PALENESS

* Cold temperature

* Simple infection

* Fright

* Pain

* Nausea and vomiting

* Anaemia

* Medical shock

Cold Temperature

When the body is cold it naturally and automatically tries to conserve heat by restricting blood flow to the skin from where heat is lost. This causes the small blood vessels under the skin to contract and shut down, which effectively blanches the skin. Children going out into the cold air, therefore, will always look pinched and pale, at least until they run around sufficiently to warm up again and develop a reassuring, healthy flush.

Simple Infection

Colds, coughs and 'flu-type infections often produce paleness in a child's skin. If a fever develops, however, the body naturally tries to lose excess heat by pumping more blood to the skin from where heat can be lost to the surrounding air. When this happens, the child looks flushed and red.

Fright

When a child becomes frightened or anxious, he produces adrenaline-like substances in the blood which suddenly cause the blood vessels in the skin to contract. This causes a temporary but noticeable pallor, sufficient to prompt the well-known remark 'you look as if you've just seen a ghost'.

Pain

A child in pain will often look pale. Babies with colic in the first three months of life can look particularly pale, but pain of any kind, will have the same effect.

Nausea and Vomiting

There are the elements of both physical discomfort and fright when a child feels nauseated or is vomiting. Blood also tends to be diverted toward the intestine and away from the skin, resulting in further circulatory shut-off in the skin itself.

Anaemia

Many people describe anaemia as 'thin blood'. In fact, the blood may indeed be 'thin' in that there are fewer red blood cells in circulation, but this is not always the case. Sometimes it is the oxygen-carrying pigment within the red blood cells themselves, the haemoglobin, which is faulty. The anaemic child is generally pale, but especially so on the inner surface of the lower eyelid, around the tongue and lips and under the fingernails. These signs are not present in a child who merely has a pale complexion or who is pale for other reasons. An anaemic child is often tired and listless with no energy, and will often seem unduly out of breath after minor exertion. Their resting pulse rate is faster than normal too.

There are a number of explanations for anaemia, one of the commonest being dietary. An infant who is entirely breast-fed after six months of age with no vitamin supplements or semi-solids whatsoever is likely to become deficient in iron. Older children who eat none of the foods which contain iron such as green vegetables, liver, eggs and nuts are also vulnerable. Alternatively, there may be sufficient iron in the diet but either the iron is not being absorbed into the body from the intestine, or else the blood is being lost through internal bleeding of some sort. There are a number of infections which can lead to anaemia, and even some medications may be responsible. Sometimes inherited or acquired blood disorders such as sickle-cell anaemia, thalassaemia or leukaemia may be the cause.

Medical Shock

Medical shock is the name given to the results of circulatory collapse. In this condition, there is sudden and severe blood loss from the body leading to a rapid pulse, an increased rate of breathing, a lower blood pressure and characteristic signs in the skin. These include intense pallor, coolness and clamminess. This type of shock is always a medical emergency and requires emergency treatment.

WHAT CAN YOU DO?

When parents notice that their child is pale, the first question to ask is whether this has always been the case or whether it is something new. If it is something new, the most likely explanation is that the child is coming down with a simple viral infection and will recover within a few days. If the child is unwell, has no energy, feels dizzy or is tired, it is worth putting him to bed, giving him plenty of fluids and keeping a close eye on him in the expectation that he will recover quite quickly. Having said that, it is also worth looking under the fingernails, at the inner surfaces of the lower eyelid and at the lips and tongue to make sure that these too do not look particularly pale or more blue than usual. Check to see that your child does not have a temperature or swollen glands in the neck which might be suggestive of a throat infection. Also ask yourself whether your child's nutrition is adequate and whether he is likely to be getting enough iron from his regular diet.

If he is definitely off colour and remains so for more than a few days, it is certainly worth having the doctor check him over to exclude any of the causes listed above which may be responsible. In the case of medical shock, there is no time to waste, and emergency treatment must be sought immediately.

WHAT CAN THE DOCTOR DO?

A doctor who sees any child who is abnormally pale needs to perform a full examination. He or she needs to ask the parents how long the problem has been going on and to take the child's natural complexion into consideration. If the pallor seems to be a new development, the doctor can check for any ear, nose and throat infection or any other obvious source of pain or discomfort.

IF YOU REMEMBER NOTHING ELSE, REMEMBER THESE THREE THINGS

1   In most cases children are pale simply because they have a naturally pale complexion.

2   Children who suddenly become pale usually do so as a result of a simple infection.

3   A child who is unduly tired or generally unwell for more than a week and who remains pale should be fully examined by a doctor.

Finally, he or she can check for anaemia, if suspected, by doing a blood test, the results of which need not take more than a few hours. If anaemia is confirmed, investigations need to be instigated to discover the underlying cause so that the appropriate treatment can be commenced. Iron-deficiency anaemia can usually be fully corrected by dietary means alone. Any child given iron supplements should ideally also take extra vitamin C, since this helps to speed up the absorption of iron from the intestine into the body.

Red, Sore Eyes

There are many conditions which can cause red, sore eyes in a child but they are rarely serious. There may be discharge, there may be itching, there may be pain and there may be lumps or bumps on the eyelids. The most important symptom, however, is problems with the eyesight (see pages 229 to 231), so if your child is not seeing properly, urgent medical attention is required.

CAUSES OF RED, SORE EYES

* Conjunctivitis due to infection

* Conjunctivitis due to allergy

* Corneal abrasion

* Stye

* Foreign body

* Uveitis

Conjunctivitis Due To Infection

This is by far the commonest cause of red, sore eyes in a child and may affect one or both eyes. It is generally caused initially by a virus and is usually seen in the context of a cold with a runny nose, sore throat and sometimes a cough. Measles is a typical example. It is highly infectious, so the infection spreads not only to the child's other eye but also to the eyes of other youngsters in close contact with him.

Typically, the eyes are gritty and the undersides of the eyelids are extremely red. There may be a greeny-yellow discharge, particularly in the inner corner of the eyes, which is most noticeable first thing in the morning.

Conjunctivitis Due To Allergy

Normally, but not always, an allergy will cause both eyes to become red and itchy simultaneously. Often the allergy goes hand in hand with irritation of the nasal passages so that sneezing and a bunged up nose or a runny nose are often seen. Hay fever is a typical example. Some babies have red eyes at delivery, and this is thought to be due to chemical irritants present in the birth canal.

Corneal Abrasion

Children are notorious for accidentally poking both themselves and their parents in the eye. Even newborn babies have particularly sharp fingernails and, being naturally clumsy, these types of eye injury easily happen. If the scratch is over the clear part of the eye (the cornea), the injury is particularly painful and the eye becomes red and watery. Treatment is important in some cases to avoid scarring and long-term visual problems.

Stye

A stye is a painful red lump on the margin of the eyelid. Styes are really tiny boils at the base of the eyelashes and occur when bacterial infection gets into the little glands situated at the bottom of each of the lashes. Sometimes infection gets into the deeper glands in the eyelids themselves, where a pea-sized, white lump can be seen, particularly with the eyes closed. This is known as a meibomian cyst. Both meibomian cysts and styes can settle down of their own accord but larger ones or recurrent ones require treatment.

Foreign Body

It is easy for bits of dust or dirt to get into a child's eye where they cause irritation and pain. Often they can be seen clearly, and if they are floating around in the fluid over the front of the eye they can generally be removed easily with a cotton bud. Sometimes the eyelid has to be lifted in order to reach the foreign body which has got underneath. If bits of heavier material such as rusty metal have embedded themselves into the surface of the eye, removal by a doctor under local anaesthetic will be necessary. For this, some special fluorescent dye may be instilled into the eye so that it may be examined thoroughly using a specially illuminated viewing instrument.

Uveitis

Uveitis is an inflammation within the eye itself (every other cause of red, sore eyes discussed here is on the outside of the eye). The characteristic feature of this condition is that the child's eyesight is affected, and in addition the eye is red and painful but shows no evidence of discharge whatsoever. It is the most serious eye condition producing a red eye, and needs urgent medical treatment.

WHAT CAN YOU DO?

For conjunctivitis producing a yellowy-green, crusty discharge, it is important to bathe away the discharge using some cotton wool soaked in sterile water. Bathe from the inner corner of the eye towards the outer corner. Because infectious conjunctivitis is contagious, the child should use separate flannels and towels to avoid it being passed to other members of the family. Also, the child should ideally be kept away from nursery or school, at least until treatment has started.

If both of your child's eyes are red and itchy and he is sneezing as well, then allergy is more likely to be the cause. Working out the cause of the allergic reaction and treating this is the best course of action.

If your child has been poked in the eye or has scratched over the surface of his eye by, for example, running through bushes in the garden, a corneal abrasion may have occurred. In mild cases this will settle quickly, but where the abrasion is deep, inflammation and infection can occur resulting in scarring. If the pain and discomfort does not settle down within an hour or two, a doctor should inspect the eye for damage. Bits of grit or dirt or small flying insects in a child's eye can often be washed out with sterile water using a simple eyebath or fished out on the end of a cotton bud. However, sometimes foreign bodies seem to embed themselves in the surface of the eye, and a local anaesthetic is required before they can be removed.

One of the most important things for a parent to do when the child's eyes are red and sore is to make sure that the child's eyesight remains unaffected. A thick discharge can temporarily blur vision, but normal eyesight can usually be restored by blinking. Where the child's vision becomes permanently distorted, and particularly where there is a red eye but no discharge, urgent medical treatment should be sought.

A tip for parents applying antibiotic ointment where the child is uncooperative is to apply the night-time dose after the child is asleep. The lower lid can be simply pulled down and a centimetre-long strip of the ointment applied beneath it. Small babies will often open their eyes reflexly if their heads are held 45° down from the horizontal.

WHAT CAN THE DOCTOR DO?

The doctor needs to make a precise diagnosis by examining the eye closely. In general, antibiotic ointment morning and evening will settle an infectious conjunctivitis within a few days. Ideally a separate tube of ointment for each eye should be used. If the doctor discovers a foreign body attached to the surface of the eye, then it may be possible to remove it with a wipe with a cotton bud, but sometimes local anaesthetic drops will be needed to allow its gentle removal with the tip of a needle. The child obviously needs to be old enough to stay still for this! For allergic conjunctivitis, eye-drops containing an antihistamine and an adrenaline-type substance will clear the redness and irritation. Other preventative drops such as sodium cromoglycate can prevent allergic symptoms in the long term. If the underlying cause of the allergy can be discovered and avoided, so much the better.

Styes are best treated with antibiotics since they may otherwise spread or become recurrent. Where the child's eyesight is affected and uveitis suspected, urgent referral to hospital is required. Inflammation within the eye itself can cause long-term eyesight damage and treatment with steroid drops is a must.

IF YOU REMEMBER NOTHING ELSE, REMEMBER THESE THREE THINGS

1   Red, sore eyes are usually due to conjunctivitis.

2   Viral conjunctivitis is very contagious amongst children.

3   Any child with red, sore eyes should always be seen by a doctor, especially if his vision is affected.

Runny Nose

Runny noses can be a nuisance in childhood because they can disturb sleep and feeding patterns and because they transform otherwise delightful-looking toddlers into snotty-nosed brats. Babies tend to develop a runny nose when they have a simple viral infection, and if they are struggling to feed or to breathe at night, sterile salt water nose-drops may be used to disperse some of the mucus. Toddlers are constantly bombarded by many different types of viruses, at nursery school, from their friends and from other members of the family, and for this reason they are almost constantly catarrhal. Their immune system has no defence against such a range of viruses, and each time they come across a different infection they develop the symptoms of a cold. The tonsils enlarge, the lymph glands at the front of the neck enlarge and the adenoids situated at the back of the nose enlarge as well. Fluid streams from the nose, and because they are poor nose-blowers, the mucus readily becomes infected with bacteria and turns greeny-yellow. This, unfortunately, is the usual scenario in most children up to the age of eight of nine.

Sometimes allergy is responsible for a runny nose, but in this case the discharge is usually watery and accompanied by frequent sneezing. Other symptoms of allergy such as wheezing and eczema may also be present. A discharge from one side of the nose only may well be due to an object which the child has forced up there. The discharge in this case is usually pretty nasty and the child may also have bad breath.

WHAT CAN YOU DO?

It is always worth seeing your doctor if the child is in any way distressed by nasal congestion, if the symptoms seem to be continuous or if the child is generally run down. It is good to encourage your child to blow his nose as much as possible, and it is well worth being on the look out for possible causes of allergy, especially if the discharge is watery and associated with red, itchy eyes and wheezing.

WHAT CAN THE DOCTOR DO?

Often the doctor just needs to reassure anxious parents that toddlers and young children can be expected to have frequently runny noses. It is a sign that they are coming into contact with new bugs, and although the results of this can be a nuisance, it also means that their resistance is likely to be increasing all the time. For troublesome symptoms, decongestant nose-drops in a paediatric formulation can be given for short periods, and antihistamine preparations in syrup or tablet form may well help to reduce the amount of discharge. Any foreign body up a nostril will need to be removed.

IF YOU REMEMBER NOTHING ELSE, REMEMBER THESE THREE THINGS

1   Many children seem to have perpetually runny noses until the age of about eight.

2   Allergy, or a foreign body up the nose, should always be considered if the runny nose is long standing.

3   Consult your doctor if other symptoms are present.

Shortness

Many parents worry unduly if their child is much shorter than other children of the same age. The commonest reason, however, is genetic or racial. Short parents will tend to have short offspring, and some races are shorter than others. However, there are also a number of relatively rare conditions which can restrict vertical growth and certainly a child whose height is below the 3rd centile or whose height velocity crosses lines on the centile chart should be seen by the family doctor.

Some babies who are born small or who suffer from intrauterine growth retardation are more likely than other children to remain small all their lives. Other children are born with a chromosomal abnormality such as Down's syndrome where average height can never be attained although in Turner's syndrome the use of growth hormone can allow the child to reach a more socially acceptable height. Sometimes social factors including poor nutrition, lack of hygiene and emotional deprivation may be responsible. Chronic infections, malabsorption of food from the intestine, congenital heart disease and hormone deficiencies may all occasionally affect growth of the skeleton. Achondroplasia, commonly referred to as dwarfism and characterised by excessively short thighs and upper arm bones and a large head, is also seen very occasionally.

CAUSES OF SHORTNESS

* Genetic and racial
* Low birth weight
* Emotional deprivation
* Chromosomal problems
* Problems in individual organs
* Chronic infection
* Malabsorption
* Hormonal problems

Causes of Shortness

Genetic and Racial:
Most children who are short compared to others of the same age have inherited their relative lack of height from their parents. This is especially true if both parents are short, and some races such as the Japanese are naturally less tall than others as well. Achondroplasia (once called dwarfism) is a rare genetic disorder affecting about 1 in 2,000 of the population in the UK, and results in very short arms and legs.

Low birth weight:
A baby who is born smaller than expected for the length of gestation is known as a 'small for dates' baby and may have been deprived of nutrients by a poorly functioning placenta or may have an anatomical defect. Either way, some low birth weight babies never fully catch up from this intra-uterine growth retardation and remain somewhat shorter as a result.

Emotional deprivation:
Children who are emotionally deprived appear to have less of a chance of ever reaching their full potential height. The reasons are complex and almost certainly include poor nutrition, bad sanitation and physical and psychological illness.

Chromosome problems:
Children born with an abnormal complement of chromosomes may suffer by restricted skeletal growth in the long-term. Down's syndrome children will never attain normal height although female children who suffer from Turner's syndrome (where an abnormality of the X chromosomes exist) can be helped by the use of growth hormone.

Problems in individual organs:
When any individual organ in the body malfunctions the full potential growth of a child may be affected. Disorders of the brain, heart, lungs, liver, kidneys or intestines are especially important here and any of these can result in abnormally short stature.

Malabsorption:
A number of disorders, notably cystic fibrosis and coeliac disease can lead to the failure to absorb dietary nutrients, minerals and vitamins at a crucial time in a child's growth and development. Short stature may therefore result.

Hormonal problems:
A child's growth is dependent on many factors but not least a hormonal system working harmoniously. Underactivity in the pituitary, thyroid and parathyroid glands will often produce abnormal shortness unless it is corrected. Similarly, any child who in the past was inappropriately given excessive doses of corticosteroids for prolonged periods may well have suffered severe stunting of growth. Thankfully, with more careful prescribing, such cases no longer occur.

WHAT CAN YOU DO?

If your child is genetically short, your most important role is to help him come to terms with it. Teasing and ridicule goes on in every school, and a sensitive child at a critical time in his life can become quite self-conscious, withdrawn and unhappy unless bolstered by sensible parental advice. Since short children tend to have shortish parents, there may well be plenty of personal experience for the parents to fall back on. Short boys are particularly prone to teasing, and even bullying, during puberty, because in addition to generally having a rather late pubescence, they tend to have their growth spurt at the end of puberty, some eighteen months after the girls. The advantage is that the same sex hormones that cause the growth spurt also fuse the growing parts on the bones, so this is why men end up taller than women. So the longer a child goes on growing before the end of puberty the better, as far as final adult height is concerned.

Any social factors which may be hindering a child's growth can be addressed, if necessary with the help of the GP, health visitor and local support groups. Where a child is unwell in other ways, further investigations and tests need to be carried out so that any underlying condition can be treated appropriately.

Finally, for children who are of such excessively short stature that their life becomes a misery, some form of medical treatment might go some way towards alleviating the problem. This would need to be discussed with a consultant paediatrician at your local hospital. Certainly, any child on long-term steroids by mouth should be under the care of a paediatrician as these have a potential to restrict growth.

WHAT CAN THE DOCTOR DO?

The doctor is in a good position to measure carefully a child's height and compare it with that of his parents. A steady rate of growth as shown by serial measurements will reassure worried parents, and an explanation about how short children may often catch up rapidly with other children when they have a particularly vigorous growth spurt towards the end of puberty may be helpful. In cases of extreme shortness, however, investigations should be carried out to exclude any underlying condition which requires treatment. If none is found, it is quite safe to 'bump start' short boys with relatively developed puberty by giving them injections of testosterone once every three months. There is no evidence that this results in any loss of final adult height.

Children who have either growth hormone or thyroid hormone deficiency tend to appear relatively overweight compared with their height, although both conditions may be treated. The use of human growth hormone in selected cases can accelerate height without accelerating the bone age at the same time, so avoiding the problem of the child ending up shorter than anticipated. In other words, the child grows faster in childhood and ends up taller than he would without treatment. An underactive thyroid gland can develop in childhood and cause failure to grow before it causes any other problems. A daily tablet of thyroid hormone can correct this.

IF YOU REMEMBER NOTHING ELSE, REMEMBER THESE THREE THINGS

1   Most cases of shortness are due to genetic and racial factors.

---

2   In a few cases, physical and emotional factors are responsible.

---

3   Treatment with synthetic human growth hormone or thyroid hormone will be effective where shortness is due to a deficiency.

Sleeping Problems

It is a fact of life that, like adults, all babies and children differ in their sleep requirements. Many normal babies will remain asleep for up to twenty hours a day when they are first born, whereas others may only sleep for twelve. As they grow older some children will sleep right through the night for a good eight or nine hours whereas others are restless or wide awake for all but four. To a large extent this is genetically determined, although the child's lifestyle may have a huge bearing on it as well. A child who is under-stimulated during the day, physically or mentally, will not be sufficiently tired at night to ensure a sound sleep. Conversely, an over-stimulated and over-excited child will not be able to settle at night either. Children with eczema, asthma, attention deficit disorder (hyperactivity) or food intolerance may also become over-active and restless at night, and others may have underlying anxieties and fears which are left unresolved.

Much depends on the child's bedtime routine. Some children stay up until very late, waiting until the parents themselves are exhausted and ready to crash out at the end of a long day before they go to bed. In some cultures children are allowed to fall asleep in their parent's arms and do not go to bed until this happens. In other households, a strict and regular bedtime routine is observed. The advantage of this is that the child soon becomes accustomed to the habit, and in addition the parents are able to enjoy some child-free time together, which is important in any adult relationship.

Waking in the middle of the night is a common problem affecting at least fifty per cent of all children under the age of five. It is quite normal, and the real problem it causes is parental lack of sleep rather than that of the child, who generally remains blissfully unaware of the repercussions and consequences the next day. The best solution if you are getting up to attend to a waking child in the night is to try and grab a little sleep during the following day, or at least to make up for it with some extra hours in bed the following night. Also, parents can, if possible, take it in turns to get out of bed when needed, thus 'spreading the load' more evenly.

Special sleep problems encountered in children include nightmares, night terrors and sleepwalking.

Nightmares

Nightmares can be extremely realistic and usually very unpleasant dreams, where the child often experiences a feeling of suffocation. They are particularly common where there is underlying anxiety or where breathing difficulties have arisen as a result of the common cold, asthma, enlarged adenoid glands or allergic nasal congestion, for example. Occasionally nightmares will arise for the first time after some kind of injury or traumatic experience. Between the ages of eight and ten they are extremely common and one of the characteristic features of nightmares as opposed to night terrors is that the child, when he wakes, is able to remember exactly what it was about.

Nightmares tend to occur in the middle part of the night or later, arising during deep sleep, otherwise known as rapid eye movement (REM) sleep. In fact, it is now well known that all dreaming occurs during this phase of sleep.

Night Terrors

These are quite different from ordinary nightmares in that the child wakes abruptly from his sleep in a terrified condition. He may be found by his parents screaming or shrieking in a semi-conscious state lasting several minutes. During this time, he is unlikely to recognise the familiar faces of his parents or his surroundings, and is not easily comforted. All the physical signs of terror are present, including a rapid heartbeat, dilated pupils, sweaty skin and rapid breathing. In fact, the child may be behaving in such an odd way that he looks quite different from the way he normally does.

Night terrors are very worrying for parents whose children experience them for the first time, and they are most likely to be seen between the ages of four and seven. Children experiencing night terrors will generally settle down again within five to fifteen minutes and drift back into deep sleep without any problem. When they wake in the morning, they will not remember the night terror nor will they have any recollection of having had a dream.

Night terrors occur in non-rapid eye movement sleep, which is the more superficial type of sleep, and they generally occur within a half to three hours after the child first falls asleep.

Sleepwalking

Otherwise known as somnambulism, sleepwalking occurs during non-rapid eye movement or superficial sleep, or during the period of waking up from it. Certain children appear to have a regular habit of sleepwalking during which they will automatically get out of bed and stroll around aimlessly before calmly getting back in again. Whilst they are walking around, they may well talk in short words or phrases which are usually meaningless, or they may urinate on the floor or even get back into the wrong bed. Very occasionally the sleepwalking may be part of a night terror, in which case the child's behaviour is more frenetic, with an abundance of screaming and thrashing around.

WHAT CAN YOU DO?

With general sleep problems it is important to remember that children always tend to sleep better and more soundly when they are tired. Physical and mental activity during the day involving play, outings and new challenges and adventures are all good ways of stimulating a child's brain. There also comes a time, usually at about three years of age, when daytime sleeping should be discontinued, as this can reduce the amount of sleep the child needs at night. A regular routine is good news for parents and good news for children too. They will always do their best to extend the time that remains before bed, but there is no doubt in my mind that they find comfort and security in the nightly ritual of being fed, having a bath, enjoying a short bedtime story and then getting into bed with the lights dimmed or turned off.

Children who have got used to a parent being present until they drift off to sleep need, at some stage, to be weaned off this habit, and in this situation a comforter in the shape of a soft toy or special piece of cloth can be invaluable. It is worth sometimes leaving a low light on in the bedroom or the corridor, or considering the use of glow plugs or dimmer switches. Sometimes a little soft music can be soothing and some parents with small babies have even been known to switch on a vacuum cleaner or other household appliance as the 'white noise' produced can have a relaxing effect on infants. A warm, friendly bedroom full of pleasant pictures to look at certainly helps, and it is worth leaving soft toys or even books with a sleepless child in the hope that he may make use of them during the night. Most parents are all too aware that rocking a baby or even taking him out in the car will generally get him off to sleep, only for him to wake again as he is placed gently back in his cot.

Really determined children may cry for hours on end when they are left alone in their cot, and conscientious parents are torn between their own need to relax at the end of a long day and the child's need for love and security. Health visitors are very well placed to give advice on this particular problem, and although nobody likes to leave their child to cry, a plan of action can be put into operation to overcome this problem. The idea is that one of the parents stays with the child initially and then reassures him that although they will be going out of the room they will not be going far or for long. The child will undoubtedly cry as the parent leaves the room, but will settle when the parent comes back in after a few minutes to again reassure the child. Each time the parent leaves the room they stay out for a few minutes longer. At first, the child may cry for as long as thirty minutes to an hour, but over the course of, say, a week, which may seem an eternity for the parents, the child gradually begins to learn that mum or dad do not go far away and always come back. Their insecurity gradually diminishes and, in an ideal world, the child suddenly gets into a routine of going straight off to sleep without any crying at all.

This sounds relatively easy, but it is harrowing for a loving parent to put into practice and presupposes that the child is in no physical discomfort. Most parents are soon able to distinguish the cry of fear, pain, thirst, hunger or discomfort from that of the child who just wants their attention. I have seen far too many parents desperate for sleep and driven to desperate and sometimes dangerous measures as a result of not sleeping. Many a child is shaken, smacked or even battered as a result of these kinds of sleeping problems, and this is a tragedy because help is always at hand to deal with this kind of situation. Obviously, it is better for a child to be left screaming than to be physically abused, so if you think there is a chance that you might harm your baby when he is screaming, lay him down, get out of the room and have a cup of tea, or anything that calms you down. Many parents feel that they would like to shake their child, but thankfully only a few do.

Many parents are lucky enough to have parents of their own who will volunteer to look after a sleepless child for a night or two in order to give the parents a break, but when no other source of help is available, professional assistance is always at hand.

A child who awakes frightened after a nightmare needs immediate reassurance and comforting. Any breathing difficulties may require medical attention since these certainly seem to herald the onset of nightmares in some children. Any worries or anxieties he might have can be discussed the following day, and sometimes merely leaving a low light on in the bedroom or corridor is sufficient to overcome his 'fear of the dark'. Most children tend to grow out of this phase by adolescence.

Night terrors, on the other hand, are much more worrying for parents since they last quite a lot longer than nightmares and the child shows real physical signs of terror. Again, the best thing for a parent to do is to sit close by and simply watch the child going back to sleep naturally since waking the child is neither helpful nor necessary.

A sleepwalking child should never be rebuked or scolded since they are not aware they are doing it. Any abrupt or physical awakening is likely to be counterproductive. The child is best steered gently back into bed without being woken. Generally speaking, he will not come to any harm even though he is walking about in a daze, although it is best to make sure that the child cannot stumble down stairs or walk into any other dangerous situation by putting up any necessary barriers. Children affected regularly by sleepwalking tend to improve as they get older.

WHAT CAN THE DOCTOR DO?

The doctor and health visitor are in a very good position to give advice on common sleeping problems. On the whole, he or she will employ the types of methods already described to solve the majority of problems. Very occasionally some doctors will consider the temporary use of a hypnotic drug to sedate a child with a severe sleeping difficulty in order to preserve the sanity of the parents. Some authorities would hold up their hands in horror at the mere thought of 'drugging' a child, but in reality, where large families sleep together in cramped accommodation, where one parent may be working shifts, where true sleep deprivation is being experienced on all sides and no other family help is available to take the child away for a night or two, drastic measures need to be taken. In fact, an appropriate dose of a mild antihistamine preparation such as Phenergan or Vallergan used for two or three consecutive nights can sometimes re-establish a sleeping pattern which will continue when the medication is stopped. Such medication should not be continued for longer than a few days because of the risk of rebound insomnia when they are withdrawn. If nothing else, it gives the exhausted parents a breather so that afterwards they can renew their efforts to establish a regular sleeping routine.

IF YOU REMEMBER NOTHING ELSE, REMEMBER THESE THREE THINGS

1   Sleeping problems are notoriously common in babies and small children.

2   A regular sleeping routine can overcome many difficulties.

3   Health visitors, doctors, self-help groups and the occasional use of hypnotics can all be helpful in severe cases.

Snoring

Snoring is common in babies and small children because their narrow nasal passages become blocked easily. A baby breathes through his nose whilst sleeping and feeding, and colds, which produce increased mucus and enlarge the adenoid glands at the back of the nose, can partially or completely obstruct the airway. This can be distressing for the baby during feeding and result in sometimes quite loud snoring whilst he is asleep. In toddlers, a blocked nose during the day can result in speech difficulties, for example the pronunciation of certain sounds such as 'M' and 'N' is affected as the mouth is closed and air cannot emanate from the nostrils. Children with blocked noses will also eat with their mouths open, as this is the only way they can breathe. They also go round with a perpetually open mouth, and the drying of the cheek linings and the mouth often results in noticeable bad breath.

In older children, enlarged adenoid glands are mainly to blame and these swell up in response to common childhood viral infections. Allergic conditions also affect the nose and adenoids, so children with asthma, hay fever and eczema are all more likely to snore. All children will develop adenoidal swelling to some degree, but some suffer more than most. These 'adenoidal' children can develop not only speech and snoring problems, but also frequent ear infections and breathing difficulties as well. The good news is that the adenoids tend to decrease in size naturally by the age of seven, but if not, or if the associated symptoms and complications are severe, surgery to remove the adenoid glands is recommended (adenoidectomy).

Enlarged adenoids are not always the problem, however, because nasal congestion from simple virus infections or from allergies is common. The bunged-up nose following a cold is usually short lived, lasting up to ten days or so in babies. Allergies, however, will continue for as long as the child is exposed to the allergen. Common sources of allergy are house dust and the house dust mite, pollen, pet fur and various environmental pollutants (see pages 278 to 280).

WHAT CAN YOU DO?

If your baby or toddler snores loudly all the time that he is asleep, it is worth getting him checked by the doctor. Sometimes no cause can be found, in which case the problem is almost certainly due to the natural narrowness of the respiratory passages in the nose and throat, causing the soft floppy part at the back of the mouth to vibrate as air moves back and forth during breathing. The problem can, nevertheless, be helped by humidifying the air in the child's bedroom, and although commercial humidifiers are available, this can be achieved more cheaply by draping a wet towel over a radiator or even balancing a bowl of water on top of it so that the water evaporates. Overweight children will certainly be predisposed to snoring, and snoring can be reduced by laying a child on his side rather than on his back.

WHAT CAN THE DOCTORS DO?

Although snoring is common, persistent, loud snoring may be a symptom of underlying medical problems. Simple colds can certainly cause distress to young babies who naturally breathe through their noses when they sleep and feed. Simple saline nose-drops in this case can help to relieve the congestion. In infants older than three months, paediatric formulation decongestant nose-drops are highly effective but should only be used for short periods, namely one to two weeks maximum.

If allergy is the problem, nasal obstruction will go on for much longer than two weeks, sometimes continuously. Attempts should

---

IF YOU REMEMBER NOTHING ELSE, REMEMBER THESE THREE THINGS

1   Snoring is very common in babies and children up to the age of seven.

2   Persistent and loud snoring is usually due to enlarged adenoids or to allergy.

3   Surgical removal of the adenoids is recommended if frequent ear infections and speech problems result.

be made to discover the cause of the allergy so that the trigger factor can be avoided or removed. Failing that, various anti-allergy preparations, both for use in the nose and orally, can be considered.

In older children, the problem is almost always enlarged adenoid glands, and if frequent ear infections, breathing problems and speech difficulties occur as a result, surgical removal of the adenoids can be carried out. Doctors, however, are reluctant to recommend this operation in younger children as the adenoid glands tend to shrink in size naturally after the age of seven, so if surgical intervention can be postponed it may never be necessary.

Sore Throat

A sore throat is an extremely common complaint in children, particularly of school age, and is usually due to infection with common viruses, although bacteria are occasionally responsible. These micro-organisms may be inhaled when we breathe or swallow the food we eat, but either way the throat is the body's first line of defence against such invaders.

The most common cause of a sore throat is tonsillitis. The tonsils

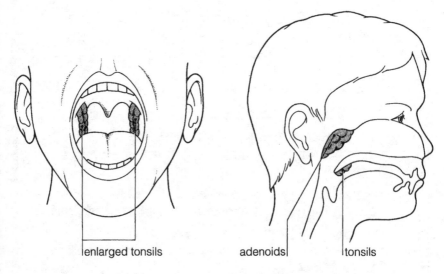

enlarged tonsils   adenoids   tonsils

Position of the tonsils and adenoids

are part of the body's defence system in the area of the throat, and are glands situated at the back of the throat on either side. They respond to infection by becoming red and inflamed, by enlarging and by recruiting large numbers of white blood cells to fight the infection.

They are the body's first line of defence, and the lymph glands situated at the front of the neck on either side represent the body's second line of defence. The function of the lymph glands is to drain infection away once it has been dealt with. Usually they are enlarged when tonsillitis is present and can be felt with the fingertips without much difficulty.

The adenoids are similar sorts of glands located at the back of the nose and have much the same function as the tonsils. There are also many smaller areas of glandular tissue which swell up and become inflamed when infection is present. Consequently, it is a complete myth that having the tonsils removed will prevent sore throats in the future, and although there are a number of good reasons for having tonsils removed, the unrealistic expectation of being able to avoid sore throats should not be one of them.

The symptoms of a sore throat may range from a trivial scratchy or tickly throat to a fairly major illness with a high temperature, sweating, shivering, vomiting, weakness and dizziness. Similarly, the duration may be just a day or two, or anything up to a week in severe cases. Often the symptoms go hand in hand with those of a common cold or 'flu, including a streaming nose, snoring at night because of nasal obstruction, coughing and bad breath first thing in the morning as a result of night breathing. Usually the child loses his appetite and lies still and quietly in whatever position he feels comfortable in. A baby cannot complain of a sore throat, but will certainly be off feeds and may cry when swallowing fluids. The child's temperature is also likely to be at or above 38°C.

Since a sore throat rarely occurs in isolation, other symptoms are usually associated with it. Earache often occurs with a sore throat, as many viruses attack the middle ear cavity at the same time as the throat. Nasal obstruction and enlargement of the adenoid glands lead to the spread of infection up the Eustachian tube to the middle ear cavity, producing fluid, mucus and catarrh as a result.

Who gets sore throats?

Sore throats are extremely common in all children, but especially in those aged from four to twelve. This is the age when children first start school. They pick up one infection after another as a result of being in close contact with other children, and many parents complain, quite understandably, that their children never seem to be free of colds or sore throats. On the positive side, it does mean that they are steadily increasing their immunity to the various germs that are causing them, and this is shown by the fact that as children get older, the number of infections they get tends to decrease dramatically. Over the age of twelve, most children have no more attacks than adults do, numbering perhaps two or three a year. On the whole, it is relatively normal for a child aged four to six to have three or four infections every year, but if it is more than seven or eight, or if the symptoms are particularly severe and the child is taking a lot of time off school, then more vigorous treatment should be considered. In certain circumstances this could include surgical removal of the tonsils and adenoids.

CAUSES OF SORE THROAT

* Tonsillitis

* Mesenteric adenitis

* Croup

* Quinsy

* Miscellaneous

Tonsillitis

Tonsillitis has a characteristic appearance. A parent can normally see a child's tonsils if the child is asked to open his mouth wide, protrude his tongue and say 'aaahhh'. If, at the same time, the parent pushes the tongue down with the flat handle of a spoon, the back of the throat and the tonsils can usually be seen clearly with a bright light, even if only for a fraction of a second before the child gags. Most viral sore throats will be red and angry in appearance, and in more severe cases there will be a number of white spots over the tonsils themselves. These, however, are more suggestive of a bacterial tonsillitis or glandular fever, and are evidence of the presence of a large number of white blood cells which have been recruited to combat the infection.

Mesenteric Adenitis

Many children also develop abdominal pain when they have a sore throat which can be quite confusing for the parents. The same germs which attack the throat are swallowed, and when they reach the intestine produce similar inflammation and swelling in the glands which protect that part of the body. As the glands swell they become painful, so much so that in some children the pain is quite severe and can even mimic the severe pain of appendicitis. This condition is called mesenteric adenitis, and is common in children of school age. It generally passes within a few days and the sore throat improves simultaneously.

Croup

Sometimes noisy breathing goes hand in hand with a sore throat. A small child whose dry cough sounds hoarse and croaky, like a performing seal, may have croup, a virus infection attacking the voice-box and windpipe. If the larynx is very inflamed, a strangled sort of noise known as stridor, present when the child breathes in, may be heard. This is a much more serious symptom which should be referred to the doctor immediately.

Quinsy

Quinsy is caused by an abscess on one of the tonsils and is often so painful that even fluids cannot be swallowed, saliva tending to dribble out from the side of the mouth. It is seen in older children and teenagers and examination of the throat shows one massively enlarged tonsil pushing right over to the opposite side. This condition needs urgent medical attention.

Miscellaneous

There are additional symptoms which may suggest the underlying cause of the sore throat. Hoarseness indicates that laryngitis or inflammation of the voice-box is the problem. A bright red rash on the face, especially the cheeks, is common in scarlet fever and some children with mumps who develop swelling of the salivary glands may also complain of a sore throat.

When a sore throat is not accompanied by a runny nose, earache or cough, allergy rather than infection may be the cause. If this is the case, it is generally much longer lasting and is commonly seen in children with other allergic symptoms such as asthma and eczema.

WHAT CAN YOU DO?

First of all think about symptoms other than the sore throat. Ask your child if he has earache, headache, tummy pain or a cough. Find out if he is feverish. Make a note of what he is able to eat and drink. Take a look at his throat using the method described on page 357 and feel for the glands at the front of the neck. What is he like in himself? Is he weak and dizzy, is he lying around with no energy whatsoever, or is he really pretty lively and healthy?

If the child is off solid food, then it is reasonable to give him liquidised meals including soup, milkshakes and ice-cream. Encourage him to drink as much fluid as possible since this not only replaces fluid loss, but may also be soothing to the throat.

Anaesthetic throat sprays are available for use with older children, as are lozenges, although these merely treat the symptoms, not the cause. Paracetamol can be given in syrup or tablet form to ease the pain and discomfort.

WHAT CAN THE DOCTOR DO?

The doctor should be consulted if the child is generally unwell or has a high temperature. He or she should be told about any noisy breathing, saliva dribbling from the corner of the mouth or earache. Similarly, the doctor should be called if the sore throat has persisted for more than four or five days.

The doctor will examine the child's ears, nose and throat, and he or she may take a swab so that a specimen can be sent to the laboratory at the hospital for a precise diagnosis. The doctor will decide whether or not to prescribe antibiotics (see page 57), and advise pain relief if necessary.

Finally, the doctor may well want to review the child in a few days time to discuss with the parents whether his infection was a 'one-off', or, if he has had many previous infections and needed a lot of time off school, whether the child should have his tonsils and adenoids removed.

Who should have their tonsils and adenoids removed?

Surgical removal of the tonsils and adenoids is often carried out in one combined operation (adeno-tonsillectomy), and tonsillectomy on its own is carried out much less frequently than it used to be. Children having surgery these days are those who suffer frequent attacks of severe tonsillits, develop a tonsillar abscess (quinsy) or have one tonsil much larger or more deeply ulcerated than the other. Adenoids are removed if nasal obstruction with recurrent ear infections or sinusitis is a problem.

Should antibiotics be prescribed?

This is a controversial area as it is impossible to tell from merely looking at the throat whether the infection is viral or bacterial. Three-quarters or more of all sore throats are caused by viruses, which do not respond in any way to antibiotics. On the other hand, the quarter of all infections that are caused by bacteria can, in a very small number of cases, produce complications such as rheumatic fever and nephritis, which may damage the heart valves and the kidneys respectively. Although these complications are extremely rare, they do still occur and antibiotics prevent their development. Contrary to popular belief, children do not become resistant to antibiotics, and bacterial resistance in the community is probably not as important as was once feared.

The swab that the doctor may take from the throat and which is examined in the laboratory is certainly helpful, but the results are often not available for three or four days afterwards, by which time it is too late to decide whether or not to prescribe antibiotics. What generally happens, therefore, is that the doctor makes a decision based on the severity and duration of the symptoms, the child's previous medical history and the parents' expectations.

It must always be remembered that prescribing too many antibiotics inappropriately can lead to problems of its own. Thrush infection, diarrhoea and skin rashes are all well-known side-effects of antibiotics and a few doctors continue to worry about the prescription of such drugs where their use is not necessarily justified.

IF YOU REMEMBER NOTHING ELSE, REMEMBER THESE THREE THINGS

1   Sore throat in children is usually caused by virus infection and antibiotics are therefore not usually necessary.

2   Call the doctor if accompanying symptoms include earache, breathing difficulties, high temperature or tummy pain.

3   Surgical removal of the tonsils does not guarantee freedom from sore throats.

Spinal Curvature

A child's spine is naturally curved front to back, beginning in a newborn baby as a single, smooth, convex curve and changing as the child grows older to the typical elongated S-shape of adult-

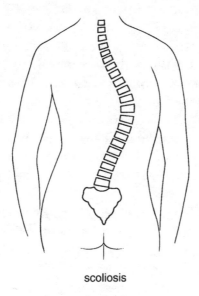

scoliosis

Abnormal spinal curvature

hood. There should be no curve, however, side to side, and when you look at a child from the back the vertebral column should lie in a vertical line. A curve to the side at any point along the spine is known as scoliosis, and mild degrees of this condition are not uncommon. Moderate to severe degrees of scoliosis, however, require treatment and this is necessary in about four children in every thousand. The problem does not occur in infants and toddlers, and most often becomes apparent at about the age of ten when spinal growth is greatest. It is usually noticed by chance when the child is in the bath or at the swimming-pool since in most cases there are no symptoms of pain or discomfort. It is rare for there to be a single curve, the spine usually compensating by curving in the opposite direction elsewhere so that the shoulders and head remain straight.

More often than not there is no apparent reason for the development of an abnormal spinal curvature. It appears to be postural, and often disappears when the child bends forward. In other cases, however, there is an identifiable physical problem. Where the child's legs are of unequal length, for example, the pelvis is tilted and the spine has to compensate for the imbalance. This leads to uneven wear and tear on the spinal joints and is probably one of the commonest causes of backache in later life. Occasionally, there will be structural problems in the bones of the spine itself, and this may be caused by either bony or muscular abnormalities. Usually, sideways curves in the lower spine tend to cause less trouble than those in the upper part of the spine between the shoulder blades, and postural scoliosis rarely causes a problem at all.

WHAT CAN YOU DO?

If you notice that your child's spine appears to have an abnormal curve in it, ask him to bend forward and touch his toes and take a look from behind. If it disappears, it is probably a simple postural problem which is not significant. If it does not disappear, there may well be a skeletal or muscular problem to account for it which requires treatment, and this is advisable to prevent any long-term problems.

WHAT CAN THE DOCTOR DO?

After a full examination to ascertain the degree of curvature and to measure leg length, X-rays should be carried out to investigate the underlying problem and the degree of scoliosis. Mild cases will require no treatment, other than perhaps providing special footwear to correct unequal leg length. Moderate to severe cases, on the other hand, may continue to develop if something is not done, resulting in permanent disability. In those rare severe cases affecting the upper spine, the ribs may be forced out of their normal position resulting in asymmetry of the chest, the development of a hump on one side and breathing difficulties in later life as respiration itself becomes affected. Treatment by specialists usually involves physiotherapy to strengthen weakened muscles, wearing a special brace to force the spine into a better position and, occasionally, surgery to realign and fuse the spine.

IF YOU REMEMBER NOTHING ELSE, REMEMBER THESE THREE THINGS

1   Side-to-side curvature of the spine is always abnormal.

2   Curvature due to posture alone will disappear when the child bends forward.

3   Severe cases require specialist treatment to prevent long-term problems.

Speech Problems

If you suspect that your child is not talking properly, it is important to find out exactly what your child should be doing at various ages. The development of speech has a great deal to do with how much you talk to your baby, because this is a valuable stimulus from his very earliest days. At first, of course, you will not notice any response, but nevertheless your baby can hear what you are saying and is becoming more familiar with the sounds of language all the time. After a while, you will find that your baby will produce voice sounds appropriate to his age in response to your voice if you allow him time to answer. This early form of conversation is very important in speech development.

From day one a child is usually surprised and startled by sudden, loud noises. By three months he is making noises like 'goo' and 'gaa' and at the age of six months he is babbling away, making repetitive noises like 'mumm mumm' or 'gaa gaaa'. At twelve to eighteen months he may use familiar words like 'ma ma' or 'da da', but it is not until about fifteen months that he restricts the use of these words to his parents. By about the same time he will have developed the use of special sounds for special objects, and will be experimenting with voice sounds all the time. My own children's first words were cat, car and digger respectively. At a year and a half most children are using about six distinguishable, single words but can understand a great deal more than they are able to say. They can also follow simple commands, and can understand tone and intonations, hence they can distinguish between anger, surprise, questioning and so on. At this time they are starting to talk about what they do when they play with their toys, and by the age of two they can use two- to three-word sentences. By three most children are using full sentences and reciting rhymes and songs. Sometimes a three year old may still be difficult to understand by strangers, although the parents can usually follow what is being said.

The important thing to remember is that just as some children learn to stand and walk late, other children may experience developmental speech delay, in which their command of speech occurs later than in others. It is also quite normal for children to mispronounce certain words until the age of two and a half to three. Obviously, it is worth encouraging your child to practise difficult words, and attending a nursery where he mixes with other children is very helpful in this respect.

If your child is not conforming to the normal pattern of speech development, then certainly you need to ask why. Sometimes it will be due to poor hearing, often as a result of frequent ear infections and glue ear (see page 268). If a child cannot hear properly, he will not be able to learn speech patterns as quickly. Often it is the consonants that he will have a problem with because in normal speech these are the quietest and softest sounds. So the child might say 'bideo' instead of 'video', or 'par cark' instead of 'car park', for example. Lack of stimulation may also be to blame, as children need a constant supply of new sounds and language to challenge them to learn. Occasionally, slow speech development will be the result of a more significant condition such as a degree of mental retardation or autism, but these conditions will usually have been identified already by their other characteristic features.

Speech may be disrupted temporarily by a blocked nose as a result of colds, allergies or enlarged adenoid glands, and children who are born with a cleft palate may have delayed speech development even after corrective surgery. It used to be thought that tongue-tie was a cause of speech difficulties. In this condition the strand of tissue which attaches the bottom of the tongue to the floor of the mouth is quite short and is attached very near to the tip of the tongue. In the past, surgeons would operate on this and snip the tissue shorter, but nowadays most doctors believe that tongue-tie is not a real cause of speech problems and that surgery is totally unnecessary.

WHAT CAN YOU DO?

It almost goes without saying that good parents will include their child in conversation as much as possible to provide him with the stimulation he needs for speech development. But bearing in mind the normal variations between children, if you still feel your child is not conforming to the general pattern of speech development, then your doctor should be consulted. By and large, if you cannot understand any words which your three year old utters, and if other people cannot understand anything he says at the age of four, you should seek advice. It may well be that the speech problem is purely temporary, being most commonly due to intermittent hearing problems. These are usually due to glue ear, and if this is the case urgent treatment is required so that the child's education is not affected.

WHAT CAN THE DOCTOR DO?

The commonest cause of speech problems in a child is poor hearing, and a full examination of the ear, nose and throat is essential. Glue ear will often respond to a three-month course of antihistamines, low-dose antibiotics and nasal decongestants, but if hearing problems persist the surgical insertion of grommets into the eardrum is generally recommended. Blocked noses due to colds or allergies may be treated with decongestant and anti-allergy nose-drop medication, and in some instances moderate to severe enlargement of the adenoid glands can be treated surgically. Where a child's speech is significantly delayed for whatever reason, and where pronunciation difficulties arise, referral to a speech therapist can bring tremendous rewards, and this is equally true for children suffering from more serious conditions such as cerebral palsy or cleft palate.

IF YOU REMEMBER NOTHING ELSE, REMEMBER THESE THREE THINGS

1 There is a normal variation in speech development in children.

2 The more you talk to your child, the quicker speech will develop.

3 Most speech difficulties are due to poor hearing.

Squint

A newborn baby has spent the first nine months of his developing life totally in the dark in his mother's womb. When he is born, light shines into his eyes for the first time, and he spends the next few months trying to make sense of everything he sees.

One of the first things a baby has to learn to do is to coordinate

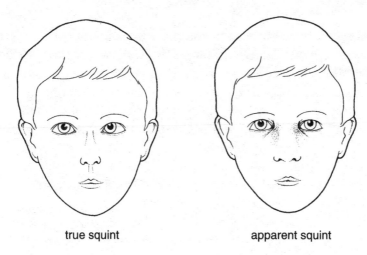

true squint   apparent squint

Squints can be misleading

the movement of his eyes. Although the newborn baby cannot do this, most babies have learnt the trick by about six weeks of age. One eye may still continue to wander a little, but certainly there is no need to worry about this in a baby less than three months old.

Sometimes parents may suspect a squint – in which the two eyes do not look in the same direction at the same time – because their child looks cross-eyed when he looks straight ahead. They may well be right, but as often as not it is simply a particularly broad bridge of the nose which conveys this appearance. The folds of skin which come down from the upper eyelid between the eye itself and the nose are called epicanthic folds, and when these are very wide the child may look as if he has a permanent squint. However, when these folds are pinched inwards towards the nose the illusion disappears, and both eyes can be seen to move together equally in every direction.

In a true squint, one eye wanders and this is usually more obvious when the child is looking to the extreme right or left. There is often a family history of the condition, and therefore a special watch should be kept on children whose parents or siblings suffered from a squint. It is usually caused by an imbalance of one of the six eye muscles which move the eyeball about in its socket, although an eye which is long-sighted or short-sighted may also be responsible. One way of detecting a squint, is to observe the

367

reflections of a bright, distant object such as a window in each of the child's eyes. If the child has a squint, they will not appear in exactly the same place in each eye.

The problem with a squint is that, apart from the cosmetic appearance, the lazy eye affects the child's vision. In order to make sense of what is being seen, the brain automatically blots out the sight from the lazy eye in order to concentrate on the sight from the good eye. Eventually, if the lazy eye is left untreated, amblyopia or blindness in that eye will result. It is therefore imperative that as soon as a squint is noticed, further testing and treatment are started.

The type of squint just described is the most common form of squint, and it will tend to come and go. Sometimes the eyes can look coordinated, fixing on an object with a parallel gaze, and sometimes the lazy eye will rove around. A much more rare situation is a fixed squint where the affected eye moves independently of the good eye all the time. This is a more urgent situation since it may signify disease within the eye itself or disorders of the nervous system within the brain.

WHAT CAN YOU DO?

First of all, if you suspect a squint, take a look to see if the bridge of the nose is particularly wide. The squint may simply turn out to be an apparent squint and not a real one at all. At any rate, your child should be having pre-school eye checks annually from an optician, and if either you or the optician are worried about a squint, this should be reported to your doctor. The optician or doctor can carry out tests to confirm the presence of a squint, in which case referral to an ophthalmologist or eye specialist is appropriate.

WHAT CAN THE DOCTOR DO?

The most common cause of squint is weakness in one of the muscles which move the eyeball. The resultant lazy eye can be forced to work a bit harder by means of a patch placed over the good eye. Like any other muscle which is 'trained up', the lazy eye muscle will strengthen and within a few weeks or months will be able to follow the movement of the good eye. In severe cases or where the patch is insufficient, some orthoptic exercises can be organised which further train the lazy eye to function properly.

In the worst cases, an operation can be performed to alter the length of the weak eye muscle, bringing the eye more into alignment with the good eye and again forcing the lazy eye to function normally. A squint operation is not usually performed before the age of two years, by which time exercises have had a chance to work. It must, however, be performed by the age of six or seven to prevent permanent blindness in the lazy eye.

In cases of long- or short-sightedness, glasses may be prescribed to correct the visual defect responsible.

IF YOU REMEMBER NOTHING ELSE, REMEMBER THESE THREE THINGS

1   All newborn babies squint before the age of three months.

2   In most cases a genuine squint can be corrected by patching the good eye, through eye exercises or by wearing glasses.

3   Operations for squints must be done before the age of six or seven to prevent blindness in the lazy eye.

Stammering

At the age of three to four, most children are speaking in full sentences and are learning new words all the time. They can become so excited at times, however, that their speech becomes jerky, the fluency being interrupted as they struggle to get out the next few words. This leads to a kind of stammering that is entirely normal and, as any parent knows, can initially be delightful to hear.

However, if noticeable stammering continues after the age of about six years, as it does in about one in twenty-five children, real problems can begin. It is noticed by other children, who might ridicule and tease the affected child. What happens next is that the self-conscious, stammering child clams up and refuses to use any words which he finds difficult. This perpetuates the problem and simply increases anxiety, so that before long the stammering can become a permanent feature. There is also no doubt that stammering tends to run in families. The good news is that speech therapy can be highly effective.

WHAT CAN YOU DO?

First of all, make sure that your child is not suffering from any kind of anxiety or tension. This will inhibit fluent and confident speech and must be avoided. Though some stammering at the age of three can be delightful, it becomes far from delightful for the child at the age of six, and certainly speech therapy should be commenced by this time. It is important always to avoid teasing or ridiculing a child with a stammering problem, and try to resist the natural temptation to say words on behalf of the child when he is struggling to get them out. Encourage your child to slow down a little, to pause and collect their thoughts before deciding on what it is they want to say. Interestingly, stammering children can often speak completely fluently when they are singing or reading poetry, so if you can encourage them to get into a kind of rhythm when they speak so much the better. Before you try to encourage your child yourself by getting him to repeat difficult words and to practice certain sounds, always consult the speech therapist, as drawing too much attention to problem areas in the wrong way can be counter-productive.

WHAT CAN THE DOCTOR DO?

The doctor basically needs to decide whether a child's stammering is part of the normal, hesitant speech which occurs at the age of three. If the doctor can see that the child is having to make an undue effort to get his words out, and if he is anywhere near the age of six, then immediate referral to a speech therapist is required. A speech therapist will work with both the child and the parents so that exercises designed specifically to address individual problems can be practised at home.

IF YOU REMEMBER NOTHING ELSE, REMEMBER THESE THREE THINGS

1 Stammering is a normal part of speech development between the ages of three and four.

2 Never draw attention to your child's stammering.

3 If stammering continues until the age of six, speech therapy is required.

Sticky Eyes

It is very common for newborn babies to develop sticky, discharging eyes. One or both eyes may be affected and the yellowy-green substance produced is often enough to stick the baby's eyelids together during the night so that he cannot open his eyes in the morning. The eyes themselves are not red, nor is the baby in any apparent discomfort. Just occasionally the eyelids and surrounding skin of the affected eye can become red and swollen, suggesting the spread of infection to other areas. Antibiotics should be prescribed urgently if this is the case.

Part of the problem is the narrow tear duct which normally drains tears out of the eye and down into the lower part of the nose. The duct is situated at the inner corner of the lower eyelid and often does not function properly until the baby is a few weeks old and has grown somewhat bigger. It is the failure of this duct to work properly which causes tears to build up and encourages infection. The bacteria which normally live on the skin thrive in a warm, moist environment so the front of the eye is a favoured location. These germs and the inflammation they cause give the discharge its yellow-green colour.

WHAT CAN YOU DO?

Bathe away any discharge from the eyes with some cotton wool moistened in sterile, warm water. A gentle sweep with a cotton bud is ideal for the purpose. When you do this, wipe from the inner corner of the eye to the outer corner to keep germs away from the tear duct as much as possible. Some doctors advise firm massage of the inner corner of the eye to encourage the proper functioning of the tear duct. If this is done, it is essential to make sure your fingertip is scrupulously clean, and it may cause some sticky material which is present in the tear duct to spill out onto the lower eyelid. The good news is that within a few weeks of birth, a sticky eye generally settles of its own accord.

WHAT CAN THE DOCTOR DO?

Where massage of the tear duct alone does not solve the problem, antibiotic eye-drops or eye ointment will generally clear the discharge within a few days and may need to be repeated from time to time to prevent recurrences. In babies, ointment is often more effective than drops as, being greasy, it stays in the eye for longer without being washed away.

If a baby is still getting recurrent sticky eyes after six months of age, he should be referred to a specialist who can syringe the duct with a fine cannula to open it up and encourage it to drain properly. However, this is no guarantee against further recurrences.

IF YOU REMEMBER NOTHING ELSE, REMEMBER THESE THREE THINGS

1   Sticky eyes are common in newborn babies.

2   The condition is caused by a narrow tear duct which becomes infected.

3   Antibiotic drops and ointment are usually effective.

Stings

Stings from whatever source including insects, jellyfish and plants produce local irritation and pain. Occasionally, in sensitive children, a major allergic reaction can occur leading to the potentially life-threatening condition of anaphylaxis. Most stings are trivial and short lived, and can be treated easily at home. However, with overwhelming allergic reactions, multiple stings or stings in the mouth, urgent medical treatment is essential.

Usually a child who is stung cries out suddenly with pain and is perhaps frightened when he spots the creature responsible. You may be able to see a sting at the tip of an area of swelling, and soon after the child will begin to itch. As the skin reddens and swells the pain increases, and if allergy occurs there may be swelling of the whole limb, breathing difficulties, a rise in the pulse rate, clammy sweaty skin and loss of consciousness. These last symptoms occur only in very severe cases and are highly unusual.

WHAT CAN YOU DO?

The child will be reassured if his parents stay calm. If the sting is still visible in the skin in can be scraped off with the sharp edge of a knife or a fingernail, taking great care not to squeeze the poison sac still attached to the end of it. If this happens, more poison will enter the child's blood stream. It is useful to apply a cold compress in the form of cold water or ice, but in the case of wasp stings dilute vinegar is better, and in the case of bee stings, bicarbonate of soda. Another tried-and-tested home remedy is the application of meat tenderiser, which you may have in your kitchen. When this is applied to the skin in a ratio of one part tenderiser to five parts water, it can be effective immediately in relieving pain.

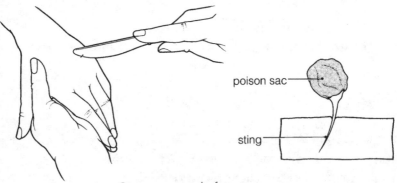

Correct removal of an insect sting

Extra care must be taken with stings inside the mouth. Again, any visible sting should be removed taking special care not to squeeze the poison sac, and ice should be either applied directly to the area or sucked. If swelling of the lips, tongue or back of the throat occurs, the child should be placed immediately in the recovery position (see page 102), and emergency help sought.

Children at the seaside who are stung by jellyfish will experience quite severe discomfort. Any bits of jellyfish remaining on the surface of the skin can be removed by rubbing with sand, and the histamine substance left by the jellyfish can be bathed off with ordinary soap and water. Later, calamine lotion or ice may be applied. Really cautious parents can make sure they carry oral non-sedating antihistamine preparations with them on holidays and picnics, which are very effective in reducing pain and irritation. Aerosol sting relievers are also available from the chemist. Those children known to have severe allergic reactions should carry some form of identification bracelet noting their particular condition. The Medic Alert Foundation (see page 468) is an organisation which can provide such items.

IF YOU REMEMBER NOTHING ELSE, REMEMBER THESE THREE THINGS

1 Most stings merely cause local irritation and pain.

2 Severe allergic reaction, multiple stings or mouth stings should be referred to the doctor.

3 Careful removal of the sting and the use of soothing lotions and/or antihistamines are usually all that is required.

WHAT CAN THE DOCTOR DO?

Most stings can be treated by the parents at home. However, when stings occur in the mouth, where multiple stings have been inflicted or where anaphylactic shock occurs, urgent medical help may be required. Antihistamines may be given orally, in tablet or liquid form, but they can also be given by injection for much quicker effect. Anaphylactic shock requires emergency treatment with antihistamines and sometimes adrenaline and steroids, followed by immediate admission to hospital for stabilisation.

Sunburn

Sunburn is caused by excessive exposure to sunlight, where the ultraviolet radiation produces an intense inflammation of the skin. The skin becomes red, slightly swollen, tight and acutely tender to the touch. In severe causes there may be blistering, cracking and bleeding too. If large areas of the body are sunburnt, dehydration and circulatory problems otherwise known as heat stroke can occur.

Since children are unaware of the dangers of exposing their skin to direct, strong sunlight, it is necessary for the parents to be extra vigilant. Most cases of sunburn are the fault of a careless parent. Prevention is the key – not only to avoid the acute symptoms of sunburn which may ruin a holiday and produce a great amount of pain, but also to reduce the possibility of any long-term damage which includes not only premature ageing of the skin but malignant change as well. Malignant melanoma, a cancer of skin occurring in moles, is a well-known and often fatal effect of excessive exposure to sunlight over many years, particularly in childhood. Furthermore, there is evidence that this condition is becoming very much more common with the thinning of the ozone layer.

WHAT CAN YOU DO?

The most important message is one of prevention. Any child with a pale skin who is not accustomed to sunlight must be protected by all means possible. This is particularly important if he is playing near water, snow or sand, each of which reflects the ultraviolet radiation even if the sun is not shining on it directly. It takes time for melanin, the dark pigment in the skin, to start to be produced in response to exposure to sunlight, so for the first few days of sunshine the child should be covered with tightly woven, light clothing and use a strong, high factor sunblock. Areas such as the lips, nose and ears are particularly vulnerable as they are continually exposed to sunlight, so a wide-brimmed hat should be worn and sunblock reapplied after swimming. Exposure to the sunshine should be increased gradually day by day, and because skin can still be sunburnt through ordinary clothing, the child should be encouraged to wear colourful, closely-woven UV-filtering outfits such as Zootz suits (see page 470).

If sunburn does occur, the use of calamine lotion or a cold compress on the skin is soothing. The child will feel more comfortable if left unclothed when indoors, and only puts clothes on to go outside. Paracetamol to ease the discomfort of any blistering is fine, and this, coupled with tepid sponging, will also help if the child develops a temperature. The sunburnt child should be kept well away from any further sunshine for at least two to three days and given plenty of clear fluids to drink to prevent dehydration.

WHAT CAN THE DOCTOR DO?

In general, the doctor will not need to see mild cases of sunburn, but he or she should certainly see any child who has become unwell, feverish or who has extensive blistering. Very occasionally, a confused and drowsy child with very dry skin is seen who might possible have heat stroke. This is a medical emergency which requires hospital admission. Other than the soothing creams mentioned above, moderate cases of sunburn may respond more quickly to anti-inflammatory creams in the form of mild steroid preparations.

IF YOU REMEMBER NOTHING ELSE, REMEMBER THESE THREE THINGS

1   Sunburn prevention is important to avoid both short- and long-term problems.

2   Treat sunburn with fluids, paracetamol, calamine lotion or anti-inflammatory creams.

3   A child with extensive blistering, a temperature or who is confused may be suffering from heat stroke and needs emergency treatment.

Swollen Neck Glands

When a child develops a cold or sore throat, there is redness and soreness at the back of the mouth and the tonsils may enlarge and be covered with white spots. These symptoms are due to the reaction of the tonsils and adenoids – the body's first line of defence against incoming infection. The second line of defence is the lymph glands, which form an organised network throughout the body, including the head and neck, and which also enlarge in response to infection. Special white blood cells are concentrated in the lymph nodes when infection strikes so that antibodies can be made to destroy the invaders. This is why children with upper respiratory infections develop tender lumps, particularly at the sides of the neck next to the windpipe and sometimes down the back of the neck and behind the ears too.

The position of the major lymph glands in the neck

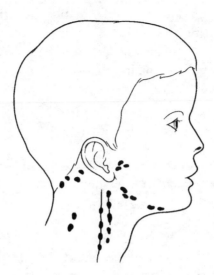

The lymph glands feel soft or rubbery and smooth, and are slightly tender to touch. They generally remain enlarged for up to two to three weeks until the infection has completely cleared up. When they are only enlarged on one side of the neck, this is often because they are draining infection from a particular site on that side only, such as an inflamed ear, an infection in a certain area of the skin of inflammation on one side of the throat only. If there is an obvious cause, such as a head cold, and the swelling lasts for less than two to three weeks, this is normal and acceptable. On the other hand, if the glands remain swollen for longer than this, or if only one single gland is enlarged and there is no obvious infection to explain it, the doctor should be consulted. Lymphoma, such as Hodgkin's disease, may be present as a painless, enlarged single gland, as can tuberculosis, an infection which is once again rearing its ugly head in large cities.

WHAT CAN YOU DO?

Whenever your child complains of painful, swollen glands it is worth establishing the extent of the problem, by feeling not only the glands in the neck, but also those under the armpits and in the groin as well. The next thing to do is to make a mental note of how long the glands remain swollen. If an obvious infection is discovered, this is good news as the glands are simply doing their job – namely reacting to infection and combating it. On the other hand, if the glands remain swollen for more than two to three weeks, if there is only a solitary gland involved or if the child has a high temperature, the doctor should be consulted.

WHAT CAN THE DOCTOR DO?

In general terms the doctor does very much what the parent should be doing, namely observing, examining and investigating the cause of the swollen lymph glands. He or she may also feel the child's abdomen to check for an enlarged spleen or liver which might indicate more widespread infection or, rarely, malignancy. In the vast majority of cases, the glands will settle down within two to three weeks, however where a single gland remains swollen for no obvious reason, further tests need to be carried out to exclude more serious conditions, and any appropriate treatment needs to be carried out urgently.

IF YOU REMEMBER NOTHING ELSE, REMEMBER THESE THREE THINGS

1   Swollen lymph glands in the neck are extremely common.

2   Glands remaining swollen for more than two to three weeks should be seen by the doctor.

3   If only a solitary gland is enlarged, the doctor should again be consulted.

Tallness

Most children who are very tall tend to have tall parents. In the vast majority of cases the reasons for excess height are genetic and racial, although in a few cases rare syndromes such as Marfan's syndrome where the fingers are greatly elongated, the skeleton double-jointed and the heart and eyes affected may be to blame. Cases where excess growth hormone is produced are even rarer. Children who develop early sexually may be tall to begin with compared with their friends, but end up in adulthood being rather shorter. The reason for this is that the sex hormones produced before puberty stimulate the skeleton to grow but prematurely age the cartilaginous growing ends of bones, preventing them from developing any further. Overweight children are often tall as children but of similar height to everyone else after puberty for the same reason.

WHAT CAN YOU DO?

Excessive tallness in boys is rarely a problem. For girls, however, it can create psychological difficulties stemming from the importance placed on physical characteristics by the culture in which we live. Helping your child come to terms with her problem, possibly drawing on personal experience, is the best you can do.

WHAT CAN THE DOCTOR DO?

If the child's parents are very tall, and if serial height measurements indicate that his ultimate height is likely to be excessive, action can be taken. In boys, anabolic steroids may be used to bring about an early end to the growth function of the epiphysis (the growing part at the end of the long bones) so that the child's ultimate height is limited. In girls, anabolic steroids should be avoided as they can cause virulism, making the girl physically more masculine. Girls can be treated using oestrogen, the female sex hormone, which works in the same way without the virulising side-effects, and should be used before the age of twelve. Also, the legs can be 'stapled' in a surgical operation designed to prevent the long bones from growing vertically any further.

IF YOU REMEMBER NOTHING ELSE, REMEMBER THESE THREE THINGS

1   Excess tallness is usually due to genetic and racial factors.

2   The onset of puberty can enhance or stunt growth.

3   Hormone treatment for girls should be carried out before the age of twelve.

Teething

Teething occurs when a baby's first set of teeth begin to cut through the gum. Rarely, a baby has a tooth present at birth but usually the teeth start to emerge at about three months and have all come through by three years. The milk teeth remain until they are replaced by the second set, and this begins at about six. Some babies who are teething may sail through with no problem at all, whereas others seem to get extremely irritable. They cry a lot, become clingy, their sleep is affected and they dribble more. A baby might even try to thrust his fist into his mouth in an attempt to chew it. Parents may feel a tender lump over the gum which looks red and swollen, and a hard lump may sometimes be felt with the fingertip. When the larger back teeth come through, the child's cheek can look red and feel hot to the touch.

There is some controversy about whether children who are teething can develop other generalised symptoms. Some doctors believe that they do not, dismissing them as negligible, whereas others, particularly those who have been parents themselves and have witnessed the problem first hand, believe that a number of other symptoms can, indeed, arise. However, it should never be assumed that any additional problems that arise at the same time as teething are necessarily *caused* by the teething, as other unrelated causes are often more likely. For example, a child may complain of earache when he is teething because the pain being referred along the nerve feels as if it is coming from the ear. However, ear infection is a more likely cause and can coincidentally occur at the same time as the teething. Similarly, a temperature, vomiting or diarrhoea, a reduction in appetite, convulsions and nappy rash may all coincide with teething, and although they may be made worse by it there is often some other treatable cause which warrants urgent attention.

WHAT CAN YOU DO?

It is well worth purchasing some of the products available that are designed to soothe the pain of teething. Teething rings which have been placed in the fridge and which the child can chew on are helpful, and so are teething gels which can be rubbed onto the child's gums with a finger. Sometimes a piece of apple or raw carrot to chew on is just as good. Paracetamol syrup may be used if the child seems to be in a lot of discomfort, but by and large it is not a good idea to rely on this too much as teething can go on for quite a long time.

WHAT CAN THE DOCTOR DO?

The doctor can do no more for teething than you can, except to check that there is no other explanation for the symptoms. A child who cries persistently, is irritable and fretful, is off feeds and not sleeping may well have some other problem which is not at all related to the teething. If this is the case, the doctor needs to find out what it is and treat it appropriately.

IF YOU REMEMBER NOTHING ELSE,
REMEMBER THESE THREE THINGS

1   Teething upsets some children more than
    others.

2   Never assume that other symptoms occurring
    at the same time are always due to the
    teething.

3   Objects to chew on and the occasional use
    of paracetamol are helpful.

Temper Tantrums

Temper tantrums are often referred to as 'the terrible twos'. In fact, they may begin as young as eighteen months and persist until the age of four, although by then they certainly become less common. Two to three seems to be the worst age, and something like twenty per cent of all two years olds have two tantrums daily for one reason or another.

The main problem is the intense frustration the child experiences at not being able to express himself as well as he would like. Children are very aware at this age of what is going on around them and they naturally want to manipulate things to their own advantage. When they are unable to make it clear exactly what they want and when they cannot get their way, their anger shows itself as a temper tantrum. Parents can find these episodes not only embarrassing when, for example, they happen in shops and supermarkets but almost impossible to deal with without bribery or smacking. Fortunately, there are a number of more appropriate means of controlling temper tantrums that can be tried.

WHAT CAN YOU DO?

First of all, try to avoid the situations where temper tantrums tend to happen. For example, if your child has temper tantrums when he is hungry, then have healthy snacks available for him to eat at all times – this is far preferable to having to resort to buying unhealthy sweets or sugary drinks in an emergency. Tiredness can also cause tempers to fray, so make sure your child still gets a daytime sleep if he needs one. A child can sometimes be distracted in the early stages of a tantrum by something more interesting or particularly different going on around them. This requires a little guile and effort from the parents but is well worthwhile.

Screaming fits born out of jealousy of a brother or sister are tiresome, but the child will respond best to extra care and attention rather than punishment, and it is as well to remember that the anger the child is experiencing is usually directed against you rather than anybody or anything else.

If the tantrums always seem to occur in crowded shops where the maximum possible embarrassment is caused, try making shopping trips shorter and postponing any form of discipline until later. Try to stay calm and ignore the child's behaviour. Do not worry about what onlookers apparently think of you – most will have had children and know what they are like! It is best to remain firm and consistent and, above all, not to back down once you have made a stand. Giving in to your child or offering bribes will merely encourage worse behaviour in the future. Occasionally, tantrums may reach such a pitch that breath-holding attacks occur, but thankfully this is rare (see pages 188–190).

Children having tantrums are best held firmly on your lap so they cannot wriggle too much and obviously any breakables or sharp objects should be removed from the immediate vicinity. Children who simply refuse to budge when you are unable to carry them because you have armfuls of shopping, for example, can be left on their own as you walk away, although obviously they should never be allowed completely out of your sight. This common situation then becomes a battle of wills, but even the most determined child will usually give in and run to catch up with his mum or dad as he watches them disappear into the distance – after all what is the point of putting on a show if there's no audience. However hard it may seem, you cannot afford to let your child win because if you do it will be all the harder next time round.

WHAT CAN THE DOCTOR DO?

On the whole there is nothing the doctor needs to do, as temper tantrums are common and a normal part of childhood development. However, when a child is having very frequent and regular tantrums or where these persist after the age of five years, a further assessment should be carried out. There may be stresses and strains within the family or home situation to account for this abnormal behaviour which are not always immediately obvious. In these cases, referral to a child psychologist may be warranted.

IF YOU REMEMBER NOTHING ELSE, REMEMBER THESE THREE THINGS

1   Temper tantrums are worse at the ages of two to three.

2   Tantrums require firm and consistent handling.

3   Frequent tantrums in a child over five should be referred to a child psychologist.

Testicular Problems

Testicular Pain

Although the vast majority of cases of testicular pain are due to a direct injury or blow, sometimes no obvious reason will be apparent and yet the pain and swelling are considerable. This can be just as serious as an injury and the doctor should certainly be consulted.

CAUSES OF TESTICULAR PAIN

* Injury
* Torsion
* Infection
* Miscellaneous

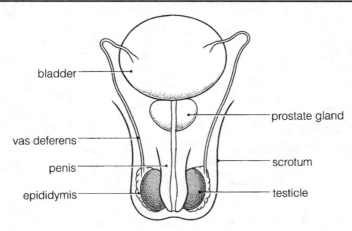

Cross-section of the male genitalia

Injury

This is the commonest reason for a child to complain of pain in the testicle. Boys can be rough when they play or fight, and any direct blow to the testicle will be extremely painful. Another fairly common accident is when a child falls astride a hard object such as a fence or the crossbar of a bicycle. These type of injuries can severely bruise or split the tough outer layer of the testicle, producing swelling of the scrotum with discoloration.

Torsion

Torsion occurs when the testicle twists on itself within the scrotum. Normally the testicles are fixed securely to the back of the scrotum by fibrous strands of tissue which function like the guy ropes on a tent. In some boys, however, the testicle is not adequately tethered and twisting can occur spontaneously. When this happens, the blood vessels twist with it and the blood supply may become completely cut off. The testicle reacts by suddenly becoming acutely painful and tender to the touch, inflamed and swollen. Often nausea and vomiting occur too. Urgent surgical treatment to untwist and permanently fix the testicle in position is essential to prevent it from becoming destroyed. The unaffected testicle is usually treated at the same time to prevent the problem occurring again.

Infection

Older boys approaching puberty can sometimes develop an infection in the sperm-collecting tube on either side of the testicles called the epididymis. This infection is known as epididymitis and causes the testicle and one side of the scrotum to become hot, red, tender and swollen. Another infection, mumps (see page 358), which normally produces swelling of the salivary glands, can also produce swelling of the testicle although rarely before puberty. Treatment with steroids is important to minimise the small risk of infertility which may result.

Miscellaneous

Other important conditions of the testicle or scrotum, none of which are normally painful and are dealt with elsewhere, include a hernia (page 169), fluid collection in the scrotum (hydrocele) (page 257) and a missing or undescended testicle (pages 390 and 256 respectively).

WHAT CAN YOU DO?

Any child who has damaged a testicle in an injury or accident will need comforting. The pain may be agonising at first but normally diminishes within the first few minutes. Pain relief in the form of paracetamol is suitable and the child should rest quietly. In the very early stages, the application of ice for short periods can reduce bruising and swelling, but after the first few hours more comfort can be achieved by relaxation in a warm bath. This has the additional effect of encouraging the circulation which in turn helps reduce the bruising.

Where swelling and discomfort have occurred without any sign of injury, torsion should be considered. If the blood supply to a testicle has become cut off, surgery needs to be performed within six hours in order to save it. Any parent who suspects the possibility of torsion should therefore consult the doctor urgently or take the child immediately to casualty for examination by a paediatrician. In older children it is difficult to distinguish between torsion and an infection, so if in doubt take your child for an urgent medical opinion.

WHAT CAN THE DOCTOR DO?

In most cases, bruising and swelling after an injury will settle down spontaneously. In severe cases, however, any free blood in the scrotum may need to be removed through a needle. Torsion needs to be recognised immediately so that surgical treatment can offer the possibility of a cure without losing the testicle. Where infection is responsible, appropriate antibiotics will resolve the situation, although mumps is due to a virus and will therefore not respond. In rare instances, where older children suffer swelling of both testicles as a result of mumps, steroids may be used to prevent infertility.

IF YOU REMEMBER NOTHING ELSE, REMEMBER THESE THREE THINGS

1   Pain in the testicle is usually due to injury.

2   Treatment involves pain relief, rest, ice immediately and hot baths later.

3   Torsion of the testicle requires surgical treatment within the first six hours or the testicle will be irreparably damaged.

Missing Testicle

Sometimes parents will notice that their little boy may apparently be missing one or both testicles. The fact is they almost always are there, but they may not be in their proper place in the scrotum. As a baby develops in the womb the testicles are first formed inside the baby's abdomen near the kidneys. As the baby develops they move downwards towards the groin and usually find their way into the scrotum shortly before birth. Part of the normal baby check carried out by the paediatrician shortly after the birth is to make sure that both testicles can be felt in the correct place. They feel soft and about the size of a small broad bean, but if they cannot be felt at that time further checks will be required as the child becomes older. Sometimes a parent can only feel a testicle if the child is examined with warm hands following a hot bath. This has the effect of relaxing the tension in the scrotal skin and allowing the testicle to descend slightly.

Although a little boy notices no problem whatsoever if the

testicle has not descended, it is important that surgery is carried out by the time the child is five or six to avoid problems in the future. An undescended testicle will not produce sperm nor will it normally produce testosterone, the male sex hormone responsible for male sex characteristics such as a deep voice and body hair when the child reaches puberty. (The other testicle, provided it is in the scrotum, will still produce sperm and sex hormone on its own.) By far the greatest reason for surgery, however, is the small risk of cancer developing in the testicle if it remains permanently within the abdomen.

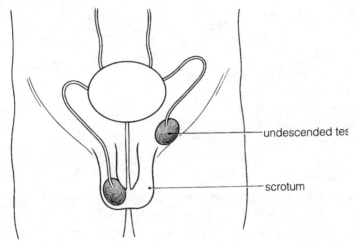

The male genitalia showing the position of an undescended testicle

WHAT CAN YOU DO?

If the baby is checked shortly after birth and is found to have an undescended testicle, the parents should ensure that the doctor carries out regular further checks on an annual basis to determine whether surgery will be required. Occasionally the testicle can be brought down by careful manipulation with the fingers after the child has relaxed in a hot bath.

WHAT CAN THE DOCTOR DO?

The doctor needs to make regular checks to determine the position of the testicles. Sometimes the testicle is partly descended and is lying in the inguinal canal, a channel just behind the fold of muscle at the top of the leg where it joins the abdomen.

Ideally, all children should be referred for a surgical opinion by the age of one year. This is essential before the age of five or six to avoid long-term complications of infertility, delay in the appearance of secondary sex characteristics or malignant change. Surgical treatment is very effective, although a two-stage operation is sometimes necessary as it is not always possible to bring the testicle down into the scrotum in a single procedure.

IF YOU REMEMBER NOTHING ELSE, REMEMBER THESE THREE THINGS

1 The testicles normally descend into the scrotum shortly before birth.

2 Long-term problems may arise if the testicles remain undescended.

3 Surgery to position the testicles correctly needs to be carried out before the age of five or six.

Tiredness

CAUSES OF TIREDNESS

* Intense activity

* Simple infection

* Diabetes or hypoglycaemia

* Chronic infection and anaemia

* Miscellaneous

Intense Activity

There is a world of difference between normal and abnormal tiredness. Children's energy levels rise and fall dramatically – they may be full of energy and vitality one minute and sitting or lying down exhausted the next. This kind of 'stop-start' behaviour is typical in two to five year olds, and the tiredness that results from such periods of intense activity is entirely normal. It is also only to be expected that if children stay up late at night and have less sleep than normal, they will feel more tired the next day. If anything disturbs their normal sleep pattern, such as a noisy brother or sister or travelling through the night on holiday, uncharacteristic lethargy will again be seen.

Simple Infection

Probably the second commonest cause of sudden tiredness is a simple cold or cough virus, particularly of the type that produces sore throats and earache. Sometimes bacteria are responsible for these infections, and one in particular, the haemolytic strepto-coccus, can cause intermittent tiredness for weeks.

Diabetes or Hypoglycaemia

Occasionally, tiredness is associated with loss of weight, excessive thirst and passing large amounts of urine, and these symptoms together are highly suggestive of diabetes. If this is the case, consult your doctor immediately.

A few children develop a low blood sugar level (hypoglycaemia) just before mealtimes which can manifest itself as recurrent but temporary tiredness.

Chronic Infection and Anaemia

There are a number of physical disorders which should always be considered in cases of excessive tiredness in children, including infections and anaemia where the ability of the blood to carry oxygen is reduced. It is common for a child to be more tired than usual after a simple virus infection, but some viruses seem to produce the protracted and debilitating tiredness known as post-viral fatigue syndrome or ME. Recent surveys suggest that ME, (myalgic encephalomyelitis) now affects up to 26,000 children in this country, and it produces tiredness, lack of concentration, muscle weakness, poor balance and other features. Glandular fever is another viral infection which starts with a sore throat but produces a protracted period of post-viral lethargy. Sometimes, a child with a persistent dry cough who is also very tired may turn out to have a patch of pneumonia on one of the lungs, but, rarely, other infections such as tuberculosis, kidney and tooth infections can cause tiredness as the major symptom.

Miscellaneous

Generally speaking, children never stay tired for long, and when they do it is first of all worth making sure that they have no anxi-eties or worries which might be at the root of it. Fear of school or interrupted sleeping patterns need to be ruled out. The child's personality should be taken into account too, because undoubtedly there are some children who simply prefer to read books than to rush around outside playing football. Some young children become listless because they are bored, and others who are naturally clumsy may appear to be unduly fatigued simply because they wish to avoid playing games that expose them to the ridicule of others. There is no doubt, also, that children approaching puberty and at puberty can experience reduced vitality. Finally, medicines which the doctor has prescribed may occasionally be responsible for drowsiness. In more obvious cases the child can become 'difficult', irritable and even aggressive with sweating, palpitations or loss of concentration.

WHAT CAN YOU DO?

Parents who are worried that their child is abnormally tired should try to keep a diary of their activity. They may be reassured to find that the apparent tiredness is interspersed with bouts of frenetic physical exertion. Ask yourself if your child generally has a quiet personality. Could he be bored, in which case he is likely to perk up whenever something exciting happens. Make sure that your child gets to bed at a reasonable time at night and is not disturbed. If he has had a recent cold then you can anticipate a period of up to ten days when he will be uncharacteristically listless, but tiredness going on for longer than that and which came on after a respiratory infection could be due to an infection such as hepatitis or even ME.

If your child's fatigue comes and goes but is especially noticeable just before mealtimes, it is possible that his blood sugar may be dipping (hypoglycaemia), in which case a between-meals healthy snack could solve the problem. More importantly, if there are any other symptoms along with the tiredness that concern you, such as loss of weight, diminished appetite and an abnormal thirst, these could suggest diabetes, especially if they occur together. If your child looks particularly pale and washed out, he could be anaemic, and a temperature, shortness of breath and coughing are suggestive of a viral infection.

By and large, children are not generally tired for very long, and if tiredness lasts for more than ten days or if there are other symptoms present, the doctor should be consulted.

WHAT CAN THE DOCTOR DO?

The doctor needs to reach a precise diagnosis as to the cause of the tiredness. If personality, social and environmental factors have been ruled out then physical causes need to be investigated. Where tiredness lasts for more than ten days after a cold, cough or earache-type infection, then a full physical examination is advisable. Diabetes can be excluded through urine and blood tests, but other infections may require a little more detective work.

IF YOU REMEMBER NOTHING ELSE, REMEMBER THESE THREE THINGS

1   Persistent tiredness in a child is unusual.

2   Acute ear, nose and throat infections are usually responsible.

3   Long-term tiredness, particularly when associated with other symptoms, requires further investigation and treatment.

Toothache

Dental caries, or tooth decay, is the underlying cause of toothache, although gum disease caused by plaque formation may also contribute. Plaque is formed by the build-up of food residues and bacteria which mix with saliva and stick to the surface of the teeth. These micro-organisms thrive when a child eats a very sugary diet, and there is no doubt that children brought up on such a diet are much more likely to suffer toothache and require more dental treatment than others.

When teeth are allowed to decay the outer protective layer of the tooth, the enamel, is eaten away and the sensitive nerves in the softer centre of the tooth are exposed. This results in pain and discomfort, particularly when anything cold, hot or sweet comes into contact with the tooth.

Some degree of plaque formation is almost unavoidable, but there are a number of things which can reduce or delay it. Fluoride certainly makes teeth more resistant to the effects of plaque, and this chemical may be added to the local water supply and is present in various toothpastes. Plaque can also be kept to a minimum by regular, correct brushing, which needs to be carried out by the parents until at least the age of four or five and then supervised until the age of seven.

WHAT CAN YOU DO?

The main job of the parents is to prevent tooth decay in the first place. The most effective way to do this is to ensure your child's fluoride intake is adequate and reduce the amount of sugar in the child's diet. Sweets, cakes, biscuits, chocolate and any kind of fizzy or sugary drink will increase the risk of dental caries and should be kept to a minimum. One of the worst things to do is to dip dummies in honey or sugary fluids as this will concentrate sugar on the teeth over a long period of time. Older children who are allowed to have cups or bottles of sweetened drinks during the night are similarly at risk. Sweet drinks, if given at all, should be made up very dilute. Where sweets themselves are enjoyed as an occasional treat, the teeth should ideally be brushed soon afterwards.

Many areas of the country provide fluoride in the local water supply, but not all do. Ask your dentist what he or she recommends – it may well be that you should be using fluoride-containing toothpastes or supplementary fluoride tablets instead. It is important to find out, since too much fluoride can badly discolour teeth.

Taking your child to the dentist regularly from an early age, and long before any toothache should occur, is likely to reduce his chance of developing a fear of the dentist (dental phobia). The visit can become a fun time for the child, and dentists are much happier seeing a young child with healthy teeth than an older child with rotten ones. Check-ups should begin at about the age of four and then be repeated regularly every six months.

If toothache does occur, make an appointment with the dentist straightaway, and in the meantime give the child paracetamol syrup to ease the pain. A hot flannel applied to the cheek may be comforting as well.

WHAT CAN THE DENTIST DO?

It helps a lot if the dentist can establish a good rapport with the child at an early age and before any problems begin. He or she should advise about fluoride, toothpaste, toothbrushes and brushing technique. At the age of about seven or eight, when the permanent teeth have come through, he or she might use a technique called fissure sealing. In this, a special plastic coating is applied to the teeth which seals them and prevents plaque from reaching the surfaces which bite together. The dentist will also discourage the use of too much sugar in the child's diet.

By and large, the dentist will aim to save decayed teeth as far as possible. Regrettably, even these days, far too many children have to lose their teeth through neglected decay, and it is the secondary permanent teeth which are lost as often as the milk teeth. A second complication of tooth decay is misalignment of the teeth which survive, and the dentist will also need to correct this. Early decay simply means drilling the teeth and filling the cavities, but where an abscess has formed through infection, antibiotics may well need to be given first. For young children, local anaesthetic injections are inappropriate and extractions may need to be carried out under general anaesthesia in hospitals.

IF YOU REMEMBER NOTHING ELSE, REMEMBER THESE THREE THINGS

1   The major cause of tooth decay is too much sugar in the diet.

2   Dental care in childhood ensures good dentition – and a wonderful smile – in the future.

3   Adequate brushing with fluoride toothpaste and/or the use of fluoride drops means fewer visits to the dentist for treatment.

Tummy Pain

When your child complains of tummy pain, two thoughts probably occur to you. First, is it genuine, and second, if it is, is it serious? The problem is that both of these questions can sometimes be very difficult to answer, even for experienced doctors. The symptom is extremely common in childhood and there are many causes of both long-standing and recurrent abdominal discomforts as well as sudden and short-lived ones.

A lot can be learned from asking yourself a few simple questions:

1 How long has the tummy pain lasted? If it has been going on for two or three weeks it is definitely not acute appendicitis warranting emergency treatment. On the other hand, if your child is curled up in agony, the pain having started suddenly only three hours ago, then he could well need urgent surgical treatment.

2 Is the pain continuous or intermittent? Pain which comes and goes ('colicky' pain) is often associated with constipation or wind, whereas the pain of acute inflammation in the abdomen is more continuous and made worse by movement.

3 Is the pain in the same place each time? If the child is pointing to different areas of the tummy on different days, it is unlikely to be due to any serious problem. If, however, he constantly points to one particular place, he may well have a genuine problem.

4 Finally, are there any associated symptoms? These can be helpful in finding the cause of the pain. Regular headaches with the tummy pain could constitute abdominal migraine, for example. A fever suggests infection and diarrhoea or wanting to pass urine more often than usual suggests a tummy bug or cystitis respectively.

There are several causes of both long-standing and sudden-onset abdominal pain, and these are dealt with separately.

SUDDEN-ONSET TUMMY PAIN

Pain which comes on out of the blue is common in children of all ages. However, if the child is generally ill with abdominal pain and this has persisted for more than three hours, it should be regarded as an emergency until proved otherwise. Appendicitis and other conditions requiring urgent treatment are too common to be disregarded for any period longer than this.

BABIES

CAUSES OF SUDDEN-ONSET TUMMY PAIN IN BABIES

---

* Colic

* Intussusception

Colic (see pages 24 to 26)

Although common, colic is a mysterious and poorly understood condition affecting many babies up until the age of six to nine months. This is irrespective of whether they are breast- or bottle-fed. Babies suffering from colic often scream in apparent agony in the early evening, drawing their knees up to their chests in a convincing display of discomfort. The good news is that these apparent symptoms disappear as mysteriously as they began independent of what measures the parents take to alleviate them.

Intussusception

In this condition one piece of bowel becomes telescoped into the next piece. It occurs commonly in children aged between five and nine months and is very unusual after the age of two. The pain comes on very suddenly and occurs in waves and the child looks pale and may vomit. Later on, blood may be passed in the motions and the doctor may be able to feel a distinct lump in the abdomen. The condition can settle by itself without treatment, although sometimes it requires surgery to relieve the obstruction.

OLDER CHILDREN

CAUSES OF SUDDEN-ONSET TUMMY PAIN IN OLDER CHILDREN

* Wind and over-eating

* Tummy bug

* Colds and sore throats

* Appendicitis

* Muscle strain

* Kidney infection

* Swollen testicle

* Infectious hepatitis

* Chest infection

* Sickle-cell disease

Wind and Over-eating

Probably the commonest cause of all for abdominal pain is wind and over-eating. These distend the bowel leading to a dull, colicky pain which comes and goes. At times the pain can be very intense and many a child who has simply over-eaten has been admitted to hospital for observation. Some have even been operated on, much to the embarrassment of the surgeons who in retrospect realise there was nothing more than hot air to explain the symptoms.

Tummy Bug

The germs which cause gastroenteritis usually produce symptoms which start either with nausea and vomiting or with a fever and dull pains that last between one and two minutes and which come and go over a period of a few days. Any diarrhoea tends to occur a little later on. The pain is often worse just before an episode of diarrhoea or immediately after eating. Often, other members of the family will have similar symptoms.

Colds and Sore Throats

In toddlers, colds and sore throats occur several times a year. The viruses and bacteria which cause them lead to enlargement not only of the lymph glands in the neck, which can be felt as mobile rubbery lumps, but also of the glands in the abdominal area. These can sometimes cause continuous, fairly intense pain, a condition known medically as mesenteric adenitis (see page 357). When severe, it can even mimic the pain of appendicitis and occasionally children are misdiagnosed and operated on unnecessarily. Glandular fever, another more chronic cause of sore throat, can also produce abdominal pain since both the spleen and the liver may enlarge and cause discomfort.

Appendicitis

Inflammation of the appendix, the redundant finger-like projection attached to the first part of the colon, affects one person in every six. Surgical removal of the appendix (appendicectomy) is therefore one of the commonest operations performed in childhood, although it is unusual for a child under the age of two to develop it. In the younger child, it is by no means easy to spot the early signs of appendicitis (and in rare cases even the late ones) as it can show itself in a number of different ways. One of the problems is that some children with only mild inflammation experience severe symptoms straightaway, whereas other children may remain relatively well right up until the moment the appendix bursts, releasing pus into the abdominal cavity. This leads to peritonitis, a serious and life-threatening condition where the outer-lining membrane of the abdomen itself becomes infected.

Having said this, there are a number of classic and unmistakable signs which are often but by no means always present. A child with genuine appendicitis will lose his appetite and feel sick. He will be tired and lethargic and may have a slight temperature. During the onset of these symptoms he complains of a pain around the bellybutton which stays there for a few hours before becoming more sharp and severe and then moving to a different place, slightly lower and to the right. This pain is often bad enough to make walking painful and some children will lie in bed with their knees raised to take any pressure off their abdomen. Constipation or slight diarrhoea may accompany appendicitis. If the child's tummy is felt, there will be distinct tenderness in the bottom right-hand corner. Any child with this constellation of symptoms should be referred to the doctor immediately.

Muscle Strain

Children can strain their tummy muscles through exercise, or even just vigorous and persistent coughing or vomiting. The difference here is that the pain is only present when the child moves or sits up, and it is a sharp, sudden pain as opposed to the dull, colicky pain which arises from an inflamed intestine. The child's appetite is normal and he is generally fit as a fiddle.

Kidney Infection

Kidney infections, which are commoner in girls than boys, can sometimes start off with pure abdominal pain, although discomfort is usually experienced in the side of the tummy or even in the back. Additional symptoms may include passing small amounts of strong-smelling urine frequently, nausea and vomiting and a fever.

Swollen Testicle

A child with a swollen testicle may often complain of pain in the tummy. This is 'referred' pain, meaning that the pain is carried along the nerves supplying the testicle that run up into the tummy. The commonest causes are injury to the testicle, a strangulated hernia or testicular torsion where the testicle twists upon itself cutting off the blood supply (see pages 387–390).

Infectious Hepatitis

Infectious hepatitis is a virus infection of the liver. It starts as a form of food-poisoning and is picked up through swallowing contaminated food or drink. The child feels unwell for a few days and then develops mild jaundice, in which the whites of the eyes and the skin turn yellow and at the same time the urine turns dark. The membrane which surrounds the liver is stretched as the liver becomes inflamed and mild abdominal pain results.

Chest Infection

Sometimes an infection in the lowest part of the lungs can produce tummy pain in children. There may be little to show for the chest infection at first other than a slight dry cough, but as the condition progresses other symptoms occur and the cause of the abdominal discomfort usually becomes apparent.

Sickle-cell Disease

Afro-Caribbean children who have this inherited blood disorder may develop tummy pain as a result of deformed red blood cells blocking the blood vessels supplying the intestine. The parents of such children will almost always be aware of the underlying condition and realise that this constitutes a medical emergency which requires hospital attention.

LONG-STANDING TUMMY PAIN

CAUSES OF LONG-STANDING TUMMY PAIN

---

 * Psychological problems

 * Constipation

 * Abdominal migraine

 * Dietary intolerance

 * Kidney infection

 * Sickle-cell disease

Psychological Problems

Some ten per cent of all schoolchildren, especially those between the ages of twelve and fifteen, complain of ongoing tummy pain which waxes and wanes with tiresome regularity. In ninety per cent of these cases, however, no physical cause is ever found and the trouble may be due to the effect of worry, stress and other psychological factors. Generally, children describe a dull pain which comes and goes, and which is felt mainly around the belly-button. Affected children may become pale and feel sick and it is not uncommon for some to complain of headache and fatigue as well. Although the vast majority of cases settle spontaneously as the child grows older, it is important not to dismiss the symptoms out of hand as this might lead to a genuine physical disorder being overlooked. In any case, tummy pain resulting from psychological factors can sometimes be extremely severe and therefore still warrants attention and sympathy. Clearly, the root cause needs to be discovered and resolved.

Constipation

Constipation is a common cause of long-standing tummy pain in childhood. Since it interferes with the normal functioning of the intestine, colicky tummy pain can occur, and distension of the rectum with hard, immovable stools can sometimes lead to quite severe discomfort.

Abdominal Migraine

Tummy pains which are only ever accompanied by vomiting are often the first sign that a child has inherited migraine from one of his parents. Most children with this condition will go on to develop the typical one-sided headaches in adulthood which are usually accompanied by nausea, vomiting and visual symptoms.

Dietary Intolerance

Although any number of dietary components can produce food intolerance, one of the commonest is lactose in milk. Tummy pain, bloating, nausea and diarrhoea are all commonly reported, and since it is the enzyme required to digest lactose that is deficient in this condition, improvement usually occurs when milk is removed from the child's diet. Other foodstuffs may also contain lactose as a 'filler', so there remains the need to check the labelling on packages to guarantee a lactose-free diet.

Kidney Infection

Kidney infections do not always produce sudden-onset symptoms. Infection which ascends to the kidney from the bladder can occur gradually over many weeks and months. As the kidney tissue becomes inflamed, fever, backache and abdominal pain may occur. The child does not necessarily need to pass urine more frequently, and there need not be any discomfort when he does.

Sickle-cell Disease

This inherited blood disorder is common in Afro-Caribbean children, and may sometimes start with abdominal pain as blood vessels in the tummy become clogged and obstructed with abnormal blood cells. Since sickle-cell disease is hereditary, the parents of such children will normally be well aware of the symptoms, and will therefore know that this kind of abdominal pain can occur in this condition.

WHAT CAN YOU DO?

It can be incredibly difficult to work out the true cause of tummy pain. It is one of the symptoms which even paediatric specialists fear because it is so easy to be proved wrong. In fact a great deal depends on experience as well as basic common sense, so the important thing for any parent to remember is to not hesitate in seeking professional help if you are worried. Any child who is generally unwell with a sudden-onset tummy pain lasting for more than three hours should be regarded as an emergency case until proved otherwise.

A child who tucks into a tasty snack and then runs about energetically, and who only remembers to complain about tummy pain when it suits him, is unlikely to be too ill. In addition, a child who only gets tummy pain just before school and never at weekends or during holidays may be using the symptom to avoid school because of school phobia or a fear of bullying. But a child with genuine tummy discomfort may be given relief in the form of a hot-water bottle and, initially, a little paracetamol. For real intestinal problems, however, this type of pain relief is relatively ineffective.

WHAT CAN THE DOCTOR DO?

Because of the enormous number of possible causes of abdominal pain in a child, the doctor has to try to establish a diagnosis. Having said that, however, the vast majority of tummy pains will never have an identified physical cause, and many of these are truly psychological. But for the cases that remain, the diagnosis can only be established by listening carefully to both the child and his parents and then carrying out a thorough physical examination. This examination should, in some cases, include a rectal examination to determine whether the tip of the appendix is inflamed. In boys, it should also include an examination of the scrotum as testicular problems can result in abdominal symptoms too. The doctor may want to feel the child's abdomen, watching the child's face carefully as he or she does so to see where any pain is being felt. Listening to the abdomen with a stethoscope will determine whether the normal rhythmic movement of the bowel, with its characteristic gurgling, is going on. Samples can be taken of urine, to check for kidney infection, or of stools, to test for tummy bugs or the presence of blood. Blood tests may be required to check for hepatitis or sickle-cell disease.

Occasionally, a child may need to be admitted to hospital for observation, especially if the doctor is unable to make a firm

IF YOU REMEMBER NOTHING ELSE, REMEMBER THESE THREE THINGS

1   The cause of tummy pain is notoriously difficult to diagnose.

2   Tummy pain may be psychological or physical in origin, or a combination of both.

3   Tummy pain in an ill child lasting more than three hours should be regarded as an emergency until proved otherwise.

diagnosis and it is not wise to keep the child at home because of the risk of rapid deterioration. In the vast majority of cases, either medical treatment will result in a cure or the tummy pain will get better on its own. Surgery is usually reserved for intussusception in a baby or appendicitis or testicular torsion in older children.

Urinary Problems

There are a number of different urinary problems encountered in childhood, although the symptoms may be very similar. The commonest complaints are of frequency and pain, or a combination of both.

'Frequency' means that the child feels a need to pass urine more often than normal, or else regularly wets himself or starts wetting himself again after he has been dry during the day for some time. Where small quantities of urine are passed and any discomfort is experienced, a urinary tract infection will often prove to be the cause. On the other hand, where large quantities of urine are passed it could be that the child is drinking a great deal more than usual either out of habit or because he is being encouraged to do so due to having a cold or a mild temperature. One important condition that might be responsible for a child producing large quantities of urine is diabetes. A child developing diabetes will also be constantly thirsty, will lose weight and become tired and listless. If tested, the urine will contain abnormally high amounts of sugar.

Any discomfort experienced by a child when passing urine may be due to an infection. A urinary infection can occur in any part of the 'waterworks' system but is most serious of all when it affects the kidney itself. When it does, the child is usually quite unwell with a high temperature, tummy or back pain, and significant fatigue. Infections lower down the system can irritate the bladder (cystitis) and the tube which drains the bladder, the urethra, and the resulting inflammation causes a stinging sensation as the urine is passed. But irritation of the tip of the penis or the vaginal lips can also occur as a result of the skin inflammation caused by nappy rash or allergy (see pages 135 and 137). Any sore skin in the nappy area will always be more uncomfortable when urine is passed.

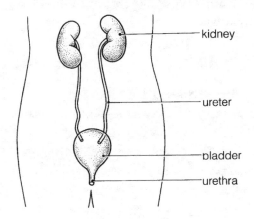

Cross-section of the kidneys and urinary system

When pain and frequency are suffered together, this combination of symptoms is almost always due to a urine infection. A child who was previously dry during the day may start to wet himself again, and the urine may take on a cloudy or milky appearance and smell particularly strong. Sometimes the child may have a temperature, and in advanced cases high temperatures with sweating and shaking can occur together with low abdominal or back pain.

Younger children with a urinary infection often have none of the symptoms described above and only come to the doctor's attention because they are tired or lethargic, because they have lost their appetite or have gained very little weight. Any child with these non-specific and rather vague symptoms should always have a urine sample tested for abnormality. This is particularly important in children under five because reflux (of urine up the ureters to the kidney) is more common, and this reflux of infected urine can lead to kidney damage. Progressive or newly-occurring damage after five is extremely unlikely.

After the age of one, urinary infections are much commoner in girls than boys. Their urethra is much shorter than that of boys, and the passage of germs from the outside upwards into the bladder is therefore much easier. Some two per cent of all girls will experience the symptoms of a urinary infection at some stage during their childhood, and at any one time five per cent of school-girls have significant numbers of bacteria in their urine with no symptoms whatsoever.

WHAT CAN YOU DO?

Check the child's temperature. The first thing to do when your child complains of any of the above symptoms is to check for any fever. Kidney infections are very likely to produce a rising temperature, whereas cystitis (inflammation of the bladder) or discomfort right at the opening of the tube from the bladder to the outside (the urethra) usually do not. They are also unlikely to cause kidney damage. Bear in mind that a child with a fever caused by other conditions may suffer urinary discomfort so the situation can often be confusing.

Look at the urine. Sometimes examining the urine in a glass jar can suggest the presence of an infection, particularly if the urine is cloudy, milky or particularly strong smelling. Strong odours, however, may also be the result of dehydration or dieting.

Take a mid-stream specimen to the doctor. A sample of the urine is extremely useful to the doctor since he or she can send it off to the laboratory to test for any bacteria present. This, in turn will help the doctor to choose the antibiotic which is most likely to eradicate the infection quickly. It is vital that the sample is collected in a completely sterile container – one that has not been washed out with soap or any other form of detergent, but has merely been sterilised using boiling water. It should also be processed by the lab as soon after collection as possible.

The urine sample should be a mid-stream specimen (MSU in medical terms) which means that when the child passes urine the first part of the stream should be discarded since this is likely to be contaminated with the bacteria normally present on the surface of the skin, and the middle part of the stream collected instead.

Ease the pain. Discomfort in the lower abdomen or back may be relieved by a hot-water bottle and paracetamol.

Parents can do a lot to prevent urinary infections and urethral discomfort and inflammation by keeping an eye on genito-urinary hygiene. Little girls can prove rather lazy in wiping themselves properly after going to the toilet, and they should certainly be trained to always wipe from front to back to prevent any faecal matter from entering the urinary system. In the case of urethral problems, it is also important to avoid bubble baths, synthetic pants and biological washing powders, and to use a regular barrier cream.

WHAT CAN THE DOCTOR DO?

The doctor can explore all the relevant symptoms and examine the child for any obvious sources of discomfort. Kidney tenderness can be felt, in some cases, by the doctor placing his or her hands on the child's abdomen, but where this is absent there may be signs of nappy rash with redness and inflammation at the vaginal lips or the tip of the penis which could identify the underlying problem. The child's blood pressure should also be taken as this may be raised if kidney disease is present. A mid-stream urine specimen should also be collected and sent to the laboratory for investigation and identification of the bacteria responsible for the infection. The results of these tests will help the doctor decide which is the most appropriate antibiotic to prescribe. Laboratory test results can, however, take a few days to come through, so sometimes, if a clinical diagnosis has been made, antibiotics can be started and subsequently changed if the lab results warrant it. Early treatment with antibiotics is important, especially in children under the age of four, since untreated kidney infection can lead to permanent damage with long-term problems.

The doctor needs to take a particular interest where urinary infections keep coming back again. Occasionally this may be because the antibiotic being used is ineffective, in which case a further sample of urine needs to be tested to identify the organism responsible. However, in a small proportion of children there will be an underlying problem such as a congenital abnormality of the kidney or its draining tubes, reflux of urine back up from the bladder towards the kidneys, or undiagnosed scarring of the kidneys themselves. These recurrent infections are more common in girls than boys because their shorter urethra makes ascending infection more likely, but boys too can have congenital abnormalities such as those of the valves in the tubes leading from the kidneys and bladder which can predispose them to urinary and kidney problems. Most cases of urinary reflux can be satisfactorily treated with low-dose, long-term antibiotics, but occasionally surgical intervention to correct the anatomical abnormality and prevent permanent damage to the kidneys is required.

IF YOU REMEMBER NOTHING ELSE, REMEMBER THESE THREE THINGS

1   Kidney infection is the commonest important urinary problem of childhood and always requires antibiotic treatment.

2   Frequent passing of large amounts of urine may be the first sign of diabetes.

3   All infections under the age of four and recurrent infections over the age of four need to be investigated fully and treated to prevent permanent kidney damage.

Vaginal Soreness

Many little girls complain of vaginal soreness or irritation from time to time.

CAUSES OF VAGINAL SORENESS

* ❋ Nappy rash
* ❋ Vulvitis
* ❋ Intestinal worms
* ❋ Foreign body
* ❋ Sexual abuse

Nappy Rash

Nappy rash is a common cause of vaginal soreness in children up to the age of thirty months. The sensitive wet skin becomes inflamed as bacteria get to work on the contents of the nappy, producing ammonia, which is an irritant, as a by-product.

Vulvitis

In older children who are out of nappies, other contaminants such as dirt, dead skin flakes and faecal matter can set up a local inflammation of the vaginal lips known as vulvitis. Using perfumed soap, talc, bubble bath and detergents can make these problems worse, and may also irritate sensitive skin in their own right.

Intestinal Worms

Any vaginal soreness which is intensely itchy may be a sign of intestinal worms, though these more frequently cause intense irritation at the anus (see page 53).

Foreign Body

Where a vaginal discharge is present in any girl prior to puberty, the possibility of a foreign body inside the vagina should be considered. Most little girls are curious about their anatomy and it is by no means unheard of for them to probe with their fingers or insert small objects such as beads or sweets inside their vagina. Such foreign bodies will eventually set up an infection with a discoloured or blood-stained discharge.

Sexual Abuse

Finally, all parents should be aware that sexual abuse is an occasional cause of vaginal soreness. This is not to say that any child taken to the doctor will be suspected of having been sexually abused, but if all parents and doctors are alert to the possibility, however remote, steps may be taken to make enquires designed to protect the child from further physical and psychological damage.

WHAT CAN YOU DO?

Parents can play an important role in teaching their children the value of thorough personal hygiene. Small girls need only have the visible parts of their external genitalia cleaned, although it is quite all right to gently part the vaginal lips and wipe the skin just inside. Barrier creams can be helpful in preventing nappy rash in babies, and all children are better off in cotton knickers or no knickers at all to allow the air to keep the skin dry. Older girls should be taught to wipe from front to back rather than the other way round to prevent any faecal contamination of the vaginal area.

When a child does complain of soreness 'down below', the parents should take a look to see if there is any obvious redness or swelling. Discharge is unusual, and when it occurs it is worth asking a child sufficiently old to understand whether there is any possibility of a foreign body having been poked inside. A simple check can be made for the presence of intestinal worms merely by inspecting the child's stools. The worms resemble slender, white threads which wriggle slightly. Finally, any undue concern and preoccupation with vaginal symptoms may predispose a little girl to embarrassment, awkwardness or other sexual difficulties in later life, so early treatment and reassurance is important.

WHAT CAN THE DOCTOR DO?

Although it is not quite true to say that every doctor taking a glance at a child's perineum can come up with an instant diagnosis, a physical examination will often be sufficient to discover the problem and its solution. A conscientious doctor should therefore always carry out such an examination. Where heavy discharge is present and there is the least suspicion of a foreign body within the vagina, a gentle internal examination by either the GP, paediatrician or gynaecologist can be performed and the offending object removed. Antibiotic treatment will then cure the condition.

Nappy rash and vulvitis, of whatever cause, will respond to a selection of soothing anti-inflammatory, antifungal or antibiotic creams or ointments, with or without the use of barrier creams as well. The treatment of worms involves taking an oral anti-worm preparation, not only by the child affected but by the whole family as well to prevent cyclical re-infection. A second dose ten to fourteen days later is recommended.

Finally, where sexual abuse is suspected a sensitive but thorough investigation should be instigated involving parents, the GP, the health visitor, the consultant paediatrician, the social services and any other relevant authorities. However, it should be remembered that definite signs of sexual abuse are not usually present, even in proven cases.

IF YOU REMEMBER NOTHING ELSE, REMEMBER THESE THREE THINGS

1   Vaginal soreness is a common and usually short-lived symptom.

---

2   The teaching of simple but thorough hygiene to small girls is an important preventative measure.

---

3   Where soreness is associated with discharge, the possibility of a foreign body in the vagina needs to be eliminated.

Vomiting

All babies gently regurgitate their feeds from time to time (posset-ting), but some do so more frequently than others. Vomiting, on the other hand, means that the stomach contents are brought up more forcibly. Vomiting in a child may have a very sudden onset, but this is not always indicative of a serious underlying condition. In most cases the child is sick and that is the end of it. There are no more episodes, the child perks up and is soon running around as though nothing had happened. If, on the other hand, the vomiting persists for more than several hours and the child is generally unwell, and if there is also a high temperature, diarrhoea or pain, there may well be some more serious underlying disorder requiring referral to the doctor. Similarly, if there has been any gradual loss of weight or if the child becomes increasingly drowsy or floppy, then again urgent medical care is needed. In addition, newborn babies and infants run a very real risk of dehydration, even within a relatively short space of time, so in this case medical help should be sought urgently.

Nausea as an isolated symptom is rare in children and they seldom complain of it. However, there are a number of hidden infections which produce little in the way of symptoms apart from a feeling of sickness. Kidney infection or a very mild liver infection (infectious hepatitis) are two examples. Any medicines that your child might be taking could also be responsible. Certain antibiotics can produce a feeling of sickness in their own right, as do anticonvulsants used in the treatment of epilepsy.

The most likely cause of vomiting depends very much on the age group of the child. Both parents and doctors should be aware of the different problems associated with different age groups, so it is useful here to consider newborn babies, infants and older toddlers separately.

VOMITING IN THE NEWBORN BABY

CAUSES OF VOMITING IN THE NEWBORN BABY

---

* Normal possetting

* Infection

* Intestinal blockage

* Birth injury

* Metabolic problems

* Kidney problems

Possetting

Bringing back small amounts of the last milk feed is absolutely normal in a newborn baby, and may even persist into toddlerhood. Some babies bring back very little, if any, and others bring back what appears to be the entire feed. But the critical question is whether or not the baby is gaining weight. It may appear, for example, that nothing has stayed down for an entire week, but if the baby is putting on weight nicely, sufficient absorption of the milk must be taking place for adequate nutrition.

Possetting is due largely to a floppy valve at the junction between the lower end of the gullet and the stomach which allows swallowed milk to come up again. As the child grows older, the valve becomes tighter and more efficient, so possetting eventually stops. What is really significant is persistent vomiting of large amounts of milk, particularly if it is stained green. This suggests the presence of bile due to obstruction of the intestine or some form of infection. A drowsy baby who is not sucking well and does not appear to be hungry is also a worrying sign. If his weight is falling, if the tummy is distended, if the baby looks dry and dehydrated or has a temperature, then again the situation is more urgent and a doctor should be consulted. Finally, if the newborn baby has passed none of the dark-green solidus black motions called meconium in the first twenty-four hours of life, or if the soft spot on the top of the baby's head is bulging, there may well be significant underlying problems which require urgent medical attention.

Infection

Vomiting is often triggered by the presence in the blood of certain toxins released by infective agents. All newborn babies are vulnerable to infection as their immune systems are not yet mature and they are wholly reliant on the antibodies passed on to them by their mother. Infection can come from a septic umbilical cord stump, from gastroenteritis, meningitis or, more commonly, from more mundane infections including those of the kidneys, ear and throat.

Meningitis.
Meningitis is one of the biggest killers of all in children, so it is important for parents to be aware of its symptoms and signs. Any newborn baby with symptoms that suggest meningitis should be admitted to hospital without delay for further investigation and treatment. Often this will necessitate a lumbar puncture which enables the doctor not only to make a diagnosis, but also to identify the organism responsible. Once this has been done, the most effective and appropriate antibiotic can be selected to eradicate it.

As most of the bugs that cause meningitis are sensitive to the antibiotics normally used to treat them, some doctors will now start a child on a course of antibiotics before performing a lumbar puncture because of the small risk involved in the procedure itself.

SIGNS OF MENINGITIS IN A SMALL BABY

* Vomiting

* Drowsiness and floppiness

* Failure to take feeds

* Convulsions

* Bulging soft spot (fontanelle) on top of head

* High-pitched cry

* Sometimes a purply-red rash

Intestinal Blockage

A newborn baby can be expected to pass meconium, a black-green sticky substance, within a few hours of birth. Very occasionally, however, a thick plug of meconium can block the intestine. This is commonly seen in cystic fibrosis where the intestinal secretions are much stickier than usual. There may be a family history of this condition, and an older sibling may well suffer from it as well. It is also seen in Hirschsprung's disease, in which part of the lower bowel is devoid of the normal nerve connections responsible for moving the intestinal contents along. Both these conditions can produce a blockage leading to distension and vomiting, since anything swallowed by the baby cannot easily pass through.

Birth Injury

Occasionally, a newborn baby can suffer a small brain haemorrhage or develop slight swelling of the brain tissue itself as a result of a very difficult labour and delivery. As well as vomiting, the fontanelle, the soft spot at the top of the baby's head, may bulge, the child may be drowsy, have a high-pitched cry and twitch or have convulsions. Treatment of the vomiting in this case depends on the underlying cause. Significant head injuries in older children can also produce vomiting.

Metabolic Problems

Vomiting may sometimes be the result of an inherited disorder affecting the baby's metabolism, but this is very rare. Most parents will remember witnessing, perhaps with some trepidation, the heel prick test performed on their baby within a few hours of birth by the midwife or health visitor. This tests for the metabolic disorder phenylketonuria and for a thyroid disorder. These conditions, along with others such as lactose intolerance and galactosaemia, are examples of metabolic disorders in which the body is unable to handle certain food substances in the gut as a result of a deficiency in key enzymes. Unless the condition is identified at an early age, abnormal by-products of metabolism may build up in the bloodstream producing vomiting and other side-effects.

Kidney Problems

Again, very occasionally, a baby may be born with anatomical kidney, bladder or genital problems which mean that abnormal or no urine is produced. There is a build-up of by-products in the baby's body and vomiting occurs. This is why parents and midwives always check that the baby's nappy is damp in the first few hours of life.

VOMITING IN INFANTS

CAUSES OF VOMITING IN INFANTS

∗ Air swallowing

∗ Infection

∗ Constant crying

∗ Travel sickness

∗ Pyloric stenosis

∗ Hiatus hernia

∗ Appendicitis

∗ Intussusception

∗ Coeliac disease

∗ Medicines and poisons

∗ Migraine

∗ Miscellaneous

Air Swallowing

The regurgitation of part of a milk feed in a newborn baby (posset-ting) is replaced by different kinds of vomiting as the infant matures. An infant who is breast-fed may swallow a lot of air if he sucks for too long on an empty breast. Similarly, a bottle-fed infant may swallow a lot of air if the hole in the teat is too small or the baby's lips don't seal the base of the teat properly, even where the hole in the teat is the right size (see page 20). After sucking on the bottle for any length of time, a vacuum is formed and until it is released by removing the baby's mouth from the teat, any increased sucking merely draws in air from the sides of the mouth. Also, some mums get into the habit of resting the bottle on a pillow so that the baby can suck away merrily while she rests or gets on with other things. This practice is never recommended due to the risk of the child inhaling the bottle's contents and choking. It is also likely to increase the amount of wind in the baby's stomach and make him more likely to regurgitate milk along with the wind. Most babies should take about ten to fifteen minutes to feed properly, so a baby who is vomiting and is taking forty-five to sixty minutes to feed may well be very windy.

Sometimes it is the way the feed is made up which is responsible. The instructions on the tin or packet should be followed to the letter – formula milk is specially modified to supply the correct amounts of all nutrients providing it is made up accurately. Never be tempted to add an extra scoop. Also avoid careless or over-vigorous handling of the baby after feeds – he should not be bounced on a knee too energetically or held over a shoulder and burped too strenuously.

Another reason for 'sicky' babies is that some are given lumpy or too solid food before they can chew. A baby learns chewing at the age of about six to seven months, and until that time foods should be puréed. Conversely, if a baby is quite capable of taking solids but is only fed milk, the large quantities of liquid required to satisfy the baby's hunger are just too much for the baby's stomach to take and they are more likely to come back up.

Occasionally, vomiting is due to a dietary intolerance. Increasingly, allergy to cow's milk is being reported. Cow's milk is not recommended as part of an infant's diet until the age of one year. True allergy, such as an anaphylactic reaction to a small amount of milk, is rare, but food intolerance, producing vomiting, irritability and continual crying or other changes in a baby's behaviour and physical health, does occur. These symptoms can respond quite dramatically to a change in milk to soya-based infant preparations.

Finally, teething occurs during the first year of life and some babies are definitely more prone to vomiting at this time (see page 383). Pain and increased saliva production contribute, and babies who are teething often put their hands in their mouths which can cause gagging. Sometimes, babies like the sensation of regurgitated food in their mouths and this can become a learnt habit.

Infection

Infection is probably the most common, serious cause of vomiting in infancy. Straightforward problems like ear infections and tonsillitis are often associated with vomiting, partly due to the fever and partly to the pain itself. A tummy bug, or gastroenteritis, may produce vomiting before diarrhoea occurs. There may be abdominal pain too, characterised by the child drawing his knees up under his chin and crying. Whooping cough is another infectious illness that classically produces vomiting after persistent bouts of coughing lasting up to two minutes or more.

Kidney infections and meningitis are serious infections that must never be ignored as possible reasons for an infant vomiting. The signs to look out for in kidney infections are urine being passed more frequently and having a stronger odour than usual. In meningitis, a child will also have a high fever, may or may not have a stiff neck, will become uncomfortable looking at bright lights, be off feeds and become increasingly drowsy. Vomiting in association with these symptoms always warrants the urgent attention of a doctor, with emergency hospital admission if necessary.

Constant Crying

Infants cry for a number of reasons, often because they are hungry, thirsty, too hot, too cold or simply have a dirty nappy. They can also cry merely to attract the attention of their parents. This may or may not be forthcoming, but any child left to cry for any length of time can work himself up to such an extent that he is duly sick.

This can be alarming and, without doubt, makes some parents feel guilty – the child then usually gets his way and is picked up and comforted. If vomiting does not return and the child settles down nicely, there is usually nothing to worry about.

Travel Sickness

Vomiting in association with some form of travel can occur at any age, but it tends to be worse in toddlers and older children. There are various ways of dealing with it, as described on page 432.

Pyloric Stenosis

This condition is usually seen in infants between three and six weeks of age, although it occurs a little later in premature babies. Boys are about five times more often affected than girls, with something like twelve children in every thousand developing it. In this condition the whole feed is brought up, often so dramatically that it can shoot several metres across the room. This is called projectile vomiting, and even when seen for the first time it is quite unmistakable. If untreated, this type of vomiting will continue for two to three days, the baby becoming constipated and dehydrated as a result. A doctor may feel a very small lump, about the size of a walnut, just above and to the right of the navel during a feed, but this is not always the case. Sometimes an abdominal ultrasound scan may be done to confirm the presence of the lump. To correct this condition, a small surgical operation to divide the thickened muscle at the base of the stomach is required.

Hiatus Hernia

A hiatus hernia occurs when there is a weakness in the diaphragm, the muscular, dome-shaped structure which separates the abdomen from the chest. The top of the stomach pushes up through the weakness, upsetting the function of the delicate valve which is found at the junction of the gullet and stomach. This causes milk to be regurgitated from the stomach, often tinged with a little blood due to irritation and inflammation of the sensitive lining of the gullet. Confirmation of the hiatus hernia can be achieved by using a special X-ray known as a barium swallow.

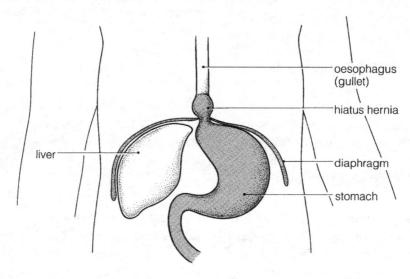

oesophagus (gullet)

hiatus hernia

liver

diaphragm

stomach

The position of a hiatus hernia

Appendicitis

Appendicitis in very small babies is rare and easily misdiagnosed, but it is a lot more common in toddlers and older children (see pages 403–404).

Intussusception

In this condition one part of the baby's bowel telescopes into an adjacent part. This causes interference with the formation of normal stools, producing blood-stained mucus which strongly resembles redcurrant jelly. The baby shrieks with pain at intermittent intervals and later on the characteristic appearance of the stools is usually enough for the doctor to be confident about the diagnosis. Surgery may be required, although sometimes water or air pushed up the child's bottom in a diagnostic barium enema can correct the condition.

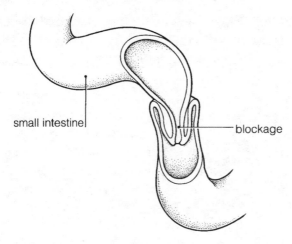

small intestine

blockage

'Telescoping' of the intestine inside itself

Coeliac disease

Coeliac disease is due to a dietary intolerance to gliadin, the protein part of gluten, present in wheat and rye flour. The symptoms begin when the infant is first given cereals, usually at about three to six months of age. Vomiting may begin almost at once but the infant also loses his appetite, becomes miserable and irritable and develops loose, pale, bulky, smelly motions. The doctor might first consider gastroenteritis as a possible cause, but when the weight loss becomes severe and prolonged and the typical fatty motions become obvious, a diagnosis of coeliac disease will become likely. A jejunal biopsy – where a tiny sample of the lining of the small intestine is taken for analysis – will confirm the diagnosis, and after that a gluten-free diet can be started, resulting usually in the child immediately gaining weight and height. This diet needs to be continued throughout the child's life.

Medicines and poisons

Vomiting sometimes occurs as a result of accidental poisoning. Many an infant, through curiosity, has accidentally poisoned himself with domestic chemicals and other such substances, and prescribed medicines can also produce vomiting when taken inappropriately. All of these potential poisons should therefore be kept well out of reach of prying hands.

Migraine

There is no doubt that vomiting associated with migraine can start even in the first year of life. There is often a strong family history of migraine but despite this the diagnosis is often not made until the child is older, when it becomes obvious that the vomiting is associated with the headache and visual symptoms typical of this condition.

Miscellaneous

There is a group of general disorders which may produce nausea and vomiting in the infant, including diabetes, kidney disorders, raised pressure of the cerebro-spinal fluid which surrounds the brain within the skull and metabolic disorders such as phenylke-tonuria which is tested for in the first few days of life. Although rare, they are always at the back of any doctor's mind when no other reason for infant vomiting can be found.

VOMITING IN TODDLERS AND OLDER CHILDREN

CAUSES OF VOMITING IN TODDLERS AND OLDER CHILDREN

---

* Psychological factors

* Infection

* Travel sickness

* Appendicitis

* Medicines and poisons

* Miscellaneous

Psychological Factors

Toddlers may vomit for many of the same reasons as younger babies, but in this age group psychological factors also become important. Some children get so excited at the idea of something like a party that they may make themselves sick. Fear and anxiety related to school or domestic problems can have the same effect. Parents themselves can make a rod for their own backs by inadvertently causing their impressionable child to feel sick merely by suggesting the idea to him. By fussing about anticipated travel sickness, for example, they make the problem more likely – the less parents remind their child that he may feel sick, the less likely it is to occur.

Occasionally, vomiting may be brought deliberately on by attention-seeking toddlers. They recognise just how anxious and protective their parents become when they are sick and soon learn

431

how to make it happen. Children with tonsillitis may jam their fingers down the backs of their throats, promptly producing the gag reflex and retching.

Infection

All of the infectious causes of sickness affecting infants also apply to toddlers (see page 426). Ear, nose and throat infections and gastroenteritis are the commonest. Meningitis, when it occurs in the older child, shows slightly different symptoms from that in babies and infants (see pages 421–422). Vomiting in this case is usually accompanied by a high fever, but in addition to the dislike of bright lights and decreasing consciousness, there may well be neck stiffness. This is manifested by discomfort and resistance to movement when the head is pushed forward towards the chest when the child is lying flat on his back in bed (see page 325).

Travel Sickness

Many toddlers suffer from travel sickness, particularly if they are sitting in the rear seat of a vehicle and are unable to see through the car window. Booster cushions help enormously, and games which distract and entertain may prevent the problem altogether on short journeys. Motion sickness is also commonly experienced on aeroplanes and boats.

Antihistamine syrup is useful in preventing travel sickness provided it is given at least an hour or two before the journey is started and continued at the prescribed intervals whilst it continues. The most effective types of antihistamine used for this purpose do however cause drowsiness and sleepiness so parents should always be warned about that if they are considering its use for their child.

Appendicitis

About one in six of the population have to have their appendix removed, and most of these are children and young adults. Any vomiting seen during appendicitis is accompanied by the more usual symptom of abdominal pain which begins around the navel and then moves downwards slightly and to the right, an area which is particularly tender if pressed upon. The child is completely off his food, may have a temperature, and may experience either constipation or diarrhoea. When vomiting goes hand in hand with abdominal pain, a doctor's opinion should always be sought.

Medicines and Poisons

Toddlers are notorious for getting into the medicine cabinet or raiding the cupboard under the kitchen sink where bleach, carpet cleaner and other toxic domestic substances are kept. It is surprising just how much of a foul-tasting cleaning fluid a toddler can swallow during his first chemical-tasting session! Adult pills and tablets which closely resemble sweets may also be the cause of accidental poisoning. In both situations, child locks must be used as a matter of priority.

Vomiting may take place immediately or a bit later on, and other symptoms in the child such as drowsiness, abdominal pain or breathing difficulties may also be seen. If you find your toddler being sick and suspect he has sampled some medicinal or domestic substance, take him to casualty immediately, along with whatever substance you suspect he may have taken. This will help the doctors decide on their best mode of action on admission to hospital.

Some medications which are prescribed for children can cause nausea and vomiting as a possible side-effect. Examples include antibiotics (especially Erythroped), antiepileptic medicines, tranquillisers, antihelminthics used to treat intestinal worms, and anticancer drugs.

Miscellaneous

All of the physical problems which affect infants can also affect the older child (see pages 424–430). In addition, vomiting in older children is common following dietary indiscretion (at birthday parties etc.) and is also experienced in asthma attacks (see page 445).

WHAT CAN YOU DO?

The first thing to do when your child is being sick is to get him into a comfortable position, which may be sitting up in bed or lying down, and provide him with a bowl. Stroking and reassuring him has a calming and soothing effect, particularly in the younger child who may be vomiting for the first time. Cool your child's brow with a dampened flannel and take the nasty taste caused by the stomach acid away from the mouth by gently brushing his teeth. Encourage him to drink small amounts of cool liquid which is more likely to be kept down than anything else. It also staves off the possibility of dehydration in the younger child if the vomiting promises to be protracted. Avoid milky drinks after any bout of sickness as the fat content is absorbed only slowly and therefore makes further vomiting more likely. Also, some children may develop a transient protein or lactose intolerance following a tummy bug and may need a soya milk for up to two months to avoid further diarrhoea. In the early stages of sickness, therefore, use clear fluids only for a few hours such as pleasant-flavoured fruit juice or pure water. Specially formulated rehydrating powder is available from the chemist, such as Dioralyte, which is made up with water and contains an ideal balance of fluid, salts and sugars, but because of its low calorie content it should be used for no more than 48 hours. Later, reintroduce bland, liquidised food followed by ordinary solids after several hours when the appetite has returned.

WHAT CAN THE DOCTOR DO?

The first thing the doctor needs to do when confronted with a vomiting child is to find the cause. There are so many possibilities that any action will depend entirely on the underlying problem.

Let us consider babies first. The normal phenomenon of possetting is the commonest cause of vomiting in the newborn baby during the first year of life, and usually requires only reassurance and advice for the parents. If it becomes clear that there is a more serious underlying problem such as infection, then it is vital to identify the nature of that infection.

The doctor's examination will typically be carried out to look for a red eardrum or any discharge from a middle ear infection. He or she will want to look at the throat for tonsillitis. The doctor will also look out for the dehydration seen in gastroenteritis, the kidney tenderness seen in kidney infection, the oozing, infected stump of an inflamed umbilicus, or the bulging, soft membrane at the top of the head and the sunken, staring eyes of a baby with meningitis. In most instances, the cause will turn out to be fairly trivial in which case treatment may be administered by the parents at home. But in more severe cases, such as severe gastroenteritis, meningitis or head injury, urgent hospital admission is required.

Older children are also susceptible to a large number of problems which may cause vomiting, and again the medical examination is vital in achieving a diagnosis.

Sometimes the diagnosis cannot be made instantly, but is made over a period of, say, 24–48 hours as the clinical picture emerges. It may be necessary for the doctor to visit the child at home the next day after seeing the child in the surgery, or it may be that a sudden deterioration in the middle of the night warrants a much more urgent re-examination. At the outset, there is often little to distinguish vomiting as a result of swallowed mucus due to head cold from the earliest signs of meningitis.

The bottom line is, if in doubt then consult your doctor not just once, but a second time too if you are worried. Generally speaking, when the vomiting is associated with other symptoms or persists for more than six hours, ask your doctor for help. The treatment of underlying conditions and the prevention of dehydration is paramount, particularly in the younger child.

IF YOU REMEMBER NOTHING ELSE, REMEMBER THESE THREE THINGS

1   All children vomit, but some seem more prone to vomiting than others.

2   Vomiting in children is usually short lived, but if it persists for more than six hours and is associated with other symptoms, call your doctor.

3   Vomiting and diarrhoea together in a baby can cause serious dehydration, and early fluid replacement is vital. If your baby is having two wet nappies a day, then he is extremely unlikely to be significantly dehydrated.

Watery Eyes

Newborn babies do not usually produce tears until the age of about two months, unless the eye is injured in some way. Later, tears are produced more abundantly and watery eyes are common in the first year of life, often as a result of a partially blocked naso-lacrimal (tear) duct. This tiny passageway runs from a very small hole just visible at the inner margin of the lower eyelid down to the middle part of the nasal cavity into which the tears drain. This is why crying tends to make the nose run. This partial obstruction is extremely common in babies, and often sorts itself out as the child grows older and the duct enlarges naturally.

Watery eyes can be made worse if low-grade infection with viruses or bacteria sets in, and an infective conjunctivitis with a sticky, greeny-yellow discharge often occurs. Allergic conjunctivitis, on the other hand, can cause watering of the eyes with redness under the eyelids, but unless infection also occurs the tears will usually remain clear.

Babies often scratch their eyes by mistake with their fingernails, and this or any other injury can result in watering. Dry, flaky eyelids (blepharitis) which irritate the eyes can occur in eczema, and sore, red, watery eyes are often seen in both measles and chickenpox.

WHAT CAN YOU DO?

If your baby's eyes are watering badly there is an increased risk of infective conjunctivitis. If you notice any greeny-yellow discharge from either eye, your doctor can prescribe antibiotic drops or ointment which will almost always resolve the problem. Since this kind of conjunctivitis can quickly spread to other small children, they should be kept away from them for a day or two and should use a separate flannel and towel for washing. In recurrent cases there is almost certainly a narrowed nasolacrimal duct, but since this is usually self-correcting, surgery would not normally be considered until the child is somewhat older.

WHAT CAN THE DOCTOR DO?

The doctor's main role is to protect a watering eye from further inflammation or infection by the use of appropriate antibiotic drops or ointment. Viral conjunctivitis is particularly contagious amongst small children and babies and minor epidemics do occur, especially in nurseries where a number of children are all together under one roof. Affected children should really be kept away from the nursery or school until they are no longer likely to be infectious.

If a child is found to have a partially blocked nasolacrimal duct,

437

he should be kept under review to make sure that normal growth results in spontaneous opening of the duct and that any attendant infection is treated.

IF YOU REMEMBER NOTHING ELSE, REMEMBER THESE THREE THINGS

1 Newborn babies do not produce tears when they cry until the age of about two months.

2 In most cases, watering eyes are due to partial blockage of the nasolacrimal duct.

3 A sticky, yellow-green discharge from the eye should be treated with ointment and antibiotic drops.

Weight Loss

It is unusual for children to lose weight, but when it happens it is usually short lived. Often it is due to a simple infection, and reduced dietary intake, excess fluid loss through perspiration, vomiting and diarrhoea all contribute. In most cases the weight loss will prove temporary, with any weight rapidly being put back on within a few days. Sometimes, however, there is a more serious underlying cause which requires full investigation by the doctor.

It seems obvious, but it is always worth checking the accuracy of the scales you (or your health visitor) use to weigh your child, as some domestic scales may be up to half a stone out. It is a bad idea, too, to compare weight readings on different sets of scales, since these can often give an impression of weight changes when none exist. A simpler method of assessing weight changes is to see if your child's regular clothes have become too big for him. If the clothes look more baggy and the waistband is looser than it used to be, this is quite often a definite sign that a problem is present.

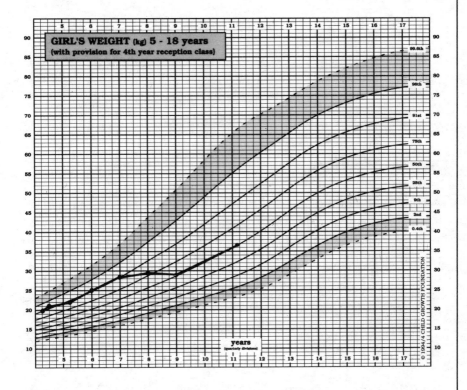

Centile weight chart showing a cessation of weight gain over a 2 year period at the age of 7 to 9

CAUSES OF WEIGHT LOSS

* Acute infection

* Intestinal problems

* Diabetes

* Chronic infection

* Asthma

* Emotional problems

* Malignancy

Acute Infection

A child will often lose weight in response to a severe sore throat, a persistent cough, an episode of gastroenteritis with diarrhoea and vomiting or a bad earache. The problem is compounded by the presence of a temperature, but generally speaking weight loss is minimal (less than five per cent) and all the weight is regained within a few days of the infection settling as most of it is due to fluid depletion.

Intestinal Problems

Fluid loss or malabsorption of food will cause a child to lose weight. In severe cases of gastroenteritis, persistent vomiting and diarrhoea will have this effect, but more chronic inflammation such as colitis or Crohn's disease, both of which produce malfunction of the bowel, may also be responsible. Cystic fibrosis and coeliac disease prevent the absorption of certain constituents of the diet, and weight loss is again a frequent symptom. Here, tissue loss in addition to fluid loss will be partly responsible.

Diabetes

There are two distinct types of diabetes, in both of which large volumes of urine are passed as a predominant symptom. In the commonest type, diabetes mellitus, there is a lack of insulin in the blood, the hormone necessary to allow the passage of glucose from the bloodstream into the cells of the body tissues. Lack of insulin means that sugar builds up in the bloodstream and 'spills over' into the urine because the mechanisms for reabsorbing it in the kidneys are overwhelmed. The sugar takes large quantities of water with it, causing the volume of urine produced to be greatly increased. At the same time, the body tissues are deprived of glucose, which is their fundamental energy supply, and water, so the tissues waste away and the body becomes dehydrated. The signs of weight loss, thirst, lethargy and passing a lot of urine are highly suggestive of diabetes mellitus. The other form of diabetes, diabetes insipidus, is much less common, but thirst and passing a lot of urine are the cardinal features here too, although glucose and insulin levels remain entirely normal.

Chronic Infection

Some infections may start so slowly that neither the child nor his parents are immediately aware of it. Not all infections cause immediate pain and discomfort in the way that an ear infection or sore throat might, which are often also accompanied by an obvious temperature. The child with a persistent, dry cough could turn out to have a patch of pneumonia on his lung, and another child with pain in the back or side could have a kidney infection. There has recently been an increase in the number of cases of tuberculosis in this country, and any of these three chronic infections, amongst many others, can produce weight loss.

Asthma

Children who suffer with severe or chronic asthma may lose weight because of the difficulty they have with their breathing. Their appetite is often affected and they may use a large amount of energy as they struggle to get air in and out of their lungs.

Emotional Problems

Sometimes there is no physical condition responsible for the weight loss, only an emotional one. Small children separated from their parents for any length of time may become anxious and withdrawn and will not eat normally. Children who are unhappy at school may respond in the same way. Alarmingly, doctors are seeing a growing number of young girls, some as young as eight or nine, developing the eating disorder anorexia nervosa, in which complex psychological factors produce a morbid fear of fatness and a deliberate and obsessional desire to lose weight.

Malignancy

Although rare, a child who lacks energy and who loses weight may be found to harbour some underlying malignancy. This is why a child who loses weight for no obvious reason needs to undergo a thorough investigation by the doctor.

WHAT CAN YOU DO?

Parents need to check the weight of their children fairly regularly, especially if they feel that their child's clothes have become rather too big for him. Ensure that the scales you use are accurate and that you take serial measurements using the same equipment. Try to find out if your child has any emotional worries – whether he is happy at school, or whether he is affected by any problems at home. If there is no obvious explanation for the weight loss, and certainly if it persists for more than a week, the doctor should be consulted so that the cause can be found. Once the underlying problem has been diagnosed, the parents can take an active role in treatment through dietary means.

WHAT CAN THE DOCTOR DO?

The doctor needs to find the cause of the weight loss. Talking to the parents and the child himself will often be helpful, but a full examination is mandatory, especially if the weight loss has occurred over any length of time. The urine should be tested for the presence of sugar to exclude diabetes. If the child has persistent diarrhoea, a stool specimen should be sent for analysis so that any invading germs can be identified and the appropriate treatment started. If the child has chronic asthma, then this recurrent and reversible condition needs to be controlled. If no cause for the weight loss can immediately be found, then the child should be referred to the hospital for further evaluation. Treatment will depend on the underlying cause.

IF YOU REMEMBER NOTHING ELSE, REMEMBER THESE THREE THINGS

1   Weight loss in a child is usually short lived and caused by a simple infection.

2   When no obvious cause is identified and the weight loss continues for more than a few days, further investigation is essential.

3   Treatment will depend on the underlying problem.

Wheezing

A wheeze is a high-pitched whistling sound produced when air rushes through a narrowed respiratory airway. It is similar to the noise made by the reed in a wind instrument, and the narrower the gap through which the air moves, the higher the pitch of the sound. Wheezing is distinct from the more rattly sound that may be heard in the back of the throat of children who are congested with catarrh or who develop a build-up of nasal secretions in their sleep which then gurgle as the child breathes in and out. The most common and important cause of wheezing in a child is asthma, although an inhaled foreign object and an infection known as bronchiolitis may be responsible too.

CAUSES OF WHEEZING

* Asthma

* Foreign body

* Bronchiolitis

ASTHMA

The most common cause of wheezing in children is asthma, although asthma may just produce a persistent cough at night and no wheezing at all (see page 211). Where wheezing or coughing is brought about by exercise, and where breathlessness is generally worse in the early morning, the diagnosis of asthma is extremely likely. Under the child's pyjamas you may even see the skin being sucked in between the ribs as the child struggles to breathe. Asthma sufferers also tend to adopt a characteristic sitting position in which they are hunched over with their arms and shoulders supported on their knees or on a piece of furniture, as this enables them to use other muscles not normally involved in breathing.

What happens during an asthma attack?

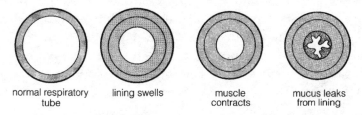

normal respiratory tube   lining swells   muscle contracts   mucus leaks from lining

The three stages of airway narrowing in asthma

The respiratory tubes which descend from the throat to the lungs are particularly sensitive in asthma sufferers. They are hyper-responsive to a number of trigger factors, any of which cause three basic things to happen:

1 First, the sensitive lining of the airways swells up, just as the lining of the nose swells up and blocks breathing when you have a cold. This has the effect of making breathing much more difficult, similar to having to breathe through a narrow straw for any length of time.

2 Next, the muscle lying in the wall of the tube contracts making the airways narrower.

3 Lastly, the swollen lining leaks fluid and produces a sticky mucus which further clogs up the air passages and makes the coughing and wheezing even worse. Usually there is a family history of asthma, and any child affected by the condition may well have brothers, sisters or at least either a mother or father who has had asthma themselves. Other allergies are also inherited, which is why eczema and hay fever are commonly seen in children who also suffer from asthma.

Who is more prone to asthma?
About 20 per cent of all young children have inherited a tendency to develop a persistent cough at night that forms part of the asthma symptoms. For some reason it seems to be about twice as common

in boys than girls, allergies clearly play a part, and children who were born prematurely and suffered breathing difficulties, especially respiratory distress syndrome, are all more likely to suffer.

Infants under one year who have had a severe bout of bronchiolitis are more vulnerable, as are children exposed to certain allergies in the first year of life, children whose parents smoke at home, and children who were bottle-fed rather than breast-fed. General environmental pollution is relevant too, so where a child lives can play a part in determining his susceptibility to asthma attacks.

TRIGGER FACTORS FOR ASTHMA

* Infection

* Allergy

* Cold air

* Exertion

* Excitement

* Irritants

* Foods and colourings

* Medicines

Infection

Viruses and bacteria of the type that normally cause colds, coughs, bronchitis and pneumonia may all start off a bout of asthma. Because the cough begins in association with other signs of a cold, it is often assumed that infection is the problem. However, when standard treatment for infective coughs fails to work and the cough persists for several weeks, then asthma should be considered seriously as a possible diagnosis.

Allergy

The persistent cough of asthma is often the result of allergy. Common causes include house dust, and the house dust mite and its faeces which are present within it. Feathers, moulds, pollens and pet fur can also irritate the lining of the respiratory passages after small quantities of them have been inhaled (see page 278).

Cold Air

Very cold air can certainly start off an asthma attack, even in people who are not normally prone to the condition. This is particularly true if the lungs are exposed to a sudden temperature drop, as happens, for example, when a child rushes out of a warm, centrally heated house into the freezing winter air.

Exertion

Vigorous exertion, especially in cold, dry air, which causes the child to pant for breath also represents quite a shock to the airways. Their sensitive lining simply does not like it, and an asthma attack may ensue.

Excitement

Some children may trigger off their asthma when they become worked up or anxious. Teaching them to remain calm and to breathe in a controlled and relaxed way is helpful.

Irritants

Cigarette smoke and other fumes are undoubtedly responsible for many attacks of asthma. Environmental pollution both indoors and outdoors is now thought to be largely responsible for the very significant increase in the number of asthma cases now being treated. Factors include an increase in house dust mite concentrations in double-glazed, draught-insulated, centrally heated, carpeted houses. Also diesel-engined cars produce far more particulate carbon matter than petrol-driven cars and may not be as 'green' as was previously thought. Photochemical smog, which produces such poor air quality during hot weather in and around large cities, occurs as a result of sunlight acting on car exhaust fumes and industrial output. Masks can be helpful, especially in older asthmatic children who spend a lot of time playing outdoors, and too much exercise in such conditions should certainly be avoided.

Food and Colourings

Very occasionally, food and drink may contain both natural and synthetic products which predispose some children to asthma. Some experts regard this as allergy, some as simply intolerance, but the effect on the child is nevertheless the same. It is worth excluding suspicious items from the child's diet and to observe whether the asthma improves.

Medicines

There are a number of medicines which are well known for making asthma worse by way of their side-effects, although these are not generally used with children. The exception is Propranolol which is used in the prevention of migraine. If a child has a persistent cough and is taking any medication, then ask your doctor if there could be any connection.

WHAT CAN YOU DO?

Clearly, if the trigger factors have been identified then it is sensible to try to avoid them. However, 'antigen-avoidance' is fine in theory but virtually impossible in practice. Infections cannot be avoided, but allergies may be reduced by avoiding contact with pets, by having hard floors rather than carpeting, by regular hoovering to remove dust and pet fur and by changing from feather-filled pillows and duvets to synthetic ones. Exertion, particularly in cold air, need not be avoided altogether, but measures such as wrapping a warm scarf around the mouth can make a difference. Dietary changes can be tried to avoid those substances which may cause increased sensitivity of the air passages. You could also ask the doctor if any medicines the child is taking could be to blame for the symptoms.

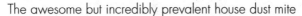

The awesome but incredibly prevalent house dust mite

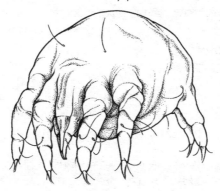

The house dust mite is a tiny creature invisible to the naked eye and which is present in huge numbers in even the cleanest of houses. The mites like to live in warm, damp, dark places where they are rarely disturbed and where food is provided. They feed on human skin scales which fall off as our skin is renewed. Consequently, they mostly live in bedrooms, particularly those with central-heating, double-glazing and fitted carpets. Something like two to five million of them live in a normal bed, and it is the inhalation of both live and dead mites and their droppings which causes the allergic reaction triggering asthma.

People who are allergic to the house dust mite, or whose children are, should follow these guidelines:

1 Old, damp houses, or houses near water contain more mites. Weekend cottages, where mites are left undisturbed contain large numbers.

2 Ventilation reduces house dust mite population. Open the window at least once a day and hang the duvet out of the window on frosty mornings to reduce the concentrations of the mites. Keeping the house cooler will also help, as warm bedrooms are an ideal breeding ground for mites.

3 Mites are killed by a hot wash, so the bed clothes should be regularly washed at high wash temperatures. Cuddly toys can be put in the hot tumble dryer, or in the deep freeze overnight every two or three weeks, vacuuming them afterwards to remove any dead mites and faeces.

4 Plastic bed covers are not very effective and not very pleasant for children. Newer covers are more effective, but more expensive (Allerayde, Advanced Allergy Technologies Ltd, Intervent – available at local chemists).

5 Smooth floors can be dusted and cleaned more easily than carpeted floors, but the new air recycling vacuum cleaners are able to reduce house dust mite quantities significantly, both from carpet and upholstery – remember the sitting room settee.

6 Generally damp dusting should be done regularly. This should include tops of curtains, the pelmet and the chest of drawers.

7 Applications that reduce the house dust mite by reducing their source of food are moderately effective and expensive. Ionisers are ineffective.

WHAT CAN THE DOCTOR DO?

The most important thing the doctor can do is to make the correct diagnosis in the first place. Something like 2,000 people still die from asthma every year in this country, and although the situation is improving, asthma is still under-diagnosed in children in whom a persistent cough at night is often the first and only sign. This is particularly true in the younger child where there is an erroneous belief that asthma cannot be accurately diagnosed. Once the diagnosis has been made, effective medication is available not only to prevent the asthma coming on in the first place, but also to treat it once it does start and should it deteriorate.

There are two main types of drugs used in the treatment of asthma.

1 'Reliever' or 'rescue' medications open up the respiratory tubes in the lungs and relieve any constriction within their muscular walls brought about by spasm. These are called bronchodilators. The most commonly used ones include Ventolin, Pulmadil, Atrovent, Bricanyl, Duovent and Alupent.

2 'Preventer' medications prevent the airway from narrowing in the first place and stop the inflammation which leads to sticky phlegm production. These are the anti-allergic drugs, such as Intal and Tilade, and the much more powerful anti-inflammatories known as steroids, which include Becotide and Pulmicort.

The above medications come in many forms – ordinary spray inhalers, powder inhalers, breath-activated inhalers and inhalers with whistles to confirm audibly that the device is being used in the correct way. It is important to remember that all inhalers need to be shaken immediately before use. Liquid and tablet preparations of many asthma drugs are also available.

Whatever treatment is chosen, some children find it difficult to coordinate the action of breathing in with squeezing their inhaler, and for them the use of a high-volume spacer or nebulizer overcomes this problem.

A typical high-volume spacer device used in the treatment of asthma

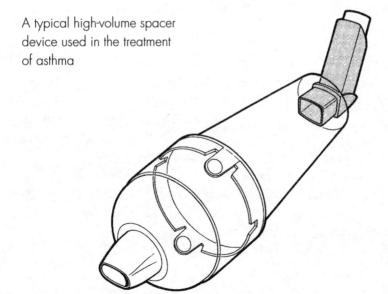

Asthma – using an
inhaler

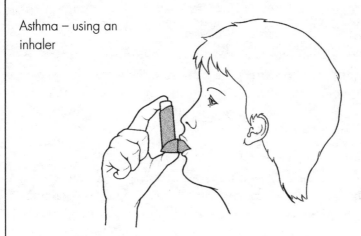

The inhaler simply fits into one end of the spacer and is squeezed until the required dose is sprayed into it as a fine mist. The child then breathes in and out of the mouthpiece at the other end at his own pace, obtaining maximum benefit but without difficulty. Two types of spacer are available on NHS prescription, namely Volumatic for use with Ventolin and Becotide inhalers, and Nebuhaler for use with Bricanyl and Pulmicort inhalers.

The choice of treatment will depend on the cause and severity of the symptoms. A typical treatment programme for a child would be tailored to his individual needs and proceed on a step-by-step basis. The first priority is simply to try to avoid the recognised trigger factors which provoke an asthma attack in the first place. Then the inhaler device which best suits the needs of the child should be selected. Finally, the doctor, child and parents should adopt a plan whereby the child himself learns about his condition and masters the ability to treat it. For children over five years of age a peak flow meter should also be prescribed so that the child can measure his response to treatment wherever necessary.

A peak flow meter is a simple device which is held horizontally to the mouth. The child takes a deep breath in, seals the mouthpiece with his lips and then blows into the meter as hard and as fast as he can. Three readings should be taken and the best of the three is recorded. When the child is well, there will be little or no

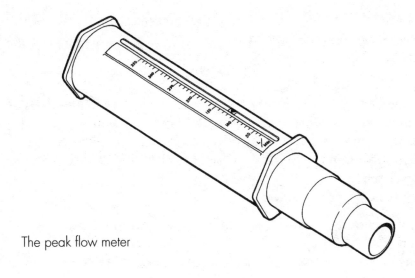

The peak flow meter

difference between readings taken several hours apart, but a difference of more than 20 per cent shows that the asthma is not controlled and that the treatment should be reviewed. The peak flow meter can therefore work as an early warning sign of worsening asthma.

A typical treatment protocol might proceed like this:

Step 1 This involves the occasional use of 'relief' or 'rescue' bronchodilator inhalers, but not more than once a day, for example Ventolin inhaler, one puff once a day.
If this fails, progress to step 2.

Step 2 Add regular anti-allergy inhaler, for example Intal inhaler, one puff four times daily.
If this fails, progress to step 3.

Step 3 Carry on using bronchodilator inhaler when required, but replace anti-allergy inhaler with a steroid inhaler, for example Becotide 100, one puff twice a day.
If this fails, progress to step 4.

Step 4 Carry on using bronchodilator inhaler when required, but increase dose of steroid and use a high-volume spacer or a dry

powder device, for example Becotide, 800 micrograms daily by spacer or Bricanyl Turbohaler.
If this fails, progress to step 5.

Step 5 Carry on with the above but use long-acting bronchodilators regularly (not just the short-acting ones used as required). In addition, bronchodilators may be more effective when given via a nebuliser. This is an electrically powered device which delivers the bronchodilator in the form of a very fine mist for inhalation and is more effective.
If this fails, progress to step 6.

Step 6 If chronic asthma is still troublesome, two other additional treatments should be considered. These are a slow-release oral bronchodilator called Theophylline and another inhaled bronchodilator which works in a different way to the others, called Ipratropium or Atrovent. Also, when asthma symptoms deteriorate at any time, a temporary increase in the dose of steroids either in inhaled or tablet form can often prove extremely effective.
If this fails, progress to step 7.

Step 7 All treatment should be reviewed regularly and immediately if asthma control is poor.

Problems With Treatment

Despite widespread worries about steroids, their use in asthma in inhaled form does not produce the side-effects sometimes seen when large doses are used in tablet form for prolonged periods. In fact, the wise use of steroids drastically improves an asthmatic child's quality of life, and undoubtedly saves lives. Many doctors now miss out step 2 altogether.

The bronchodilators are stimulants and can occasionally cause some palpitations, anxiety and shaking, especially if inhalers are over-used. For this reason, the prescribed dose should never be exceeded. When it is, it more often than not suggests that the treatment itself is no longer effective and that a review of the current therapy is required.

Having stabilised the child on the correct medication it is vital that he learns to manage his own treatment. The technique of using an inhaler correctly needs to be closely supervised to begin with, as in most cases failure of medication is due to the child being unable to coordinate his breathing correctly and the misuse of the inhalers.

Finally, the GP can advise generally regarding exercise and lifestyle, as asthma symptoms should never be a bar to normal development. Sports enjoyed by other schoolchildren should be enjoyed by asthmatic children too. Perhaps the best form of exercise for asthma sufferers is swimming, as swimming-pools often have a warm, moist atmosphere, and it can be no coincidence that several of Britain's Olympic swimmers have succeeded despite being life-long asthma sufferers.

IF YOU REMEMBER NOTHING ELSE, REMEMBER THESE THREE THINGS

1   A persistent, dry cough at night may be the first and only sign of asthma in a young child.

2   Effective treatment is available to prevent as well as relieve asthma and any child with persistent asthma symptoms needs to have his medication reviewed.

3   Asthma should be no bar to the enjoyment of sport and other normal children's activities.

OTHER CAUSES OF WHEEZING

Foreign Body

When a child develops a sudden wheeze, it is possible he may have inhaled a small object like a sweet, a peanut or a bead. Young children tend to put small objects in their mouths which, as they run round excitedly or stumble, may be accidentally inhaled and become lodged in one of the smaller respiratory passageways. This causes a partial obstruction to air going in and out, and a wheeze is produced. If the object is not removed, inflammation and infection will follow resulting in more serious symptoms.

Bronchiolitis

This is an infection caused by the respiratory syncitial virus which affects chiefly the smaller airways. It tends to occur in winter epidemics and is dangerous in children under the age of one. It starts with the symptoms of a common cold, but within two or three days breathing becomes laboured, and there is rapid panting and general distress. The child often has a high temperature and a wheeze. The problem is due largely to narrowing of the small airways – the bronchioles – caused by inflammation and large amounts of sticky mucus. Hospital admission is often needed to keep the child under observation and to provide added oxygen. Occasionally tube feeding, in which a small tube is passed down the nose into the stomach, is required because the child is too tired to feed. A small number of children will need to be fed intravenously and even ventilated artificially for a short while.

WHAT CAN YOU DO?

Every parent should be careful not to allow small children to play with toys or other objects which can be easily swallowed or inhaled by mistake. They should certainly be told never to run about with anything in their mouths – sweets included. If sudden wheezing does occur and inhalation of a foreign body is suspected, the child should be taken to a casualty department straightaway for tests and treatment.

Infants with wheezing as a result of a bad cold must always be seen by the doctor and treated promptly.

WHAT CAN THE DOCTOR DO?

Careful listening to the child's chest with a stethoscope can sometimes reveal the presence of an inhaled object in the respiratory passages since only one lung will be affected by the obstruction. Usually however, X-rays are needed to localise the offending object which is then removed under anaesthetic by use of a flexible tubular instrument called a bronchoscope.

Bronchiolitis may require no treatment other than observation at home, but in severe cases children should be admitted to hospital for observation and oxygen therapy and intravenous therapy if necessary.

IF YOU REMEMBER NOTHING ELSE, REMEMBER THESE THREE THINGS

1 An inhaled foreign body produces wheezing of sudden onset.

2 Small inhaled foreign objects may only show up when infection ensues and proves resistant to treatment.

3 An infant under one year with a wheeze should always be seen by a doctor.

CHAPTER SEVEN

SOURCES OF HELP

Every parent, with or without experience, will at some time require help and support with their children, however angelic and easy to manage they may be. The following is a list of the most useful sources of support.

The Family Doctor

The GP with whom you and your child are registered is contracted under his or her terms of service (at least for the moment) to provide round-the-clock, 24-hour cover for your medical needs. And he or she is there not just to treat illness, but also to advise and support you in every possible aspect of health. GPs, above all other healthcare professionals, can offer a holistic approach to health and medical problems, but are frequently able to help with personal and family difficulties as well. Many people imagine that doctors are only required to sort out illness and disease, but in fact it is good for doctors to see children who are healthy and happy as well, not only because a child learns that the doctor's surgery can be an interesting and fearless place to be, but because the doctor then has a 'standard' to compare the child with when he is unwell.

The doctor is able to provide advice over the telephone, he or she can sit and consult in the surgery or health centre and is available to visit the parent or child at home in an emergency. But the GP is just part of the primary healthcare team which consists also of midwives, health visitors and social workers. Many doctors now run health promotion clinics from their surgeries and are able to employ independent therapists such as counsellors and physiotherapists under the terms of newly negotiated contracts. Child health clinics partly run by doctors carry out regular health and developmental checks on babies, and incorporate immunisation clinics as well.

How to Register

Newborn babies should be registered with a GP as soon as possible. Normally, when the baby's birth is registered at the local registry office, the parents are given the standard pink card containing his new NHS number which is then signed by one of the parents and sent to the GP in question. Alternatively, if the baby needs to be seen before the pink card has been obtained, a registration form can be provided at the doctor's surgery itself. It is important that the baby is registered at all times in case of emergency, so if you move house or go to stay even temporarily in another area, make sure that a local doctor is willing to accept you.

Getting The Best Out of Your Doctor

The doctor–patient relationship is a two-way thing and there is no doubt that there are certain ways of getting the very best out of your doctor. It is by no means a certainty that you and your doctor will get on. Personalities and styles vary and there is little point persevering where there is suspicion or mistrust on either side. You are quite within your rights to change to another doctor if this suits you, but consider that your own attitude may need to change if you have found no common ground with more than two or three doctors in as many years.

When you go to see the doctor, be absolutely certain about what it is that you want to achieve. If you feel nervous or shy, write down a list of the things you wish to discuss and do not be fobbed off by dismissive replies. Yes, the doctor's time is limited, but you would not be going to see him or her if it was not important to you, and the doctor can certainly make time if it is required. Also, with limited time available with the doctor, a lot of information needs to be conveyed very quickly. It is very easy to take in only a fraction of what is said, so ask the doctor to repeat the advice he or she has given if necessary, or even record it on a tape recorder if the doctor is happy with that. Be prepared to question what you have been told. Ask about any alternatives to the treatment that has been offered and remember that you are entitled, where it is reasonable, to a second opinion.

If there is no need for your child to be present with you at the consultation, ask somebody to mind your child at home for you so that there will be less distraction and disruption when you go. If you do need to take the children, take something to keep them occupied and entertained. If English is not your first language and there are communication problems, ask your health visitor if there are any Link Workers or Health Advocates available in your area who can assist with cultural concerns or translation.

If you are new to an area then ask around for recommendations of which GPs are particularly well thought of locally. You might be able to find a GP who has a special interest in children and families. If you find one, but the doctor is unable to take you because his or her list is full or because you live outside the catchment area, your Community Health Council or local Family Health Services Authority (FHSA) will provide you with a list of doctors, and if necessary the FHSA can oblige one of them to take you on. If you live in Scotland you will have to contact your local Health Board and if you live in Northern Ireland contact the Central Services Agency in Belfast.

The Community Midwife

The community midwife will visit you and the newborn baby in the early days after you have returned home from hospital. If you had your baby at home, then you will have already formed quite a strong bond with the midwife, who may well have been present at the birth itself. She will visit whenever necessary and will usually provide a 24-hour, round-the-clock phone number to contact for urgent help.

The Health Visitor

The health visitor generally makes her first visit when the baby is ten days or so old. The health visitor is a qualified nurse who has been given extra training in health promotion of all kinds. Her main rule is the education of families in order to avoid illness and promote healthy lifestyles. She is ideally placed to answer any anxieties or concerns that a parent has about their child, and again is available at the end of a phone during working hours. Depending on where she is based, and this varies from region to region, she may be found at a health centre, at the doctor's surgery or at a child health clinic.

Child Health Clinics

These clinics are normally run by health visitors and/or doctors. Health and development checks are carried out on children at such clinics, and immunisation procedures are performed there too. They are a good opportunity to meet other parents of similarly aged children, and many are a source of contact for local self-help groups where advice on childminding and the provision of secondhand baby clothes and equipment may be obtained. Health visitors who work there can often supply infant formula milks and vitamins more cheaply than the chemist's, and, for those who are entitled, free milk and vitamins.

Community Health Councils

Community or local health councils provide information on how to satisfy your requirements from the health service and what you are entitled to by right. It may well be able to provide a list of local services as well as lists of local doctors with whom you may wish to register.

Social Workers

Social workers can assist with practical and financial difficulties and help with domestic, personal or accommodation problems. It is worth remembering, if applying for urgent accommodation, that pregnant women and parents of any child under sixteen are regarded as priority groups by the housing department, at least for the moment. Social workers are also well placed to advise about the existence of local self-help groups and other voluntary organisations. They generally work within social services departments and can provide information about playgroups, day nurseries and childminders. They are involved too in making sure that the requirements of special needs children are met. Education departments are responsible for any state-run nursery or infant school and are empowered to assess all children with special needs and to provide appropriate education for them.

Non-statutory Sources Of Help

Many people assume that the sorts of help described above are the only ones that really matter. But close family is usually the greatest source of support, followed by other relatives and friends. Certain kinds of advice and help are not the sort you want from healthcare professionals anyway, but will certainly be available from other parents, local groups or voluntary organisations. Often in the course of my own medical career, I have come across gaps in the provision of healthcare where parents or patients have been able to come to the rescue themselves. One shining example was the setting up of the support link for facially handicapped people called Let's Face It, set up by Christine Piff in 1984. She had a rare but serious illness, the treatment of which resulted in significant cosmetic disfigurement. As she recovered from the physical and emotional consequences of her treatment, she discovered that there was no immediate or long-term source of support other than the limited facilities provided at the hospital. So she simply set one up herself. This organisation now flourishes, and it is just one example of the very many which now exist to the enormous benefit of the rest of the population.

To find out about other local groups, contact your local health visitor or doctor or ask at your Citizens' Advice Bureau, the local library, the Social Services Department or the local Council for

Voluntary Service. Finally, there are hundreds of useful national organisations with local branches near you whose help and support can prove invaluable. Some of these are listed below, but contact the National Council for Voluntary Organisations for the complete list which covers a wide range of current social issues.

Useful Organisations

Association of Breastfeeding Mothers
26 Holmshaw Close
London
SE26 4PH
0181 778 4769

Association for all Speech Impaired Children
347 Central Markets
Smithfield
London
EC1A 9NH
General: 0171 236 6487

The Association for Stammerers
15 Old Ford Road
Bethnal Green
London
E2 9PJ
General: 0181 983 1003

Blisslink (for parents of premature babies in special care)
17–21 Emerald Street
London
WC1N 3QL
0171 831 9393

British Association of Cancer United Patients (BACUP)
3 Bath Place
Rivington Street
London
EC2A 3JP
Admin: 0171 696 9003
Fax: 0171 696 9002
Counselling: 0171 696 9000

Info service: 0171 613 2121
(+ free in London 0800 181199)

British Diabetic Association
HQ 10 Queen Anne Street
London
W1M 0BD
0171 323 1531

British Epilepsy Association
Anstey House
40 Hanover Square
Leeds
LS3 1BE
General: 0113 2439393
Helpline: 0800 309030

Cerebral Palsy – SCOPE
Head Office: 12 Park Crescent
London
W1N 4EQ
0171 636 5020
Helpline: 0800 626216

Child Accident Prevention Trust
18–20 Faringdon Lane
London
EC1R 3AU
0171 608 3828

Child Growth Foundation
2 Mayfield Avenue
Chiswick
London
W4 1PW
0181 995 0257/994 7625

Coeliac Society of the UK
P O Box 220
High Wycombe
Bucks
HP11 2HY
01494 37278

The Compassionate Friends (for bereaved parents)
53 North Street
Bristol
BS3 1EN
0117 953 9639

Cry-sis (for constantly crying babies)
27 Old Gloucester Street
London
WC1N 3XX
0171 404 5011

Cystic Fibrosis Research Trust
Alexandra House
5 Blyth Road
Bromley
BR1 3RS
General: 0181 464 7211

Down's Syndrome Association
155 Mitcham Road
London
SW17 9PG
General: 0181 682 4001

The Dyslexia Institute
Head Office: 133 Gresham Road
Staines
TW18 2AJ
01784 463851

Eating Disorder Association
Sackvill Place
44 Magdalene Street
Norwich
NR3 1JU
Helpline: 01603 621414
Youth helpline (under 18): 01603 765050 – every Wednesday 4–6pm

Enuresis Resources and Information Centre (ERIC)
65 St Michael's Hill
Bristol
BS2 8DZ
0117 9264920

Foundation for the Study of Infant Deaths
Cot Death Research & Support
14 Halkin Street
London
SW1X 7DP
General Enquiries: 0171 235 0965
Counselling: 0171 235 1721
Appeals: 0171 823 2216

Gingerbread (for one parent families)
16–17 Clerkenwell Close
London
EC1R 0AA
General: 0171 336 8183

The Haemophilia Society
123 Westminster Bridge Road
London
SE1 7HR
General: 0171 928 2020

Hyperactive Children's Support Group
71 Whyke Lane
Chichester
PO19 2LD
01903 725182

ME Association
PO Box 8
Stanford-le-Hope
Essex
SS17 8EX
01375 642466

The Medic Alert Foundation
12 Bridge Wharf
156 Caledonian Road
London
N1 G44
0171 833 3034

Mencap
123 Golden Lane
London
EC1Y 0RT
General: 0171 454 0452

Meningitis Research Foundation
13 High Street
Thombury
Bristol
BS12 2AE
General: 01454 281811
Helpline: 01454 413344

National Childbirth Trust
Alexandra House
Oldham Terrace
London
W3 6NH
0181 992 8637

National Children's Bureau
8 Wakeley Street
London
EC1V 7QR
General: 0171 843 6000

National Council for One Parent Families
255 Kentish Town Road
London
NW5 2LX
General: 0171 267 1361

National Deaf Childrens Society
15 Dufferin Street
London
EC1Y 8PD
General: 0171 250 0123

National Eczema Society
163 Eversholt Street
London
NW1 1BU
General: 0171 388 4097

National Meningitis Trust
Fern House
Bath Road
Stroud
Gloucestershire
GL5 3TJ
General: 01453 751738

Naevus Support Group (birthmarks)
58 Necton Road
Wheathampstead
St Albans
Herts
AL4 8AU
01582 832853

Parentline
National Office
Endway House
The Endway
Hadleigh
Essex
SS7 2AN
Helpline: 01702 559900
Admin: 01702 554782

ROSPA (accident prevention)
Cannon House
The Priory Queensway
Birmingham
B4 6BS
0121 200 2461

Sickle Cell Society
54 Station Road
Harlesdon
NW10 4UA
General: 0181 961 4006

Still birth and Neonatal Death Society (SANDS)
28 Portland Place
London
W1N 4DE
General: 0171 436 7940
Helpline: 0171 436 5881

Twins and Multiple Birth Association (TAMBA)
PO Box 30
Little Sutton
South Wirral
Liverpool
L66 1TH
0151 348 0020

Thalassaemia Society United Kingdom
107 Nightingale Lane
London
N8 7QY
General: 0181 348 0437

Zootz Australia (sun protective swimsuits)
5 Brashland Drive
East Hunsbury
Northants
NN4 0SS

INDEX

INDEX